A Clinical Guide to Kidney Diseases

A Clinical Guide to Kidney Diseases

Editor: Donald Moore

AMERICAN
MEDICAL PUBLISHERS
www.americanmedicalpublishers.com

AMERICAN
MEDICAL PUBLISHERS
www.americanmedicalpublishers.com

Cataloging-in-Publication Data

A clinical guide to kidney diseases / edited by Donald Moore.
p. cm.
Includes bibliographical references and index.
ISBN 978-1-63927-837-4
1. Kidneys--Diseases. 2. Kidneys--Disease--Diagnosis.
3. Kidneys--Diseases--Treatment. 4. Nephrology.
I. Moore, Donald.
RC902 .C55 2023
616.61--dc23

American Medical Publishers,
41 Flatbush Avenue,
1st Floor, New York,
NY 11217, USA

ISBN 978-1-63927-837-4 (Hardback)

Contents

Preface

The main aim of this book is to educate learners and enhance their research focus by presenting diverse topics covering this vast field. This is an advanced book which compiles significant studies by distinguished experts in the area of analysis. This book addresses successive solutions to the challenges arising in the area of application, along with it; the book provides scope for future developments.

Kidney diseases (or renal diseases) are a group of disorders characterized by damage to or disease of the kidney that affects the ability of the kidney to filter fluid and waste from the blood. These diseases can be classified into two categories, namely, nephritis and nephrosis. Nephritis is a condition in which there is inflammation in the kidney. There are several types of nephritis based on the site of the inflammation and it can lead to nephritic syndrome. Nephrosis is a condition without any inflammation in the kidney which can cause nephrotic syndrome. There are several causes of kidney diseases including accumulation of immunoglobulin A antibodies in the glomerulus, long term exposure to lead and its salts, long-term usage of analgesics, and administration of chemotherapy agents in the body. The diagnosis of kidney diseases involves a physical examination, and tests such as urine tests and renal ultrasonography. The topics covered in this extensive book deal with the core aspects of kidney diseases. It consists of contributions made by international experts. This book will serve as a valuable source of reference for graduate and post graduate students.

It was a great honour to edit this book, though there were challenges, as it involved a lot of communication and networking between me and the editorial team. However, the end result was this all-inclusive book covering diverse themes in the field.

Finally, it is important to acknowledge the efforts of the contributors for their excellent chapters, through which a wide variety of issues have been addressed. I would also like to thank my colleagues for their valuable feedback during the making of this book.

Editor

1

The left ureterocele and stone of calyceal diverticulum in the patient with bilateral incomplete duplex kidneys managed by flexible ureteroscopy

Yang Pan, Gang Chen*, Han Chen, Yunxiao Zhu and Hualin Chen

Abstract

Background: Duplex kidneys are one of the most common renal congenital abnormalities, mostly asymptomatic and of no clinical significance. There are little reports about the left ureterocele and stone of calyceal diverticulum in patients with bilateral incomplete duplex kidneys managed by flexible ureteroscopy.

Case presentation: A 69-year-old Chinese woman was presented with left waist pain for 1 month. A preoperative computed tomography (CT) scan and intravenous pyelogram revealed the left ureterocele which located in the left ureterovesical junction, and stone of calyceal diverticulum which located in the upper kidney of left incomplete duplex kidneys. The ureterocele was confirmed in view of ureteroscopy and the holmium laser was used for the resection of ureterocele. It took us a lot of efforts to find out the stone because of diverticular neck stenosis. Fortunately, when diverticular neck stenosis was incised internally by holmium laser, the stone was discovered clearly and removed using the holmium laser and nitinol stone basket through flexible ureteroscopy. A double-J ureteral stent was inserted and remained in place for 1 month. The symptom disappeared postoperatively and no complications were developed during the placement of the stent. There were no stone residents observed on CT scan before removing the ureteral stent 1 month later.

Conclusions: Flexible ureteroscopy with holmium laser is feasible to manage the ureterocele and calyceal diverticulum stones in patients with bilateral incomplete duplex kidneys in one operation.

Keywords: Ureterocele, Stone, Calyceal diverticulum, Duplex kidneys, Flexible ureteroscopy, Case report

Background

Duplex kidneys are common congenital malformations of urogenital system, with an incidence of approximately 1–3% [1, 2]. Duplex kidneys can be categorized as complete or incomplete according to ureteral morphology [3]. Meanwhile, such a duplication also can be bilateral or unilateral, and some studies have reported that only 0.3% of the patients are detected bilateral duplex kidneys by excretory urography [4, 5].

Most patients with duplex kidneys have no significant clinical symptoms. But some complications like urolithiasis and vesicoureteral reflux (VUR) are relevant to duplex kidneys [5]. Iatrogenic ureteral injury is a possible risk during many urogynecology surgeries, and it's more

* Correspondence: chengang2308@163.com
Department of Urology, The First Affiliated Hospital of Chongqing Medical University, No. 1 Road Youyi, Yuzhong District, Chongqing, China

likely to occur when the ureter exists anatomical varieties [6].

Percutaneous nephrolithotomy (PCNL), retrograde intrarenal surgery (RIRS) and extracorporeal shock wave lithotripsy (SWL) are now the standard treatment modalities for the majority of upper tract stone diseases [7]. SWL shows a relatively lower stone-free rate (SFR), while PCNL represents a higher risk of bleeding [8]. Flexible ureteroscope can reach the pelvicalyceal system easily, and it is beneficial to the improvement of SFR. As a result, RIRS combined with holmium laser lithotripsy has become a less-invasive and preferred procedure for the management of < 20 mm upper urinary tract stones on the basis of its high SFR and acceptable complication rates [9, 10].

We report a clinical case of the left ureterocele and stone of calyceal diverticulum in the patient with bilateral incomplete duplex kidneys managed by flexible ureteroscopy. At the same time, we conduct some literature reviews and provide some suggestions on the treatment of the ureterocele and stones of calyceal diverticulum in patients with duplex kidneys.

Case presentation

A 69-year-old Chinese woman was presented with left waist pain for 1 month. She had no fever or other pain. There were no abnormal results in the blood routine examination, renal function, and urine routine examination. And the result of urine culture was negative. A preoperative computerized tomography (CT) scan and intravenous pyelogram (IVP) revealed bilateral incomplete duplex kidney and ureter (Fig. 1). The stone of calyceal diverticulum was located in the upper kidney of left incomplete duplex kidneys by CT scan (Fig. 2). In the meanwhile, IVP and CT scan revealed that a ureterocele was located in the left ureterovesical junction (Fig. 3).

The patient had hypertension and type 2 diabetes mellitus for 5 years. The risks of surgery and general anesthesia were relatively higher. The diameter of the stone in the calyceal diverticulum was 12 mm by CT scan and it's difficult for the stone to pass out spontaneously. The patient and her family wished to remove the stone because they were extremely worried about stone-related complications. Moreover, they wouldn't like to perform second operation and anesthesia due to relatively higher risks. Therefore, we planned to make an attempt to remove the ureterocele and calyceal diverticulum stone in one operation.

The contraindications for surgery in such cases mainly included untreated urinary tract infection, severe urinary tract stricture, and anesthetic contraindications like cardiopulmonary dysfunction. Relevant examinations such as lung-function testing and Holter electrocardiogram were conducted. We also paid special attention to the results of urine routine and urine culture. When we made sure all these examination results were normal, we decided to perform the surgery.

Flexible ureteroscopy with the holmium laser was conducted for solving the ureterocele and stone of calyceal

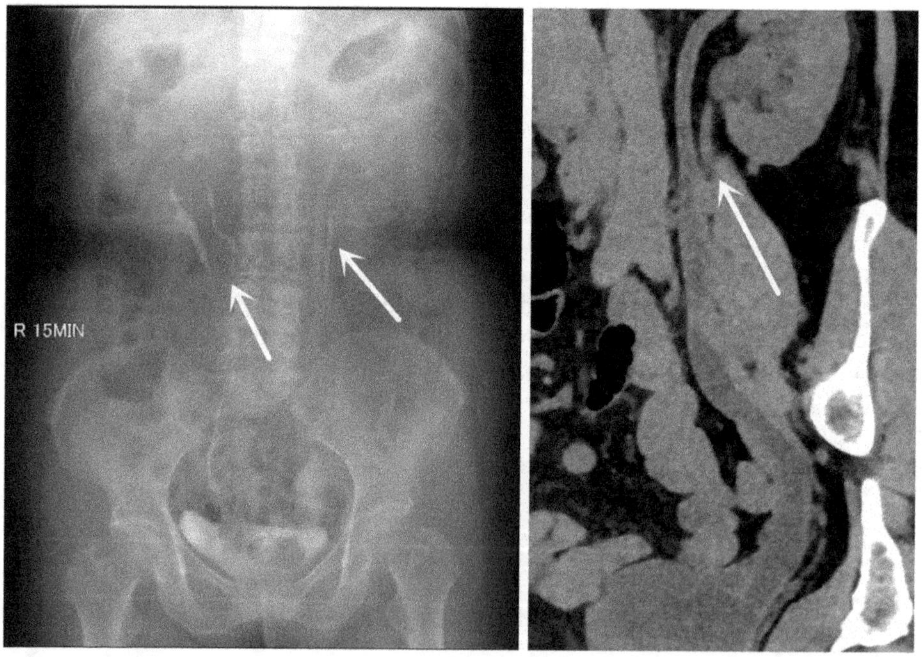

Fig. 1 Intravenous pyelogram and CT scan revealed bilateral incomplete duplex kidney and ureter

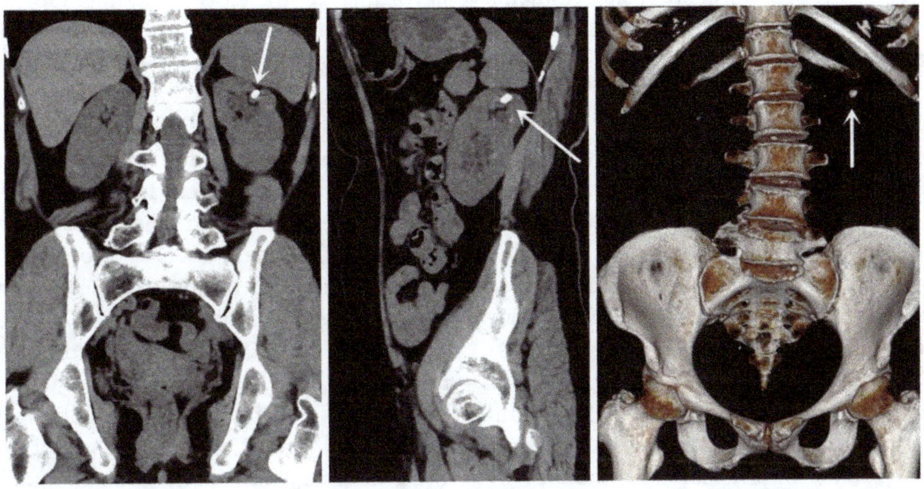

Fig. 2 The stone of calyceal diverticulum was located in the upper kidney of left incomplete duplex kidneys by CT scan

diverticulum. To begin with, the ureterocele was confirmed in view of ureteroscopy and the holmium laser was used for the resection of ureterocele. The ureterocele resection surgery was completed in 10 min and no complications like bleeding occurred intraoperatively. Then, we made an attempt to remove the stone of calyceal diverticulum. During the operation, we found the calyx neck of calyceal diverticulum where the stone was located had obvious stenosis. It took us a lot of effort to find out the stone because of calyx neck stenosis. Fortunately, the stone was discovered when calyx neck stenosis was incised internally by holmium laser. After dilatation of the narrow calyx neck, a 200-μm holmium laser through flexible ureteroscope was used to make the stone fragmented gradually and carefully. The parameter of the holmium laser was set at a power of 0.8 J and a pulse frequency of 10 Hz. Higher power and frequency might cause renal damage and hemorrhage because the calyceal diverticulum stone was near the edge of the kidney and the renal cortex was thin by CT scan. In order to prevent the formation of ureteral steinstrasse postoperatively, a nitinol stone basket was used to remove large stone fragments as soon as possible, and the smaller powdered fragments were flushed out of the diverticulum using an automated irrigation pump. At last, the pelvicalyceal system was examined once again to ensure no large remaining stones. The overall surgical time was controlled in 60 min for the purpose of preventing postoperative infections. A double-J ureteral stent was inserted and remained in place for 1 month. The symptom of left lumbar back pain disappeared post the operation and no complications were developed during the

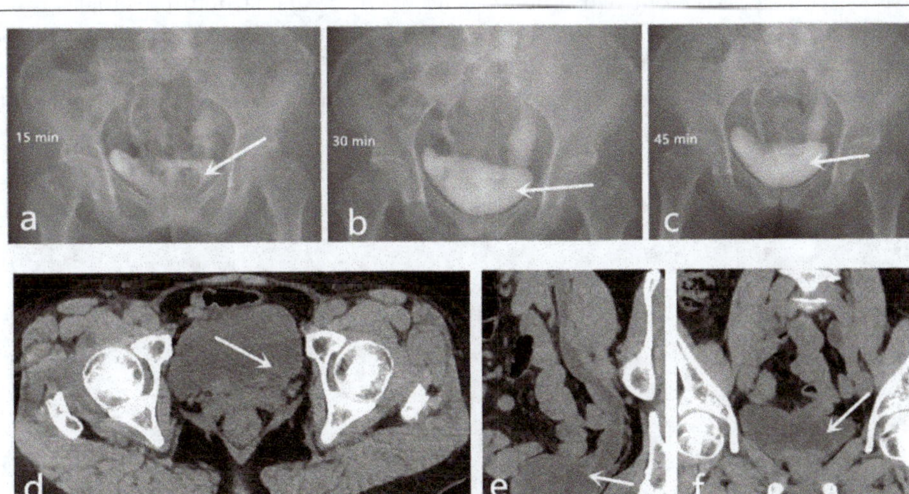

Fig. 3 Intravenous pyelogram at 15 (**a**), 30 (**b**), 45 (**c**) minutes respectively after injecting contrast medium revealed a ureterocele. CT scan (**d**, **e**, **f**) revealed that a ureterocele was located in the left ureterovesical junction

placement of the stent. There were no stone residents observed by CT scan before removing the ureteral stent 1 month later (Fig. 4).

Discussion and conclusions

Duplex kidneys refer to a kind of renal congenital anatomical malformations in which the renal unit is made up of two separate pelvicalyceal systems [11, 12]. The renal vessels, collecting system and ureter of duplex kidneys are respectively separated. The incidence of duplicate kidney and ureter is about 1~3% [4]. A few malformations can accompany ureteral ectopic opening or ureteral protrusion. Most patients with duplex renal and ureteral malformations have no specific clinical symptoms. It was often found in physical examination, or complicated with stone, hydronephrosis, infection and other symptoms.

At present, some studies have shown that ultrasound is a major imaging examination for the survey of duplex kidneys [13]. Ultrasound is extremely conducive to diagnose because of its simplicity and convenience. Furthermore, it is not radioactive to the patient. IVP and CT are also important imaging methods to diagnose the disease, moreover, the sensitivity of CT is better than the former two. According to the studies, the diagnostic coincidence rates of urinary system for B ultrasound, IVP and CT were 44.7, 60.0 and 100%, respectively. At the same time, the diagnostic coincidence rates of CT for hydronephrosis, calculi, ectopic ureteral orifice and ureterocele were also higher than those of B ultrasound and IVP.

Duplex kidney and ureter malformations can be divided into complete and incomplete according to ureteral morphology. The former refers to two independent pelvicalyceal systems derived from two ureteric buds of the mesonephric duct [14, 15]. Two resulting ureters have a respective fusion to the mesenchyme and cause isolated drainage of ipsilateral kidney. These two ureters were identified as lower or upper moiety according to the corresponding location. The opening position of ureter conforms to the Weigert–Meyer rule [16]. It means that the ureter from the upper moiety of the complete duplex kidney usually opens below and medial to the one from the lower moiety [2, 15].

Incomplete duplex kidney and ureter are derived from a premature division of the ureteral bud before fusing with the renal mesenchyme. Bifid moieties form at the proximal of 'Y-shaped' ureter, however, a confluence occurs at the distal of the ureter eventually. The confluence occurs in the upper and lower ureters respectively accounting for 25% and the middle ureter accounts for 50% [17].

Due to the unique anatomical abnormalities of duplex kidney and ureter malformations, it is easy to appear urine drainage [18]. The drainage can result in upper urinary tract obstruction, infection, calculi and other complications. The treatment of duplex renal and ureteral malformations combined with upper urinary calculi, is mainly based on the size of the calculi, location, degree of obstruction, whether combined with lumbago, hematuria, infection, kidney damage or not. If it is a small duplex kidney stone, without clinical symptoms, and don't cause hydronephrosis or renal function damage, it can be observed or conservative treatment.

Most patients with duplex kidneys have no significant symptoms, but complications are relatively frequent [19]. The complications of duplex kidneys can be classified as the upper moiety complications and lower moiety complications, and the former is significantly more common according to a few current literature [1, 4, 14]. Upper moiety complications are related to the ureteral ectopic insertion, usually complicated with a ureterocele or multi-cystic dysplastic moiety kidney. Males may occur a pelvic mass if urine gradually drains into an accessory sexual structure; Females can experience urinary incontinence when the inserting position is under the urethral sphincter [18, 20]. The most common upper moiety complication is urinary tract obstruction due to a ureterocele [4].

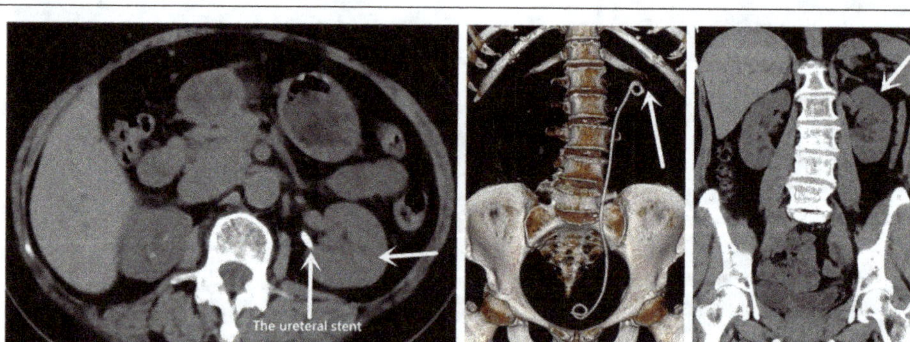

Fig. 4 There were no stone residents observed on CT scan 1 month later postoperatively

Lower moiety complications are mainly caused by the lateral shift of the ureters insertion into the bladder and consist of VUR, renal scarring and pelviureteric junction (PUJ) obstruction [18]. The most prevalent lower moiety complication is VUR and it can lead to recurrent urinary tract infections (UTIs) which may have a permanent impairment on renal function [21, 22]. Saddle reflux is a special complication unique to duplex kidneys and it means that the reflux occurs from one proximal end of the bifid ureter of incomplete duplication [4]. PUJ obstruction in duplex kidneys was found to be less than 1% according to current literature [23].

At present, a variety of minimally invasive surgeries have gradually replaced the traditional open surgery. If surgical treatment is required, clinicians can provide individualized minimally invasive treatment for patients according to the size, location, degree of hydronephrosis, renal function, patient willingness, operator experience and so on. Nowadays, the minimally invasive surgical methods for duplex kidneys with upper urinary stones mainly include ESWL, PCNL, Ureteroscope lithotripsy (URL), laparoscopic ureterolithotomy, etc. Although ESWL has the advantages of no anesthesia, simplicity, safety and small trauma in the treatment of duplex kidneys stones, however, the rate of re-treatment is as high as 58.6% [24]. PCNL, on the other hand, is relatively minimally invasive, with high lithotripsy efficiency and rapid postoperative recovery. But the risk of bleeding and injury to surrounding organs should not be ignored. Laparoscopic ureterolithotomy is suitable for patients with large upper ureteral calculi when other minimally invasive methods don't work. It can replace open surgery; however, relatively large trauma and ureteral stenosis are easy to occur. The ureteroscopy can only handle middle and lower ureteral calculi, while the flexible ureteroscopy lithotripsy can handle upper ureteral and renal calculi with great advantages. To some extent, it can overcome the poor effect of ESWL lithotripsy, the need for multiple treatments, puncture trauma and high risk of bleeding of PCNL, and it is also a better choice for teenagers [25].

Combined with our surgical experience, we choose flexible ureteroscopy with holmium laser for the management of upper urinary tract stones in patients with duplex kidney and ureter malformations. And we conclude the following experience:

First, due to the anatomic abnormality of duplex kidney and ureter malformations, choosing a small size ureteroscope as far as possible to reduce the difficulty to enter ureteral lumen and the damage to ureter wall while there exists ureteral stenosis. For upper ureteral calculi, ureteroscopy and holmium laser lithotripsy can be used firstly. After the calculi fall into the renal pelvis, flexible ureteroscopy can be utilized. This can shorten the time of using flexible ureteroscopy and reduce the consumption of machines. Although the image of the electronic flexible ureteroscope is clearer, the diameter is larger than the fibrous flexible ureteroscope. When choosing the electronic flexible ureteroscope, it may be difficult to enter the lateral half kidney with the calculi. Moreover, during the process of lithotripsy, the outflow from the ureteral catheter sheath is extremely slow, and the pressure in the renal pelvis is high, which increases the risk of urosepsis after surgery. As a result, the fibrous flexible ureteroscope is recommended.

Second, for patients with incomplete duplex kidney malformations, making sure that the ureteroscope gets to the double ureteral fusion position firstly. After identifying the bifurcation of two ureters, the specific location of the calculi can be determined according to the preoperative examination results. Then, the guidewire is placed in the side of the ureter with the calculi. It can also avoid unnecessary damage when entering the non-calculous ureter. Usually, the distal end of the ureteral catheter sheath should be placed to the ureteral fusion position, which can avoid the ureter bifurcation avulsion caused by the passive expansion of the sheath.

Third, for patients with complete duplicate renal and ureteral malformations, the position of calculi should be found combining with preoperative IVU or CTU in order to avoid the embarrassing situation that the calculi can't be found. And the ureteral openings should be found according to Weigert-Meyer's rule. The upper kidney and ureter are usually lean inward and downward, while the lower kidney and ureter are usually located outward.

Forth, for a small number of patients with incomplete duplicate kidney and ureter malformations, the stricture could exist at the bifurcation of the double ureter. As a result, the internal incision and balloon dilatation of ureteral stricture can be conducted through ureteroscopy firstly. Then, flexible ureteroscopy lithotripsy can be performed, and two double J ureteral stents can try to be retained to avoid ureteral stricture postoperatively.

Fifth, the angle between the repeated ureter and the corresponding lower renal calyx should be carefully evaluated before the operation when the calculi are located in the lower renal calyx. PCNL can be considered in the case of the following conditions: 1) flexible ureteroscope can't enter the lower renal calyx with an extremely small angle; 2) the ureteral catheter sheath can't be placed because the ureter is narrow or distorted severely; 3) the calculi are too large with the diameter of greater than 2 cm.

Duplex kidneys and ureter are one kind of common urological malformations, which are often of no obvious symptoms. Whereas there are nearly half of patients with duplex kidneys who need to be managed because of all kinds of comorbidities. A ureterocele and VUR are considered as the most frequent upper moiety complication and lower moiety complication, respectively. While the patient has the ureterocele and bilateral incomplete duplex kidney and ureter combined with calyceal diverticulum stones, flexible ureteroscopy and holmium laser lithotripsy might be a feasible and effective choice.

The patient in our report had four special comorbidities including the left ureterocele, calyceal diverticulum stone, diverticular neck stenosis, and bilateral incomplete duplex kidney and ureter. It's relatively rare that four comorbidities occurred in one patient. What's more, we conducted a minimally invasive surgery for the resection of ureterocele, the dilatation of diverticular neck, and the removal of calyceal diverticulum stone. Therefore, the special features of our report were made up of the rare four coexisting diseases and one endoscopic operation for solving three problems.

In conclusion, it appears that flexible ureteroscopy and holmium laser is a feasible, effective and minimally invasive way for managing the ureterocele and stones of calyceal diverticulum in patients with bilateral incomplete duplex kidneys in one operation.

Abbreviations

VUR: Vesicoureteral reflux; PCNL: Percutaneous nephrolithotomy; SWL: Extracorporeal shock wave lithotripsy; RIRS: Retrograde intrarenal surgery; SFR: Stone free rate; CT: Computerized tomography; IVP: Intravenous pyelogram; UTIs: Urinary tract infections; PUJ: Pelviureteric junction; URL: Ureteroscope lithotripsy

Acknowledgements

Not Applicable.

Authors' contributions

YP was a major contributor in writing the manuscript. GC provided the initial idea, financial aid, the report design and revised the final manuscript and gave some effective advances. HC performed initial analysis and interpretation of the data. YXZ and HLC reviewed the literature and drafted the literature review and discussion. All authors read and approved the final manuscript.

References

1. Hunziker M, Kutasy B, D'Asta F, Puri P. Urinary tract anomalies associated with high grade primary vesicoureteral reflux. Pediatr Surg Int. 2012;28(2):201–4.
2. Davda S, Vohra A. Adult duplex kidneys: an important differential diagnosis in patients with abdominal cysts. JRSM Short Rep. 2013;4(2):13.
3. Varlatzidou A, Zarokosta M, Nikou E, Theodoropoulos P, Kakaviatos D, Piperos T, et al. Complete unilateral ureteral duplication encountered during intersphincteric resection for low rectal cancer. J Surg Case Rep. 2018;2018(10):rjy266.
4. Privett JT, Jeans WD, Roylance J. The incidence and importance of renal duplication. Clin Radiol. 1976;27(4):521–30.
5. Papageorgiou D, Kyriazanos I, Zoulamoglou M, Deskou E, Kalles V, Stamos N, et al. Incomplete bilateral duplication of the ureters identified during cytoreductive surgery for ovarian cancer: a case report. Int J Surg Case Rep. 2019;60:213–5.
6. Selzman AA, Spirnak JP. Iatrogenic ureteral injuries: a 20-year experience in treating 165 injuries. J Urol. 1996;155(3):878–81.
7. Mehmet NM, Ender O. Effect of urinary stone disease and its treatment on renal function. World J Nephrol. 2015;4(2):271–6.
8. Akman T, Binbay M, Tekinarslan E, Ozkuvanci U, Kezer C, Erbin A, et al. Outcomes of percutaneous nephrolithotomy in patients with solitary kidneys: a single-center experience. Urology. 2011;78(2):272–6.
9. Turk C, Petrik A, Sarica K, Seitz C, Skolarikos A, Straub M, et al. EAU guidelines on interventional treatment for urolithiasis. Eur Urol. 2016;69(3):475–82.
10. Yang B, Ning H, Liu Z, Zhang Y, Yu C, Zhang X, et al. Safety and efficacy of flexible ureteroscopy in combination with holmium laser lithotripsy for the treatment of bilateral upper urinary tract calculi. Urol Int. 2017;98(4):418–24.
11. Hartman GW, Hodson CJ. The duplex kidney and related abnormalities. Clin Radiol. 1969;20(4):387–400.
12. Horst M, Smith GH. Pelvi-ureteric junction obstruction in duplex kidneys. BJU Int. 2008;101(12):1580–4.
13. Ladwig SH, Older RA, Foster WL, Korobkin M. Computed tomographic diagnosis of the obstructed duplex kidney in adults. N C Med J. 1982;43(6):429–31.
14. Whitten SM, Wilcox DT. Duplex systems. Prenat Diagn. 2001;21(11):952–7.
15. Malek RS, Kelalis PP, Stickler GB, Burke EC. Observations on ureteral ectopy in children. J Urol. 1972;107(2):308–13.
16. Lee KH, Gee HY, Shin JI. Genetics of vesicoureteral reflux and congenital anomalies of the kidney and urinary tract. Investig Clin Urol. 2017;58(Suppl 1):S4–s13.
17. Geavlete P, Nita G, Georgescu D, Mirciulescu V. Endoscopic classification and endourologic therapy in proximal incomplete ureteral duplication pathology. Eur Urol. 2001;39(3):304–7.
18. Doery AJ, Ang E, Ditchfield MR. Duplex kidney: not just a drooping lily. J Med Imaging Radiat Oncol. 2015;59(2):149–53.
19. South Bedfordshire Practitioners' Group. Development of renal scars in children: missed opportunities in management. BMJ. 1990;301(6760):1082–4.
20. Chertin B, Mohanan N, Farkas A, Puri P. Endoscopic treatment of vesicoureteral reflux associated with ureterocele. J Urol. 2007;178(4 Pt 2):1594–7.
21. Stokland E, Jodal U, Sixt R, Swerkersson S, Hansson S. Uncomplicated duplex kidney and DMSA scintigraphy in children with urinary tract infection. Pediatr Radiol. 2007;37(8):826–8.
22. Thomas JC. Vesicoureteral reflux and duplex systems. Adv Urol. 2008;2008:651891.
23. Gonzalez F, Canning DA, Hyun G, Casale P. Lower pole pelvi-ureteric junction obstruction in duplicated collecting systems. BJU Int. 2006;97(1):161–5.
24. Tunc L, Tokgoz H, Tan MO, Kupeli B, Karaoglan U, Bozkirli I. Stones in anomalous kidneys: results of treatment by shock wave lithotripsy in 150 patients. Int J Urol. 2004;11(10):831–6.
25. Jurkiewicz B, Zabkowski T, Samotyjek J. Ureterolithotripsy in a paediatric population: a single institution's experience. Urolithiasis. 2014;42(2):171–6.

2

Kidney triplication with ectopic ureterocele

I. B. Osipov, D. A. Lebedev* and M. V. Lifanova

Abstract

Background: Kidney triplication is a rare urological abnormality. Association of triplex kidney and ureterocele is out of ordinary. Treatment of such patients usually implies heminephrureterectomy of the upper moiety. We report a case of a saved function of the upper moiety after minimal invasive surgical procedure.

Case presentations: 5-year old girl complained for continuous wetting. Examination revealed 3 - segmented left kidney with pelvi-ureteric dilation of the upper moiety, IV grade vesicoureteral reflux in the upper moiety, cervical ectopic ureteral orifice of the upper moiety and a commune ureteral orifice of the lower segments.

An endoscopic laser dissection of ureterocele was performed. Drainage of the upper moiety of triplex kidney was restored. Examination 18 months later showed no wetting and infection symptoms. Pelvi-ureteric dilation of the upper moiety and cavity of ureterocele decreased to minimal. Grade of vesicoureteral reflux decreased to I.

Conclusion: Minimal invasive elimination of obstruction of the upper moiety of triplex kidney was successful and led to regress of vesicoureteral reflux, urinary incontinence and let to avoid heminephrectomy.

Keywords: Triplex kidney, Ureterocele, Vesicoureteral reflux, Incontinence

Background

About 100 cases of renal triplication are described in scientific literature. A little over than 20 cases is associated with ureterocele. In 1870 Wrany first described triplex kidney with ureterocele that was revealed at 3-year-old girl autopsy [1, 2]. As usual ectopic ureterocele is associated with severe or critical damage of the upper moiety of triplex kidney.

Treatment of such patients usually implies heminephrureterectomy of the upper moiety [2, 3]. In case of extant function of the upper moiety there are some ways of minimal invasive treatment of obstruction. Mainly they are linked with the use of laser or electrocatheter for punction or dissection of ureterocele and upper segment decompression [4, 5]. We demonstrate successful outcome of endoscopic treatment of ectopic ureterocele in a child with kidney triplication.

* Correspondence: Urolog.Lebedev@gmail.com
Urology Department, State Pediatric Medical University, 2 Litovskaya Street, build.2, St. Petersburg, Russian Federation 194100

Case presentation

In august, 2017 5-year-old girl was admitted at pediatric urology department of Saint-Petersburg State Pediatric Medical University. The complaints were continuous wetting and recurrent urinary tract infection (UTI). Prenatal 32 weeks ultrasound revealed left pelvi-ureteric dilation. The child did not have episodes of anoxia, trauma, dehydration, hereditary pathology. By the age of 1 year the child had got over several episodes of UTIs.

At 1 year 5 months the child was examined at a local hospital. Ureterocele was revealed and an attempt to decompress it by endoscopic electric dissection was undertaken. At that time kidney triplication hadn't been revealed. A diagnose sounded as complete left kidney duplication.

Further examination and treatment were carried out at the base of Saint-Petersburg State Pediatric Medical University. Ultrasound revealed that left kidney consisted of 2 moieties with the upper moiety pelvis dilation to 30 ×

15 mm. A large ureterocele was seen in the bladder. Intravenous pyelogram (IVP) demonstrated 3 contrasted moieties of the left kidney with megaureter of the upper one. Ureters of the middle and lower moieties fused along the way (Type 2 by Smith) [1]. There was rounded contrast defect in the bladder – ectopic ureterocele (Fig. 1).

DMSA scan confirmed extant function and urinary retention in the upper moiety. Functional capacity distributed as 51% to the right kidney and 49% to the left. Left upper moiety took upon itself 23% of left kidney function, middle and lower moieties – 77%. Computer tomography (CT) showed an additional blood supply of the upper moiety of triple kidney. The collecting system of the upper moiety and the ureter were significantly expanded (Fig. 2).

Cystography revealed IV grade vesicoureteral reflux (VUR) in the upper moiety. Dilated pelvis, ureter and ureterocele were seen contrasted (Fig. 3).

In September, 2017 cystoscopy and laser dissection of ureterocele were performed. We used 10 Fr cystoscope, 4 Fr light guide, 10 W fiber tome mode Yag-Ni laser. Cystoscopy showed ectopic ureteral orifice of the upper moiety in the bladder neck, and a commune ureteral orifice of the lower segments. Ectopic orifice was wide and located in the sphincter zone. Ureterocele was large and located in the lower part of the bladder and it's neck. We saw no traces of the previous surgical treatment and ureteral orifice hadn't been deformed. We did not insert a catheter into the ureter since identification was not difficult and there was no risk of injury. A new upper moiety ureteral orifice was formed with the aid of laser at the front surface of ureterocele from the inside of it and then slightly widen from the inside of the bladder. Sufficient decompression of the upper moiety pelviureteric system was achieved. There were no complications during surgery. Upper moiety was not catheterized. Bladder was catheterized with Foley catheter for a day. There were no complications during early postoperative period.

Complex investigation was performed in 7 months. UTI had no one episode by that time. Urinary incontinence considerably decreased. Ultrasound revealed much smaller dilation of the upper moiety pelviureteric system. The pelvis size was 15 × 10 mm. Cavity of ureterocele was reduced to 5 mm in diameter. Cystography revealed II grade VUR in the upper moiety. Cystoscopy was performed to assess the local situation after surgery. A new formed upper ureteral orifice was able to discharge urine. There was no stenosis or inflammation.

Investigation 1 year 6 months after surgery showed good results. There were no complaints for UTI symptoms. Urinalyses were good and culture showed no growth. Voiding was uncomplicated and there was no wetting. Uroflowmetry showed normal voiding without residual. Ultrasound demonstrated 10 mm dilation of the upper moiety pelvis. Parenchyma was rather thinned. There was 4 mm in diameter residual cavity of ureterocele in the bladder. Upper moiety ureter was 6 mm in the distal part. IVP confirmed positive dynamics in the upper moiety dilation (Fig. 4). Grade of VUR decreased to I. DMSA scan demonstrated decreased parenchymal mass of the upper moiety but improvement of absorption and transport function. We expect that successful outcome of treatment will persist; however, we are planning to perform an examination of the patient in 3 years.

Discussion and conclusions

The described type of kidney and ureteral triplication was identified as II type by Smith [1]. Occurrence of

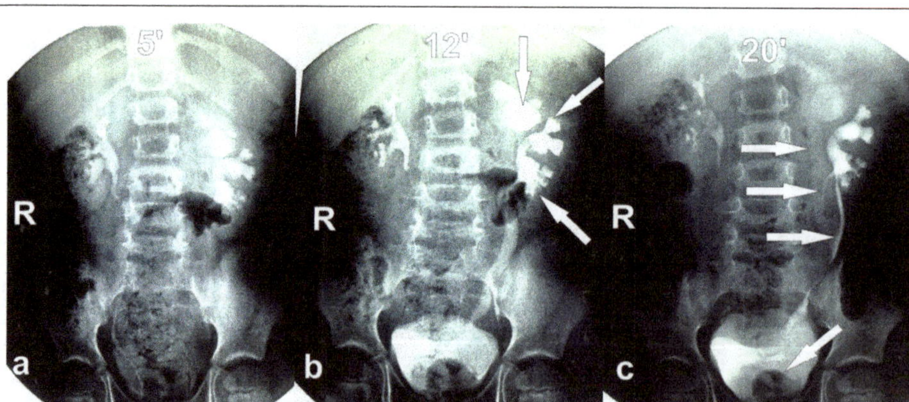

Fig. 1 Intravenous pyelogram in 5 (**a**), 12 (**b**) and 20 (**c**) minutes after the injection of contrast media revealed left kidney triplication. Arrows indicate three segments of left kidney (IVPb) and three ureters (IVPc). The ureters of the middle and lower moieties merge along the way (IVPc)

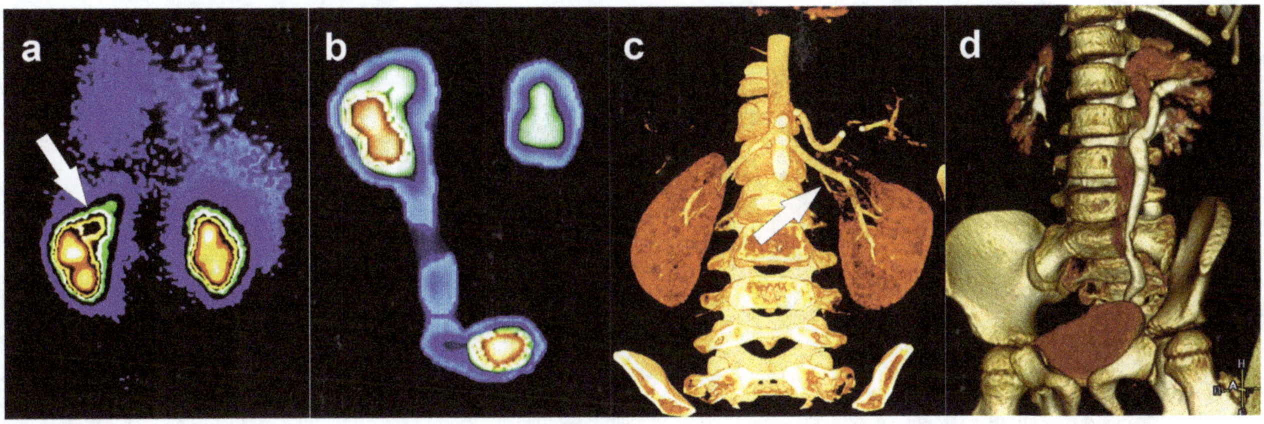

Fig. 2 DMSA scans (**a** and **b**) show decrease of functioning parenchyma volume and urinary retention in the upper moiety. CT (**c** and **d**) show an additional vessel to the upper moiety (arrow), renal triplication and dilation of pelvicalyceal system and ureter of the upper moiety

this type is 21% [6]. Existence of ectopic ureterocele negatively affects the upper moiety of triplicated kidney. Upper moiety function may be lost due to affected drainage and VUR. That may cause persistence of UTI and stones formation [7]. In this case there were significant pelvi-ureteric dilation and high grade VUR with UTI symptoms.

Contemporary trends in treatment of children with ureterocele mean conservative or minimally invasive surgical tactics with high possibility of getting good results. When we chose tactic of treatment we based on described criteria of patients selection for conservative treatment. These are lost function of upper moiety, absence of lower pole moieties obstruction, low grade VUR in the lower moiety ureter and absence of bladder neck obstruction [8]. There was no one mentioned criteria in this case. DMSA confirmed upper moiety function which was 23%. Conservative treatment was not indicated in this case and we could expect positive results of the use of minimal invasive surgical tactic. The patient had no associated congenital abnormalities which could discourage endoscopic surgery.

The second surgical procedure was necessary and successful. Decompression of ureterocele let to eliminate upper moiety dilation, VUR, urinary incontinence and UTI simultaneously. The first attempt to dissect ureterocele was unsuccessful probably because of minimal surgical impact on it.

This clinical case is an extremely rare one. In patients with large ureteral orifice in bladder neck and ureterocele the only applicable treatment is dissection of ureterocele. There is no need in orifice dilation like balloon plastic or bougieurage [9]. In case of ectopic ureteral orifice in bladder neck without ureterocele its dilation is acceptable [10]. Dissection of the front wall of ureterocele

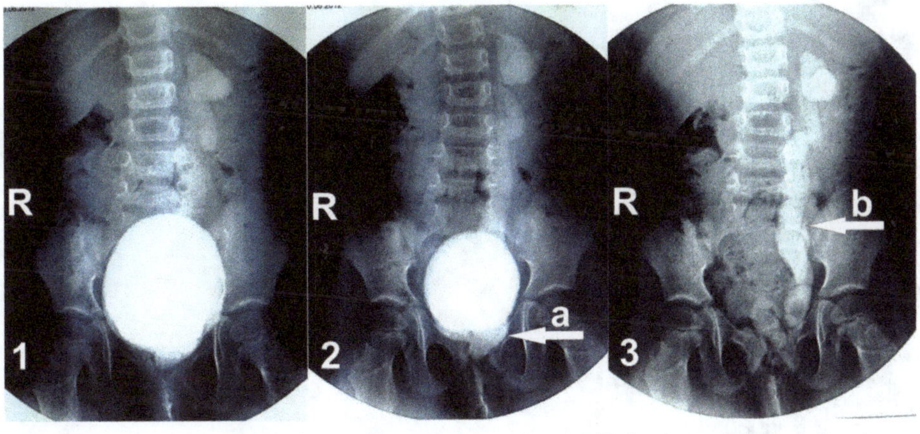

Fig. 3 Voiding cystography: IV grade vesicoureteral reflux in the upper moiety. Contrast-filled ureterocele (**a**) and dilated ureter (**b**) are seen

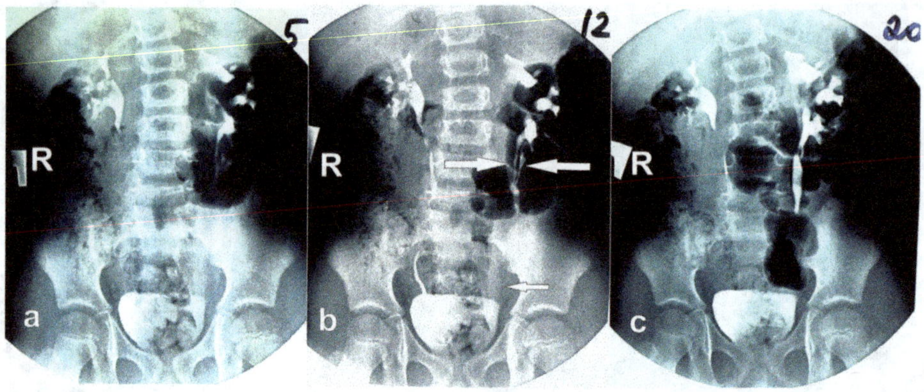

Fig. 4 Intravenous pyelogram in 18 months after endoscopic surgery revealed a significant reduction of the ureter and pelvicalyceal system of the upper moiety and improved drainage of the middle and lower moieties

from the inside of it through the ectopic orifice allowed to create a new orifice of optimal size and position without risks of damage of deep bladder wall layers.

This extremely rare case of kidney triplication with ectopic ureterocele demonstrated complete improvement of the condition after endoscopic decompression of ureterocele.

Supplementary information

Additional file 1. Video 1080 of this clinical case.

Abbreviations

UTI: Urinary tract infection; IVP: Intravenous pyelogram; CT: Computer tomography; VUR: Vesicoureteral reflux

Acknowledgements

We highly appreciate the aid of colleagues from X-ray and radioisotope diagnostic department in making correct diagnose and choosing adequate treatment tactic.

Authors' contributions

DL made substantial contributions to the conception and design of the work. He was involved in acquisition, analysis and interpretation of data, drafted the work and substantively revised it. IO substantively revised the work. ML was involved in acquisition, analysis and interpretation of data and drafted the work. All authors have read and approved the manuscript.

References

1. Smith I. Triplicate ureter. Br J Surg. 1946;34(134):182–5 https://doi.org/10.1002/bjs.18003413409.
2. Gosalbez R, Piro C, Martin JA, Jimenez A. Ureteral triplication and ureterocele: report of 3 cases and review of the literature. J Urol. 1991; 145(1):105–8 https://doi.org/10.1016/S0022-5347(17)38261-7.
3. Lee M, Lee Z, Eun D. Intraureteral and intravenous indocyanine green to facilitate robotic partial nephroureterectomy in a patient with complete ureteral triplication. Korean J Urol. 2015;56(6):473–6 https://doi.org/10.4111/kju.2015.56.6.473.
4. Maizels M, Liu D, Gong EM, Kaplan WE, Cheng EY. Endoscopic ureterocele-otomy - retrograde incision from orifice (RIO) of urethral segment of ureterocele and extending to bladder neck is a feasible and simple procedure. J Pediatr Urol. 2016;12(3):137–8 https://doi.org/10.1016/j.jpurol.2016.05.010.
5. Gander R, Asensio M, Royo GF, Lloret J. Evaluation of the initial treatment of Ureteroceles. Urology. 2016;89:113–7 https://doi.org/10.1016/j.urology.2015.11.025
6. Neisius A, Schröder A, Riedmiller H, Brzezinska R, Stein R, Thüroff JW. Ureter triplex with non-functioning upper pole due to ectopic ureterocele and refluxive third ureter bud : case report and review of the literature. Urologe A. 2008;47(11):1483–6 https://doi.org/10.1007/s00120-008-1696-3.
7. John NT, Phukan C. Triplication of ureter with ureterocoele and renal calculi. ANZ J Surg. 2015;85(3):199 https://doi.org/10.1111/ans.12858.
8. Shankar KR, Vishwanath N, Rickwood AM. Outcome of patients with prenatally detected duplex system ureterocele; natural history of those managed expectantly. J Urol. 2001;165(4):1226–8 https://doi.org/10.1016/S0022-5347(05)66494-4.
9. Parente A, Angulo JM, Romero RM, Rivas S, Tardáguila AR, Corona C. Dilatación con balón de Alta presión Como tratamiento del ureterocele ortotópico. Actas Urol Esp. 2012;36(2):117–20 https://doi.org/10.1016/j.acuro.2011.07.005.
10. Akbal C, Lee SD, Kaefer M. Minimally invasive retrograde endourological technique for obstructed ectopic ureter. J Urol. 2004;172(4 Pt 1):1445 https://doi.org/10.1097/01.ju.0000137851.67567.2d.

3

Laparoscopy combining with ureteroscopy for horseshoe kidney accompanying with duplicate kidney and a ureteral calculus

Jindong Zhang[†], Liang Gao[†], Changlong Li, Xiaokang Yang, Yusheng Lei and Chuan Liu[*]

Abstract

Background: Horseshoe kidney (HSK) is a common renal fusion anomaly, occurring in about 1 in 400–600 individuals. In addition, the incidence of duplicated collecting system is about 0.8%.

Case presentation: This report documents an extremely rare case, which was treated by multiple procedures in the same operative session to accomplish laparoscopic amputation of the HSK isthmus, resection of duplicate kidney and ureteroscopic lithotripsy.

Conclusion: Results showed that minimally invasive surgery with use of multiple endoscopes may be a feasible choice for this patient population with complicated comorbid renal conditions.

Keywords: Horseshoe kidney, Duplicate kidney, Laparoscopy

Background

Horseshoe kidney (HSK) is a common renal fusion anomaly that typically involves the lower poles of the kidney and rarely the upper poles. This anomaly occurs in about 1 in 400–600 individuals, with a 2:1 male:female ratio [1, 2]. In addition, the occurrence of duplicated collecting system is about 0.8% and the upper poles of kidney are more frequently affected as a result of hydronephrosis [3]. However, the coexistence of these two anomalies is extremely rare [4]. This case report presents a patient who was diagnosed with HSK accompanied by duplicate kidney and ureteral calculus, which were treated by laparoscopy and ureteroscopy.

* Correspondence: liuchuan100@hospital.cqmu.edu.cn
[†]Jindong Zhang and Liang Gao contributed equally and should share the first author.
Department of Urology, the Second Affiliated Hospital of Chongqing Medical University, Chongqing 400000, China

Case presentation

In January 2019, a 31-year-old man was referred for evaluation at our hospital after the diagnosis of a giant renal cyst was made at another hospital, where the patient had initially presented with a 2-week history of dull right lower abdominal pain.

On admission, abdominal enhanced computed tomography (CT) combined with CT ureterography (CTU) showed the following: bilateral lower pole fusion; a low-density region (83 × 85 × 114 mm) in the right kidney during the arterial phase without entrance of the contrast agent in excretory phase and a left ureteral calculus with a 2.9-mm diameter. The multiple diagnoses of HSK with a right renal cyst and left ureteral calculus were suspected. (Fig. 1).

Considering the abnormal shape of renal cyst, however, we thought that the possibility of right hydronephrosis could not be eliminated. Therefore, a retrograde urography study was conducted, which showed a duplicated renal pelvis and ureters with severe hydronephrosis in the

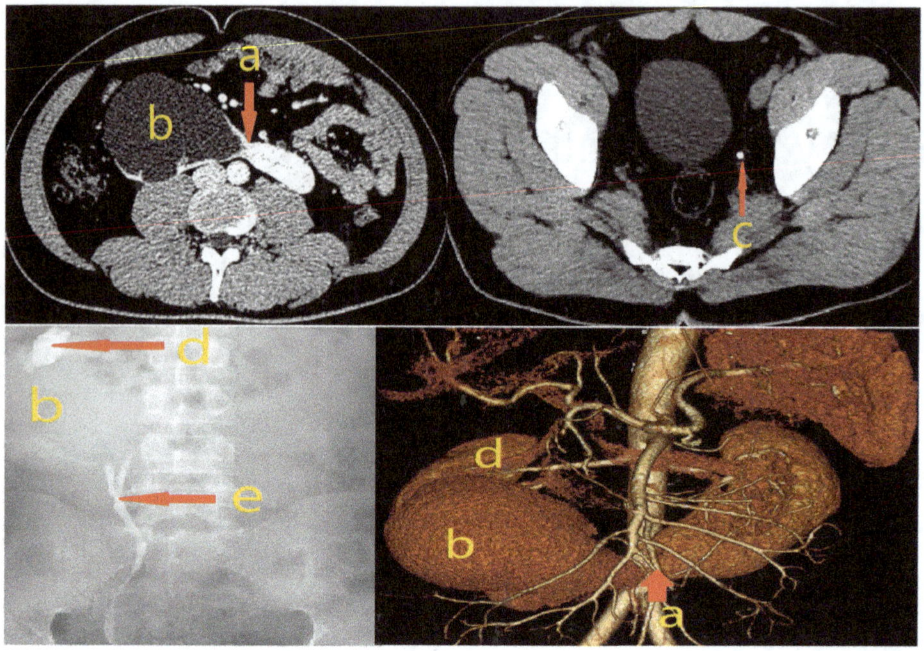

Fig. 1 Abdominal enhanced computed tomography (CT), CT ureterography and retrograde urography images show: a) fusion of the bilateral lower poles; b) right lower kidney; c) left ureteral calculus; d) right upper renal collecting system; e) confluence of the duplicate renal collecting system

right lower renal pelvis (Fig. 1). Furthermore, results of renal imaging showed that the right lower kidney had no blood supply, whereas the right upper kidney had a normal blood supply; the glomerular filtration rates (GFRs) were calculated to be 0 mL/min and 23.7 mL/min, respectively. No other abnormalities were evident on other examinations. Based on these results, the diagnosis was confirmed as HSK accompanying a right duplicated kidney, severe hydronephrosis with a nonfunctioning right lower kidney and a left ureteral calculus.

Surgery

Surgery was scheduled for the patient under general anesthesia. Firstly, the patient was placed in a bladder lithotomy position. A bilateral ureteroscope was used to remove the left ureteral calculus and stents were inserted into the ureters on each side. Secondly, the patient was placed in a modified lateral position and four puncture sheaths were inserted. After careful separation, a laparoscopic linear incision stapler was used to break off the isthmus of HSK (Fig. 2). Then, a knot-free suture (Johnson & Johnson) was used to reinforce the left side of separated section. After the inferior vessels were clamped and severed, the right lower kidney and ureter were excised.

During this procedure, however, the right ureteral stent was found to be inserted into the nonfunctional kidney. Therefore, this stent was removed through

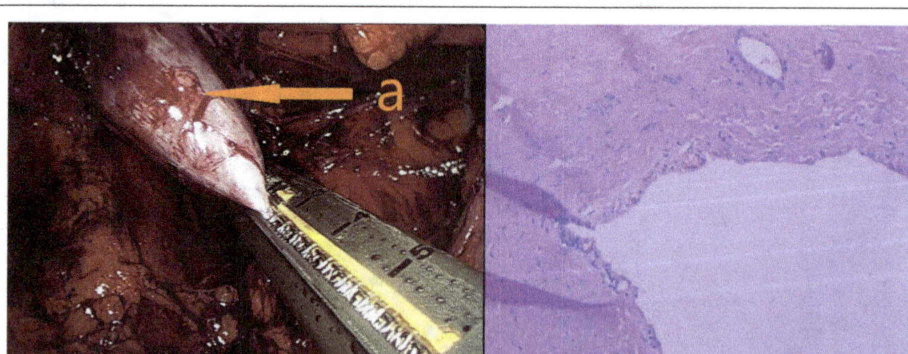

Fig. 2 Laparoscopic dismemberment of the isthmus of the horseshoe kidney shows the right lower kidney (a) with hydronephrosis. Pathologic examination shows renal cortex atrophy, interstitial inflammatory cell infiltration, pyelomegaly and mucosal atrophy

laparoscopy and then finally implanted through ureteroscopy in the bladder lithotomy position after the laparoscopic procedures.

Outcomes

The operative time was 6 h and 12 min, Pathologic examination showed severe atrophy of the renal cortex and mucosa with the infiltration of inflammatory cells in interstitium (Fig. 2).

No obvious complications were observed except for moderate incision pain, which was relieved by an intravenous analgesic. The patient's serum creatinine concentration returned to normal at postoperative Day 5, decreasing from the highest concentration on postoperative Day 2 at 125.5 umol/L. Abdominal X-ray showed that the position of the bilateral ureteral stents was normal. The patient was discharged on postoperative Day 6 after 13 hospitalisation days total.

At 3-month follow-up, the patient's renal function remained normal. Abdominal CT showed a few inflammatory changes but no hydronephrosis for either kidney. The bilateral ureteral stents were successfully removed (Fig. 3).

Discussion and conclusions

This case report presents the extremely rare anomaly of HSK comorbid with duplicated kidney. Most patients with duplicated kidney are asymptomatic and have no need for treatment [3]. However, these patients should be treated if complications occur, including hydronephrosis, calculus, infection or tumour [5]. In addition, most patients with HSK are also asymptomatic. Urinary tract infections, renal calculi and hydronephrosis are the most frequent complications, and 15–30% of patients have uretero-pelvic junction obstruction (UPJO) [6, 7]. The patient in this case had both anomalies, further complicated by hydronephrosis and a ureteral calculus, which was consistent with the complications noted in the literature.

A multicenter study reported that robot-assisted laparoscopic pyeloplasty (RALP) was a safe and feasible approach with satisfactory efficacy in children who had HSK [8]. A study by Guliev reported on 130 patients with HSK, 10 (7.7%) of whom had hydronephrosis treated with laparoscopic pyeloplasty, which achieved a success rate of 90% [9]. Minimally invasive surgery has gradually replaced traditional open surgery to shorten the hospital stay and postoperative recovery time; however. Retroperitoneal laparoscopic treatment for HSK is still rarely reported [10].

The standard treatment for duplicate kidney is surgical heminephrectomy [11]. Laparoscopic upper pole heminephrectomy was first reported in 1993, and then in several subsequent studies [12, 13]. Two different laparoscopic approaches have been used for the management of duplicate kidney, including the retroperitoneal approach in the lateral position and transperitoneal approach in the supine position [11]. Moreover, RALP is becoming a new minimally invasive method for treatment of duplicate kidney [14].

Up to now, only a few cases have been reported of HSK comorbid with duplicate kidney, but none of these patients have been treated laparoscopically. Because the experience in treating this patient population is very limited to date, the operative time and time that the stents were maintained was longer than that for more typical HSK or duplicate kidney cases. In addition, a ureteric stent was inserted to distinguish the duplicated ureter during surgery, which may serve to protect the normal ureter and avoid a possible stricture at the meeting of two ureters. Although this approach seemed to be working during laparoscopic procedure, the ureteric stent was subsequently found to have been inserted into the diseased ureter and thus had to be reinserted after the laparoscopic procedure.

This case management was performed by laparoscopy in an improved position, which confirmed the effectiveness of this method. We hope this case presentation can

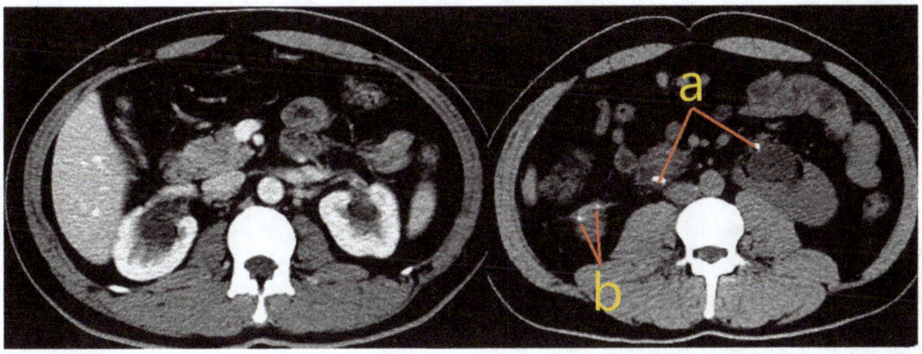

Fig. 3 Postoperative computed tomography shows a few inflammatory changes and hydronephrosis for both kidneys: a) bilateral ureteral stent. b) postoperative changes after use of a laparoscopic linear incision stapler

provide a reference for the minimally invasive treatment of this disease. Based on the literature review and considering that to date only one such case has been treated by the approach described herein, the authors recommend that a highly experienced laparoscopic surgeon is required.

In conclusion, this report documents a rare case of multiple renal anomalies that included HSK, duplicate kidney, unilateral hydronephrosis and unilateral ureteral calculus. The results showed that minimally invasive surgery combining laparoscopy and ureteroscopy may be a safe and effective approach for this disease presentation.

Abbreviations
HSK: horseshoe kidney; CT: computed tomography; CTU: computed tomography ureterography; GFR: glomerular filtration rate; UPJO: uretero-pelvic junction obstruction; PALP: robot-assisted laparoscopic pyeloplasty

Acknowledgements
Not applicable.

Authors' contributions
JZ: Data Collection, Manuscript writing and Manuscript Revision. LG: Manuscript writing and Manuscript Revision. CL1: Manuscript writing and editing. XY and YL: interpretation of data, evaluated the patient clinically and helped to operate the patient. CL2: Writing – review. All authors read and approved the final manuscript.

References

1. Natsis K, Piagkou M, Skotsimara A, Protogerou V, Tsitouridis I, Skandalakis P. Horseshoe kidney: a review of anatomy and pathology. Surg Radiol Anat. 2014;36(6):517–26.
2. Schiappacasse G, Aguirre J, Soffia P, Silva CS, Zilleruelo N. CT findings of the main pathological conditions associated with horseshoe kidneys. Br J Radiol. 2015;88(1045):20140456.
3. Liu W, Zhang L, Ma R, Wu R. The morphology and treatment of coexisting ureteropelvic junction obstruction in lower moiety of duplex kidney. Int J Surg. 2016;34:23–7.
4. Jamshidian H, Tavakoli K, Salahshour F, Nabighadim A, Amini E. Supernumerary kidney associated with horseshoe malformation: a case report and review of literature. Urol Case Rep. 2017;11:57–9.
5. Zissin R, Apter S, Yaffe D, Kots E, Hertz M. Renal duplication with associated complications in adults: CT findings in 26 cases. Clin Radiol. 2001;56(1):58–63.
6. Chaabouni Y, Guesmi R, Hentati Y, Kammoun K, Hmida MB, Mnif Z, et al. Minimal change disease in horseshoe kidney. Pan Afr Med J. 2017;26:243.
7. Yohannes P, Smith AD. The Endourological Management of Complications Associated with horseshoe kidney. J Urol. 2002;168(1):5–8.
8. Esposito C, Masieri L, Blanc T, Manzoni G, Silay S, Escolino M. Robot-assisted laparoscopic pyeloplasty (RALP) in children with horseshoe kidneys: results of a multicentric study. World J Urol. 2019;37(10):2257–63.
9. Guliev BG. Laparoscopic pyeloplasty for hydronephrosis of horseshoe kidney. Urologiia. 2016;5:58.
10. Wang P, Xia D, Ma Q, Wang S. Retroperitoneal laparoscopic management of ureteropelvic junction obstruction in patients with horseshoe kidney. Urology. 2014;84(6):1351–4.
11. Joyeux L, Lacreuse I, Schneider A, Moog R, Borgnon J, Lopez M, et al. Long-term functional renal outcomes after retroperitoneoscopic upper pole heminephrectomy for duplex kidney in children: a multicenter cohort study. Surg Endosc. 2017;31(3):1241–9.
12. El-Ghoneimi A, Farhat W, Bolduc S, Bagli D, McLorie G, Khoury A. Retroperitoneal laparoscopic vs open partial nephroureterectomy in children. Brit J Urol Int. 2015;91(6):532–5.
13. Lee RS, Retik AB, Borer JG, Diamond DA, Peters CA. Pediatric retroperitoneal laparoscopic partial nephrectomy: comparison with an age matched cohort of open surgery. J Urol. 2005;174(2):708–12.
14. Herz D, Smith J, McLeod D, Schober M, Preece J, Merguerian P. Robot-assisted laparoscopic management of duplex renal anomaly: Comparison of surgical outcomes to traditional pure laparoscopic and open surgery. J Pediatric Urol. 2016;12(1):44.e1–7.

4

The role of specific biomarkers, as predictors of post-operative complications following flexible ureterorenoscopy (FURS), for the treatment of kidney stones: A single-centre observational clinical pilot-study in 37 patients

Stephen Fôn Hughes[1,2*], Alyson Jayne Moyes[1,3,4], Rebecca May Lamb[1,4], Peter Ella-tongwiis[1,2], Christopher Bell[2,5], Ahmed Moussa[2,5] and Iqbal Shergill[1,2,5]

Abstract

Background: The number of patients diagnosed and subsequently treated for kidney stones is increasing, and as such the number of post-operative complications is likely to increase. At present, little is known about the role of specific biomarkers, following flexible ureterorenoscopy (FURS) for the surgical treatment of kidney stones. The main aim of the study was to evaluate the role of kidney and infection biomarkers, in patients undergoing FURS.

Methods: Included were 37 patients (24 males, 13 females), who underwent elective FURS, for the treatment of kidney stones. Venous blood samples were collected from each patient: pre-operatively, and at 30 min, 2 and 4 h post-operatively. Changes to kidney (NGAL, Cystatin C) and infection (MPO, PCT) biomarkers was quantified by means of ELISA, Biomerieux mini-vidas and Konelab 20 analysers.

Results: Four patients developed post-operative complications (3 - UTIs with urinary retention, 1 - urosepsis. NGAL concentration increased significantly following FURS ($p = 0.034$). Although no significant changes were seen in Cystatin C, MPO and PCT ($p \geq 0.05$) some key clinical observation were noted. Limiting factors for this study were the small number of patients recruited and restriction in blood sampling beyond 4 h.

(Continued on next page)

* Correspondence: Stephen.hughes6@wales.nhs.uk
[1]North Wales & North West Urological Research Centre, Betsi Cadwaladr University Health Board (BCUHB) Wrexham Maelor Hospital, Wrexham, Wales, UK
[2]North Wales Clinical Research Centre, Betsi Cadwaladr University Health Board (BCUHB) Wrexham Maelor Hospital, Wrexham, Wales, UK
Full list of author information is available at the end of the article

(Continued from previous page)

Conclusions: Although not confirmative, changes seen to biomarkers such as Cystatin C, NGAL and MPO in our observational clinical pilot-study may warrant further investigation, involving larger cohorts, to fully understand the role of these biomarkers and their potential association with post-operative complications which can develop following FURS.

Keywords: Flexible Ureterenoscopy, (FURS), Kidney stones, Biomarkers, Infection, Post-operative complications

Background

Flexible ureterorenoscopy (FURS) is an increasingly popular procedure for the treatment of kidney stones. The complication rate following FURS is up to 25% with this figure likely to increase [1]. Conventionally in the UK, patients have been monitored post-operatively using routine blood tests, such as the full blood count, urea and electrolyte and C reactive protein (CRP). Although these traditional blood tests are clinically useful, they are non-specific in nature, and fail to identify patients at increased risk of developing postoperative complications, such as infection and acute kidney injury.

At present, there is limited literature and evidence-based reports highlighting the role of specific biomarkers, which can monitor patients following FURS. In turn, it is anticipated, in the future, that a specific panel of biomarkers (or biomarker profile) may help aid clinicians in the monitoring of patients undergoing FURS and could help identify or predict those individuals at increased risk of developing complications post-procedure.

In the present study, we have identified specific kidney and potential infection biomarkers that may provide clinically important information that will aid monitoring and subsequent managing of these patients. Cystatin C is a cysteine proteinase inhibitor which is produced by all nucleated cells and is has gathered increasing interest as a specific marker of kidney function [2].

Due to its low molecular weight (13.3 kDa), Cystatin C is freely filtered at the glomerulus, and is neither secreted nor reabsorbed in the renal tubules [3]. Although Cystatin C has been shown to be a useful biomarker for identifying renal injury post-surgery in a critical care setting [4], at present there are no studies that have reported the role of the parameter in patients undergoing FURS. This makes cystatin C a novel and exiting prospect for the monitoring of kidney stone patients.

Neutrophil gelatinase-associated lipocalin (NGAL) belongs to the lipocalin family, predominantly found within neutrophils, but are also found in low levels in the kidney, prostate and respiratory tract [5]. NGAL is reported to be a modulator of the inflammatory response, binding and attacking small lipophilic substances in bacteria such as lipopolysaccharides and formyl peptides [6]. Several studies have suggested NGAL may be a useful kidney injury biomarker, particularly in patients with nephrolithiasis or its associated pathologies [7–10]. NGAL has been reported as a potential renal injury biomarker in the early period after surgery and has a multifaceted role in inflammation and cancer [2, 11]. Notably, in their study of urinary biomarkers in 30 patients post-FURS, Benli et al (2017) reported a significant increase in NGAL levels 2 h post-operatively [2]. This suggests that the early post-operative rise in NGAL may provide an opportunity for this biomarker to be utilised as part of monitoring patients following FURS. In the present study, we aim to expand on previous work undertaken by others and to investigate changes in NGAL amongst other biomarkers up to 4 h post-FURS.

Myeloperoxidase (MPO) is an enzyme which has been shown to be expressed within neutrophils and monocytes [12]. MPO produces hypochlorous acids (HOCl) as part of the respiratory burst process, providing a highly anti-microbial environment for bacteria and other pathogens [13, 14]. It is believed to have a role in cellular homeostasis and is associated with inflammatory disease development and progression; strong link has been established in this regard, especially in the field of cardiovascular disease (CVD) [15]. Hasmann et al. (2013) have previously reported the role of MPO activity in wound fluid, as a potential marker for infection, as it can be appreciated that this biomarker may provide a more rapid diagnosis, in comparison to traditional means of testing for infection via microbiological methods and the non-specific CRP [16]. MPO therefore warrants investigation in the present study, as a potential biomarker for infection or monitoring the respiratory burst in patients post-FURS.

Sepsis, a potential life-threatening condition can be defined as bacteriuria with systemic inflammatory response syndrome (SIRS). It can be appreciated that sepsis can be caused by an array of microorganisms such as bacteria, fungi and viruses. However, bacterial sepsis is by far clinically the most diagnosed [17]. In sepsis, pathogens enter the blood stream where they can thrive and release harmful infectious factors into the bloodstream [18]. These products can stimulate the release of mediators of sepsis from biological cells such as monocytes, macrophages, neutrophils and plasma cell precursors [19]. The body's attempt to fight the infection can involve a systemic inflammatory response (SIRS), however, the resultant activation of inflammatory proteins can result in more extensive tissue and organ damage [20]. Procalcitonin (PCT), a calcitonin precursor, is upregulated in response to such damage [21]. Raised blood PCT levels indicate systemic bacterial infection. With urosepsis a well-known complication of FURS, monitoring PCT pre and post FURS may prove beneficial in managing these patients [20, 21].

Several groups, including ours, have reported on the effect of various urological and other surgical procedures on post-operative routine and novel blood tests [22–27], However, crucially, there are few studies into the effect of FURS on kidney and infection biomarkers. Our study aimed to evaluate the role of these biomarkers in order to better establish their post-operative levels following FURS for the treatment of nephrolithiasis.

Methods

Subject volunteers

Ethical approval for this study was received from the Welsh Research Ethics Service (REC) 4 committee (REC4: 12/WA/0117) and were carried out in accordance with the ethical rules of the Helsinki Declaration and Good Clinical Practice. As this is a single-centre observational clinical pilot-study, no sample size or power calculation has been performed, and therefore all the comparisons that will be considered are exploratory in nature regardless of the significance level found. Thirty-seven consecutive patients undergoing elective FURS for the treatment of kidney stones were recruited (n = 37). Twenty-four males and 13 females aged between 28 and 87 years (median 50 years) were recruited after receiving written informed consent [23].

Flexible ureterorenoscopy (FURS)

FURS was performed as per local protocol at the Betsi Cadwaladr University Health Board (BCUHB) Wrexham Maelor, NHS hospital, North Wales, UK by a single consultant surgeon who is an expert in the field, having undertaken >1000 FURS procedures. The Olympus URF-P6 fibreoptic flexible Ureterorenoscope was used in all cases. This has a working channel of 3.6Fr, working length 670 mm, outer diameter 4.9Fr and outer diameter insertion tube of 7.95Fr. Height of the irrigation fluid was set to 80cmH2O and in all cases a 10/12Fr Coloplast ureteral access sheath was used, to standardise all operations. As a result, injury to the distal tubule was unrelated to the surgical procedure itself. The indication to treat the patient with a 25 mm stone was based on a multi-disciplinary decision which was patient centred, due to significant co-morbidities and as such not suitable for standard PCNL surgery. Clinical and surgical information pertaining to the present study are presented in Table 1. Where possible, stones were sent for composition analysis, using infrared spectroscopy at the Leicester Royal Infirmary, UK [23].

Table 1 Clinical and surgical information

Number of stones	Patients (n = 37)
1	24
2	10
3	3
Median Stone Size	9.1 mm (range: 3.0 mm–25.00 mm)
Median Hounsfield Unit (HU)	1123 (range: 240–2224)
Stone location	
Upper pole	15 patients
Mid pole	8 patients
Lower pole	14 patients
Median duration of laser lithotripsy	9.54 min (range: 30 s-54.02 min)
Average energy	3232.7 J (Joule)
Mean pulse	6272.76 (number of pulses)
Median Operating time	57 min (range: 20–175 min)
Complete stone clearance	100% (n = 37), confirmed via imaging at 3 months KUB XR if radio-opaque stone and CT if lucent
Stent insertion	24 patients

Blood samples

Pre-operative (baseline) venous blood samples were collected, with subsequent samples collected after FURS at 30, 120 and 240 min. All samples were collected using di-potassium ethylenediaminetetraacetic acid (EDTA) and serum separator tube (SST) vacutainers. An 83% compliance was obtained regarding blood sample collection at all time points, with the remaining 17% non-compliance being due to difficulty (i.e. poor veins) with the venesection.

Measurement of kidney biomarkers

Serum Cystatin C levels (mg/ml) were measured employing a latex enhanced immunoturbidimetric methodology, using a Thermo Fisher KoneLab 20 automated analyser. The Cystatin C kits were supplied from Randox Laboratories (*Cat No:* CYS4004).

Serum Neutrophil gelatinase-associated lipocalin (NGAL) concentrations (ng/ml) was measured using commercially available kits via quantitative sandwich enzyme immunoassays (ELISA) and were supplied by R&D Systems (*Cat No:* DLCN20).

Measurement of infection biomarkers

Serum Myeloperoxidase (MPO) concentrations (ng/ml) were measured using commercially available quantitative sandwich enzyme immunoassay (ELISA) kits supplied by R&D Systems (Cat No: DMYE00B).

Plasma Procalcitonin (PCT) levels (ng/ml) were measured using commercially available kits (*Cat No:* 30450) and a Biomerieux mini-VIDAS automated immunoanalyser, employing a one-step immunoassay method.

Statistical analysis

Statistical analysis was performed using SPSS (version 26). Testing for normality was carried out, and where data was parametric, repeated measures one-way analysis of variance (ANOVA) employed, using a 5% level of significance. The Bonferroni method for pairwise comparisons between means was used for post-hoc testing.

Non-parametric data were analysed using the Friedman test. Where this reached statistical significance, subsequent tests were performed with the Wilcoxon. Statistical significance was defined when $p \leq 0.05$.

All parametric data is presented as mean ± standard deviation (S.D), whilst non-parametric results are presented as median ± interquartile range (Iqr).

Results

Effect on Cystatin C concentration

The results are expressed as mg/ml and represent changes to serum Cystatin C following FURS (Fig. 1). Cystatin C was measured as means of a kidney biomarker. Cystatin C concentration did not change significantly from baseline (2.95 ± 2.53 mg/L) to 30 min post-FURS (2.95 ± 2.66 mg/L). At 120 min post FURS there was an increase in Cystatin C levels (3.8 ± 2.36 mg/L) followed by a decrease back toward basal levels at 240 min (2.94 ± 2.7 mg/L). There were no statistically significant changes in Cystatin C concentrations following FURS (p = 0.462), as determined by the Friedman test.

Effect NGAL

The results are expressed as ng/ml and represent changes to serum NGAL following FURS (Fig. 2). Initially, there was an increase in NGAL concentration from baseline (74.59 ± 9.4 ng/ml) up to 30 min (88.12 ± 11.25 ng/ml) post-FURS. At 120 min (86.45 ± 11.45 ng/ml) and 240 min post FURS (77.63 ± 8.90 ng/ml) NGAL concentration decreased toward basal levels. Friedman analysis illustrated a significant increase in NGAL following FURS (p = 0.034). Post hoc analysis employing the Wilcoxon test, confirmed a significant increase in NGAL between baseline and 30 min post-FURS (p = 0.047), although these changes did not correlate with surgical time ($p > 0.05$).

Effect myeloperoxidase (MPO) concentration

The results are expressed as ng/ml and represent changes to serum MPO following FURS (Fig. 3). MPO was measured as means of a biomarker for infection. Initially, a decrease in MPO concentration from baseline (11.66 ± 2.2 ng/ml) was seen, at 30 min (10.87 ± 2.2 ng/ml) and 120 min (9.38 ± 1.6 ng/ml) post FURS. However, a sharp increase occurred at 240 min (27.88 ± 1.3 ng/ml) post FURS. However, statistical analysis found no significant changes in MPO following FURS (p = 0.38), as determined by the Friedman test.

Effect on PCT concentration

The results are expressed as ng/ml and represent changes to plasma PCT following FURS (Fig. 4). PCT was measured as means of a biomarker for infection. Only a negligible change in PCT concentration between baseline (0.195 ± 0.002 ng/ml) up to 240 min (0.188 ± 0.004 ng/ml) post-

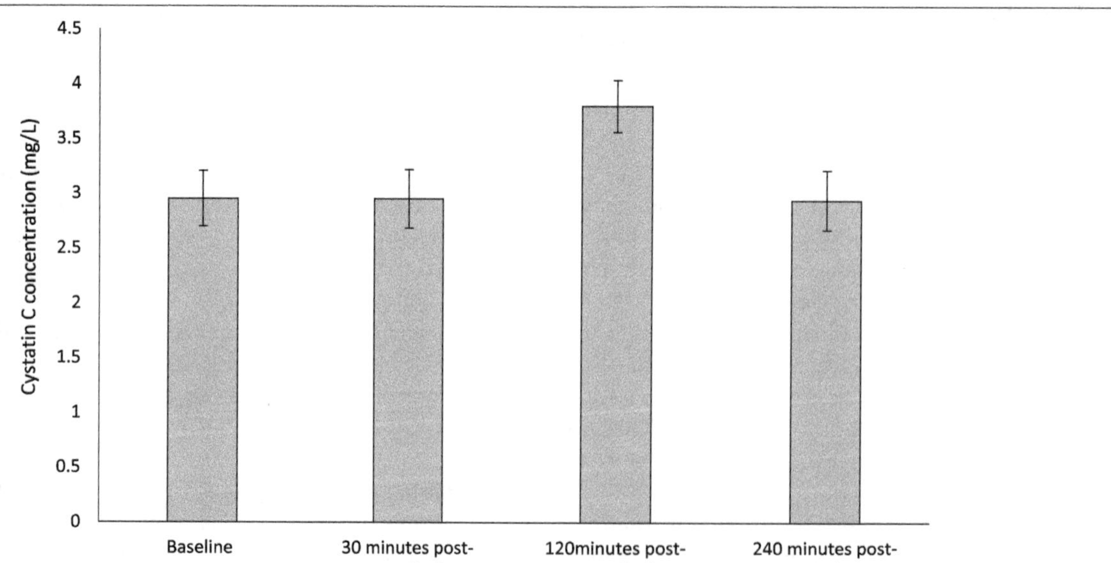

Fig. 1 The effect of FURS, for the treatment of nephrolithiasis, on Cystatin C concentration. The points represent the median ± Iqr, p = 0.462 (n = 37)

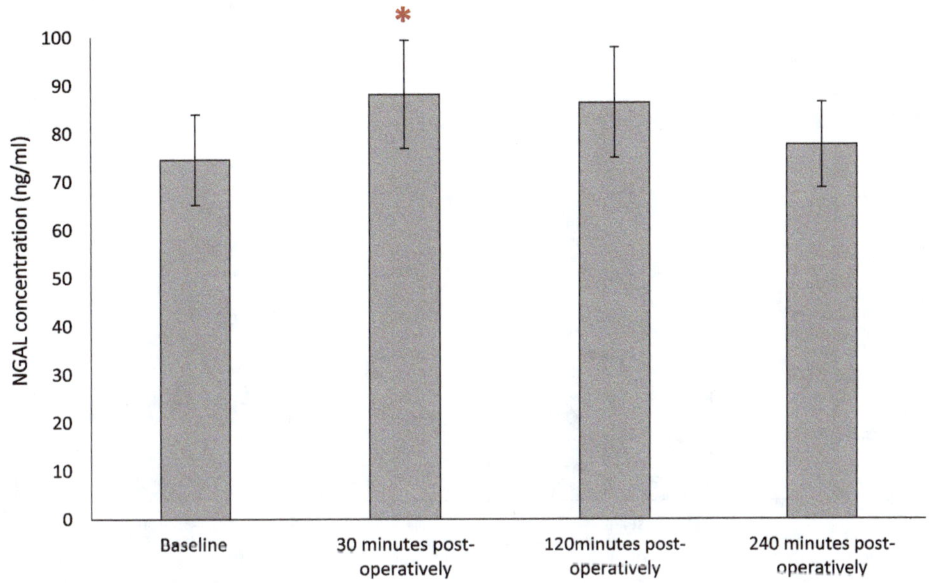

Fig. 2 The effect of FURS, for the treatment of nephrolithiasis, on NGAL concentration. The points represent the median ± Iqr, $p = 0.034$. * = Wilcoxon test showed significance ($p = 0.047$) between levels at baseline and 30 min post-operatively $n = 37$. Normal reference range = 42-177 ng/ml

FURS was demonstrated. Analysis employing a paired t-test showed no significant change in PCT concentration (p = 0.539). No samples analysis was undertaken for PCT at 30 and 120 min post-operatively, due to the high cost of purchasing assay kits and financial restrictions.

Stone analysis results

As per routine protocol, stone analysis was undertaken at the Department of Pathology, Leicester Royal Infirmary Hospital (UK). Stone composition results are presented in Table 2.

Post-FURS complications

One female and two males developed a post-operative urinary tract infection (UTI) with urinary retention. One male patient developed urosepsis. Levels of Cystatin C and NGAL for these patients are compared with the average ($n = 37$) in Figs. 5, 6, 7, 8.

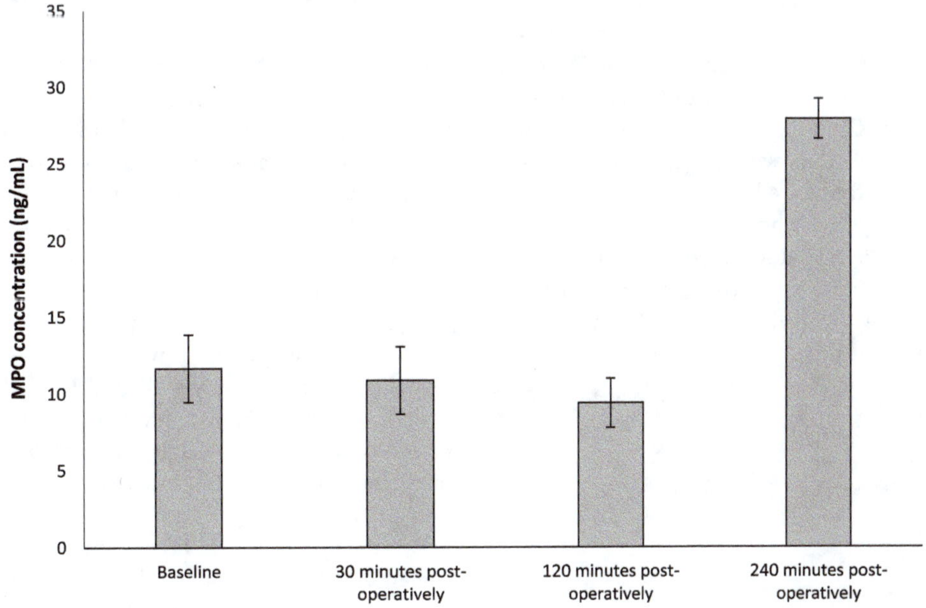

Fig. 3 The effect of FURS for the treatment of nephrolithiasis on MPO concentration. The points represent the median ± Iqr, $p = 0.38$ ($n = 37$)

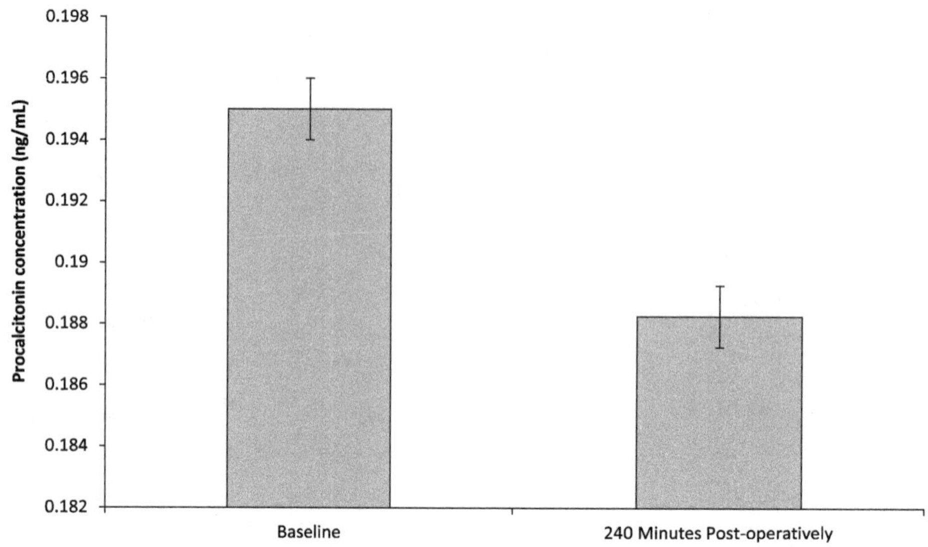

Fig. 4 The effect of FURS, for the treatment of nephrolithiasis, on PCT concentration. The points represent the mean ± S.D, $p = 0.539 (n = 37)$

A summary of the main findings from the study are presented in Table 3.

Discussion

The aim of this prospective observational study was to evaluate novel kidney and infection biomarkers, following FURS in the management of nephrolithiasis. Currently, studies reporting on the role of biological markers following FURS are limited.

Serum cystatin C is a non-glycosylated, 13.3-kDa protein belonging to cystatin protease inhibitors [28]. It has shown promise as a replacement for serum creatinine as a potential kidney biomarker [29, 30]. A 2002 meta-analysis based on 46 studies concluded that cystatin C is superior to creatinine for detection of compromised renal function, as well as subsequent renal function monitoring [31]. Although in our study there were no significant changes in Cystatin C levels following FURS, some interesting observations were noted when comparing data of those who developed complications (patients 9, 10, 12 and 32) with those who did not (Fig. 5).

Specifically, patient 9 had developed 3 stones (size 2 mm, 20 and 5 mm; comprising 100% calcium oxalate; duration of procedure 28 min); patient 10 developed 1 stone (size 20 mm; comprising 80% calcium phosphate and 20% calcium oxalate monohydrate; duration of procedure 32 min); and patient 12 developed 2 stones (size 20 and 17 mm; comprising 100% calcium phosphate; duration of procedure 98 min). With regards to patients 9, 10 and 12 none were first time stoners, none received pre-operative stents and all three received a stent post-operative. Interestingly, The Cystatin C levels of patients who developed UTIs and subsequent urinary retention (patient 9, 10, and 12) were higher to that of the normal average patient response (Fig. 5). This biomarker, therefore, shows potential promise and warrants further investigation, as for the patients who developed complications, Cystatin C levels rose sharply within a four-hour time period, thus highlighting its sensitivity and potential role as a marker of monitoring patients post FURS.

Table 2 Stone composition

Main constituent of stone(s)	Patients
Calcium oxalate monohydrate	21
Calcium phosphate stones	7
Cystine stones	3
Calcium hydroxyl phosphate	3
Calcium-oxalate dihydrate stones	3

Recent research has suggested that NGAL is a useful biomarker for measuring renal function and predicting kidney injury [32, 33]. NGAL measured in the present study demonstrated a significant increase in NGAL levels post FURS ($p = 0.034$), with levels peaking between 30 min and 2 h post treatment. Our results compliment findings from a Dede et al. (2015) findings, in 30 patients, that NGAL increased significantly 2 h post-FURS [34]. Interestingly, the present study also highlighted that patients who developed a complication post-FURS (specifically patients 12 and 32; Fig. 6), reported increased NGAL levels compared to the average patient response. Although not confirmative, these initial pilot data provide some interesting results and may warrant further investigation by recruiting larger cohorts.

With respect MPO, no significant changes were observed in this biomarker following FURS. However, and interesting trend of increased MPO levels were observed and reported in patients who developed a complication

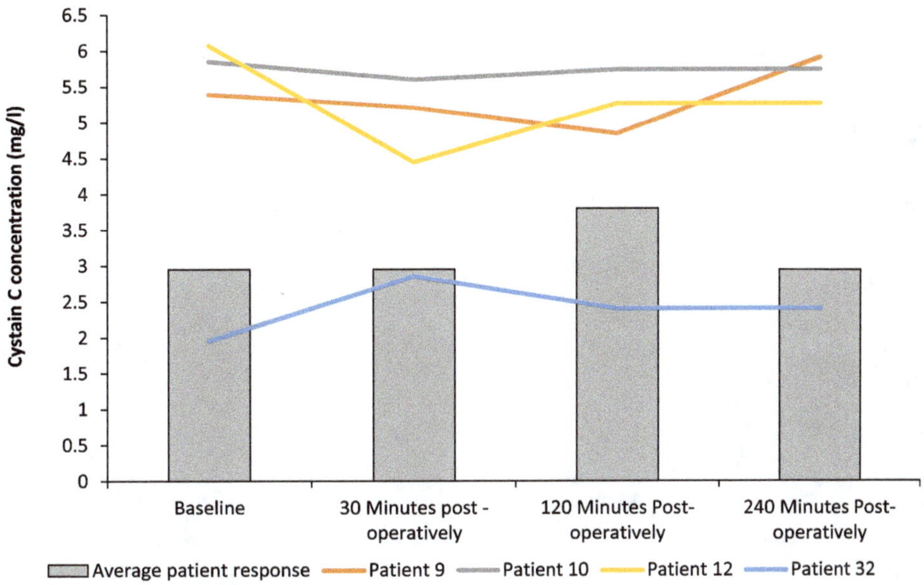

Fig. 5 Comparison of Cystatin C concentration across all patients with those developing a complication. Patients 9 (male), 10 (male), and 12 (female) developed urinary tract infection (UTI) with urinary retention. Patient 32 (male) developed urosepsis (Average patient response $n = 37$). Patients 9, 10 and 12 exhibited higher Cystatin C levels than the average group response

post-FURS (specifically, patients 9, 12 and 32; Fig. 7). Although MPO has been reported to be increased in various inflammatory conditions and is considered a risk marker for cardiovascular disease [35, 36], here we provide evidence that MPO may also be considered as a potential biomarker for identifying patients with infectious complications post FURS, although it is appreciated that studies involving larger cohorts will be needed to validate this proposition.

Although PCT is considered a reliable biomarker that displays greater specificity than other proinflammatory markers, such as cytokines in identifying patients with sepsis and aiding in the diagnosis of bacterial infections [37]. The results from our pilot study were disappointing

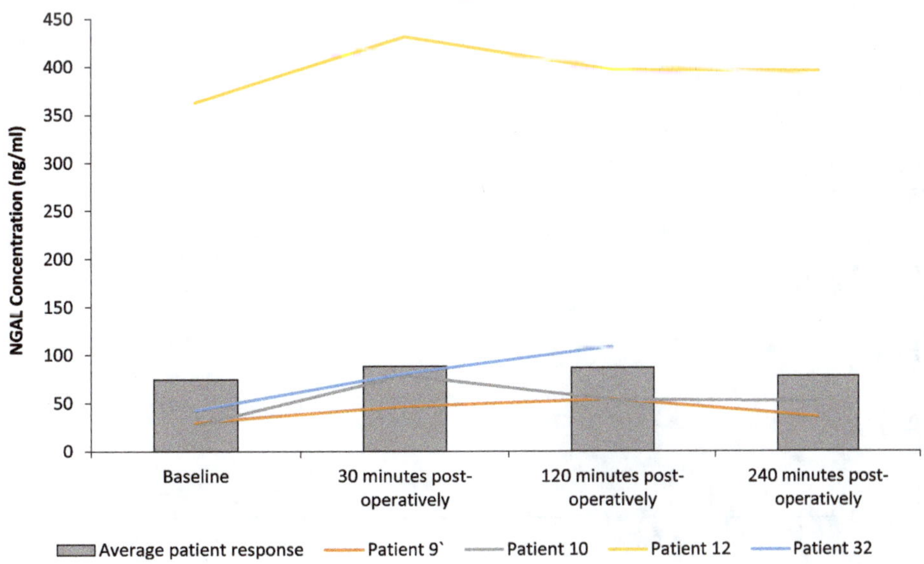

Fig. 6 Comparison of NGAL concentration across all patients with those developing a complication. Patients 9 (male), 10 (male), and 12 (female) developed urinary tract infection (UTI) with urinary retention. Patient 32 (male) developed urosepsis (Average patient response $n = 37$). Patients 12 and 32 exhibited higher NGAL levels than the average group response. Missing data is representative of no sample collection or inadequate sample volume for analysis

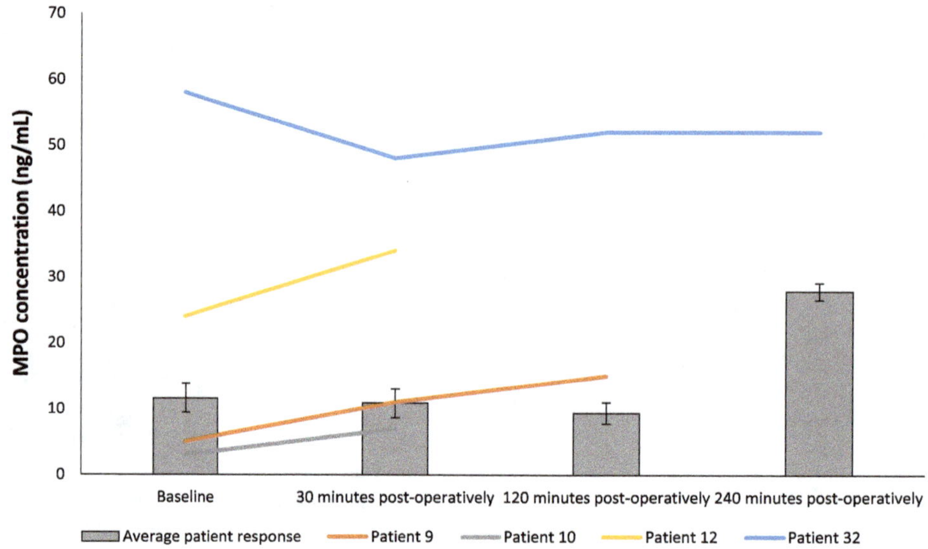

Fig. 7 Comparison of MPO concentration across all patients with those developing a complication. Patients 9 (male), 10 (male), and 12 (female) developed urinary tract infection (UTI) with urinary retention. Patient 32 (male) developed urosepsis (Average patient response $n = 37$). Patients 12 and 32 exhibited higher MPO levels than the average group response. Missing data is representative of no sample collection or inadequate sample volume for analysis

in that PCT levels did not appear to significantly increase in the four patients that developed complications. Meisner et al. (1999) have previously reported on the kinetic profiles of different biomarkers of bacterial infection, illustrating that PCT levels in plasma tend not to peak until 10–12 h following infection [38, 39]. In the present study, blood sampling was not undertaken beyond >4 h period due to ethical restirctions, which may provide an explination as to why no significant changes to PCT levels were reported. It is postulated that the time frame (and a limitation of the present study) was too short to see elevated PCT in patients with complications [38]. However, in addition, further evidence is provided here, in that that the other biomarkes

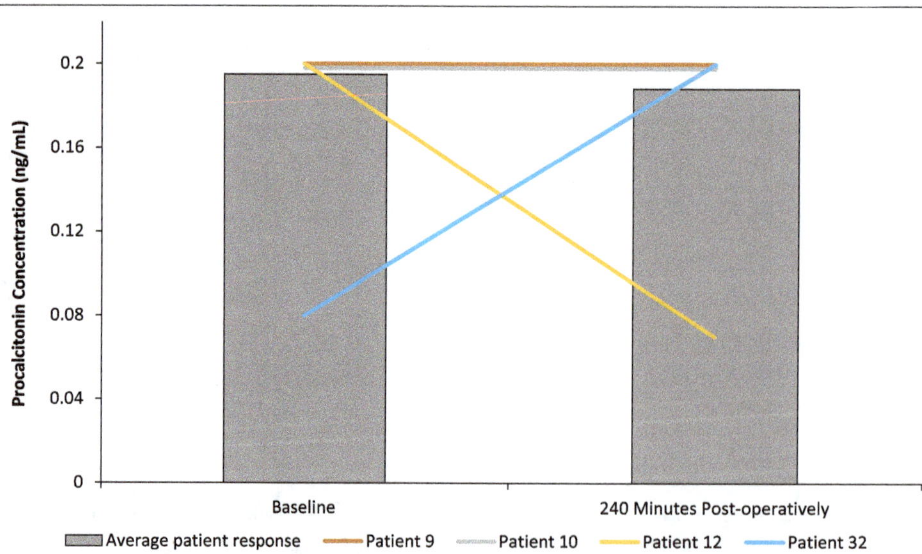

Fig. 8 Comparison of PCT concentration across all patients with those developing a complication. Patients 9 (male), 10 (male), and 12 (female) developed urinary tract infection (UTI) with urinary retention. Patient 32 (male) developed urosepsis (Average patient response $n = 37$). Patients 9, 10 and 32 exhibited higher PCT levels than the average group response

Table 3 Summary of main findings

- ➢ A significant increase in NGAL concentration post-FURS for the management of nephrolithiasis ($p = 0.034$).
- ➢ No significant differences were seen in Cystatin C, MPO or PCT concentrations post-FURS, for the management of nephrolithiasis ($p > 0.05$)

investigated in the present study (i.e. Cystatin C, NGAL and MPO) may provide more sensitivity for detecting complications ealier than PCT follwoing FURS.

A limiting factor associated with this study was the relatively small number of patients recruited and the number of sampling time points. It would have been beneficial to have obtained further blood samples at time point beyond 4 h (e.g. up to 24–48 h), but as these were day-case patients obtaining additional samples was not possible. In addition, the inclusion of a comparative control group, possibly involving patients undergoing other urological procedures such as shock wave lithotripsy (SWL) or TUR-B without fluid pressure to the controlling system (reflux out ruled) thereby identifying the potential influence of anaesthesia may have been identified. However, restriction to current ethics did not permit the inclusion of such control groups.

In summary, we report that this study provides a basis to undertake further investigations involving biomarkers for monitoring FUR patients during the post-operative period. It is envisaged that when these preliminary studies have been performed and authenticated in larger cohorts, a panel of biomarkers (or biomarker profile) may be produced that can help identify or predict those patients that will develop post-operative complications following FURS.

Conclusions

Changes seen to biomarkers such as Cystatin C, NGAL and MPO in our observational clinical pilot-study may warrant further investigation, involving larger cohorts, to fully understand the role of these biomarkers and their potential association with post-operative complications which can develop following FURS.

Abbreviations

CRP: C reactive protein; EDTA: Ethylene diaminetetraacetic acid; ELISA: Enzyme-linked Immunoassay; FURS: Flexible ureteroscopy; HOCl: Hypochlorous acid; ICU: Intensive care unit; Iqr: Interquartile range; MPO: Myeloperoxidase; NGAL: Neutrophil gelatinase-associated lipocalin; NO: Nitric Oxide; PCT: Procalcitonin; SD: Standard deviation; SIRS: Systemic inflammatory response syndrome; SWL: Shock wave lithotripsy; UTI: Urinary tract infection

Acknowledgments

The authors are indebted to the patients who kindly agreed to take part in this study. The authors wish to thank all the staff at the Department of Urology at Betsi Cadwaladr University Health Board (BCUHB), Wrexham Maelor Hospital, North Wales, UK, for their support regards our continued research activities.

Authors' contributions

Conceived concept, study designed and supervision: SFH and IS. Performed the experiments: AJM, RML and PET. Analysed and interpreted the data: AJM and SFH. Wrote the paper: SFH, AJM, CB, AM and IS. All authors read an approved the paper.

Author details

[1]North Wales & North West Urological Research Centre, Betsi Cadwaladr University Health Board (BCUHB) Wrexham Maelor Hospital, Wrexham, Wales, UK. [2]North Wales Clinical Research Centre, Betsi Cadwaladr University Health Board (BCUHB) Wrexham Maelor Hospital, Wrexham, Wales, UK. [3]School of Medical Sciences, Bangor University, Bangor, Wales, UK. [4]Department of Biological Sciences, University of Chester, Chester, UK. [5]The Alan de Bolla Department of Urology, BCUHB Wrexham Maelor Hospital, Wrexham, Wales, UK.

References

1. Skolarikos A, Gross A, Krebs A, Unal D, Bercowsky E, Somani B, de la Rosette J. Outcomes of flexible Ureterorenoscopy for solitary renal stones in the CROES URS global study. J Urol. 2015;194(1):137–43.
2. Benli E, Ayylidiz S, Cirrik S, Noyan T, Ayyildiz A, Cirakoglu A. Early term effect of ureterorenoscopy (URS) on the kidney: research measuring NGAL, KIM 1, FABP and CYS C levels in urine. Brazil J Urol. 2017;43(5):887–95.
3. Tenstad O, Roald A, Grubb A, Aukland K. Renal handling of radiolabelled human cystatin C in the rat. Scandinavian J Clin Labortatory Investigation. 1996;56:409–14.
4. Hall I, Koyner J, Doshi M, Marcus R, Parikh C. Urine Cystatin C as a biomarker of proximal tubular function immediately after kidney transplantation. Am J Nephrol. 2011;33(5):407–13.
5. Soni S, Cruz D, Bobek L, Chionh C, Nalesso F, Lentini P, et al. NGAL: a biomarker of acute kidney injury and other systemic conditions. Int Urol Nephrol. 2009;42(1):141–50.
6. Cowland JB, Borregaard N. Molecular characterization and pattern of tissue expression of the gene for neutrophil Gelatinase-associated Lipocalin from humans. Genomics. 1997;45(1):17–23.
7. Legrand M, Mari A, Mebazaa A. The elusive task of biomarkers of renal injury. Crit Care. 2013;17(3):132.
8. Peng Z-Y. The biomarkers for acute kidney injury: a clear road ahead? J Transl Int Med. 2016;4(3):95–8.
9. Zhu W, Liu M, Wang G, Che JP, Xu YF, Peng B, Zheng JH. Urinary neutrophil gelatinase–associated lipocalin, a biomarker for systemic inflammatory response syndrome in patients with nephrolithiasis. J Surg Res. 2013;187(1): 237–43
10. Kandur Y, Gonen S, Fidan K, Soylemezoglu O. Evaluation of urinary KIM-1, NGAL, and IL-18 levels in determining early renal injury in pediatric cases with hypercalciuria and/or renal calculi. Clin Nephrol. 2016;86(2):62–9.
11. Chakraborty S, Kaur S, Guha S, Batra S. The multifaceted roles of neutrophil gelatinase associated lipocalin (NGAL) in inflammation and cancer. Biochim Biophys Acta. 2012;1826(1):129–69.
12. van der Veen BS, Winther MP, Herringa P. Myeloperoxidase: molecular mechanisms of action and their relevance to human health and disease. Antioxidants Redox Signaling. 2009;11:2899–937.
13. Hughes S, Cotter MJ, Evans S, Jones K, Adams R. Role of leucocytes in damage to the vascular endothelium during ischaemia-reperfusion injury. Br J Biomed Sci. 2006;63(4):166–70.
14. Baldus LD. Myeloperoxidase and its contributory role in inflammatory vascular disease. Pharmacol Ther. 2006;111:16–26.
15. Olza J, Aguilera C, Gill-Campos M, Leis R, Bueno G, Martines-Jimenez M, et al. Myeloperoxidase is an early biomarker of inflammation and cardiovascular risk in Prepubertal obese children. Diabetes Care. 2012;35(11): 2373–6.
16. Hasmann A, Wehrschuetz-Sigl E, Marold A, Wiesbauer H, Schoeftner R, Gewessler U, et al. Analysis of myeloperoxidase activity in wound fluids as a marker of infection. Ann Clin Biochem. 2013;50(3):245–54.
17. Feldmann H, Geistbert TW. Ebola, hemorrhagic, fever. Lancet. 2011; 377(97768):849–62.
18. Livorsi DJ, Stenehjem E, Stephens D. Virulence factors of gram-negative bacteria in sepsis with a focus on Neisseria meningitidis. Contrib Microbiol Immunol. 2011;17(31):31–47.
19. Willey J, Sherwood L, Christopher JW. Prescotts's Microbiol. Chapter. 2011;8:97.

20. Rimmele T, Leli C, Payen D, Cantaluppi V, Marshall J, Gomez H, et al. Immune cell phenotype and function in sepsis. Shock. 2016;45(3):282–91.
21. Fan S, Binbin G, Hao Z, Zhang L, Zhou J, Zhang Y, Liang C. Risk factors of infectious complications following flexible ureteroscope with a holmium laser: a retrospective study. Int J Clin Exp Med. 2015;8(7):11252–9.
22. Hughes S, Moyes AJ, Thomas-Wright S, Banwell J, Williams R, Mushtaq S, et al. A pilot study to evaluate Haemostatic function, following shock wave lithotripsy (SWL) for the treatment of solitary kidney stones. PLoS One. 2015; 10(5):e0125840.
23. Moyes AJ, Lamb RM, Ella-Tongwiis P, et al. A pilot study evaluating changes to haematological and biochemical tests after flexible Ureterorenoscopy for the treatment of kidney stones. PLoS One. 2017;12(7):e0179599. https://doi.org/10.1371/journal.pone.0179599.
24. Hughes SF. The role of phagocytic leukocytes in the acute inflammatory response during ischaemia-reperfusion injury and various orthopaedic surgeries. Thesis. Keele University; 2008.
25. Hughes SF, Edwards DR, Middleton JF. Applied upper limb Orthopaedic surgery results in increased inflammation and changes to leukocyte, coagulation and endothelial markers. PLoS One. 2010;5(7):e11846.
26. Hughes SF, Hendricks BD, Edwards DR, Bastawrous SS, Middleton JF. Lower limb orthopaedic surgery results in changes to coagulation and non-specific inflammatory biomarkers, including selective clinical outcome measures. Eur J Med Res. 2013;9(18):18–40.
27. Hughes SF, Hendricks BD, Edwards DR, Maclean KM, Bastawrous SS, Middleton JF. Total hip and knee replacement surgery results in changes in leykocyte and endothelial markers. J Inflamm. 2010;7:2.
28. Murty MS, Sharma U, Pandey V, Kankare S. Serum cystatin C as a marker of renal function in detection of early acute kidney injury. Indian J Nephrol. 2013;23(3):180–3.
29. Husain A, Willey J, Moon Y, Elkind M, Sacco R, Wolf M, et al. Creatinine-versus cystatin C-based renal function assessment in the northern Manhattan study. PLoS One. 2018;13(11):e0106839.
30. Gharaibeh K, Hamadah A, El-Zoghby Z, Lieske J, Larson T, Leung N. Cystatin C predicts renal recovery earlier than Creatinine among patients with acute kidney injury. Kidney Int Rep. 2018;3(2):337–42.
31. Sharnidharka V, Kwon C, Stevens G. Serum cystatin C is superior to serum creatinine as a marker of kidney function: a meta-analysis. Am J Kidney Dis. 2002;40:221–6.
32. Slocum J, Heung M, Pennathur S. Marking renal injury: can we move beyond serum Creatinine? Transl Res. 2012;159(4):277–89.
33. Seibert F, Sitz M, Passfall J, Haesner M, Laschinski P, Buhl M, et al. Prognostic value of urinary Calprotectin, NGAL and KIM-1 in chronic kidney disease. Kidney Blood Pressure Res. 2018;43(4):1255–62.
34. Dede O, Dagguli M, Utangac M, Yuksel H, Bodakci M, Hapipoglu N, et al. Urinary expression of acute kidney injury biomarkers in patients after RIRS: it is a prospective, controlled study. Int J Clin Exp Med. 2015;8(5):8147–52.
35. Aratani Y. Myeloperoxidase: its role for host defense, inflammation, and neutrophil function. Arch Biochem Biophys. 2018;640:47–52. https://doi.org/10.1016/j.abb.2018.01.004.
36. Ndrepepa G. Myeloperoxidase – a bridge linking inflammation and oxidative stress with cardiovascular disease. Clin Chim Acta. 2019. https://doi.org/10.1016/j.cca.2019.02.022.
37. Samsudin I, Vasikaran SD. Clinical utility and measurement of Procalcitonin. The Clinical biochemist. Reviews. 2017;38(2):59–68.
38. Meisner M. Procalcitonin: experience with a new parameter for bacterial infections and systemic inflammation. Laboratory Med. 1999;23(5):263–72. https://doi.org/10.1515/labm.1999.23.
39. Meisner M, Tschaikowsky K, Palmaers T, Schmidt J. Crit Care. 1999;3(1):45. https://doi.org/10.1186/cc306.

5

Mayo Adhesive Probability (MAP) score of non-donated kidney aids in predicting post-operative renal function following donor nephrectomy

Katherine J. Cockerill[1], Amanda E. Kahn[1], Stacy M. Young[2], Colleen T. Ball[3], Martin L. Mai[4], C. Burcin Taner[4], Dana K. Perry[4] and David D. Thiel[1*]

Abstract

Background: To examine the association of preoperative Mayo Adhesive Probability (MAP) scores in the donor (MAP_d) and non-donor kidneys (MAP_{nd}) with post-donation renal function.

Methods: Three hundred thirty-one patients undergoing hand assisted laparoscopic donor nephrectomy (HALDN) were reviewed. MAP_d and MAP_{nd} were obtained. Estimated glomerular filtration rate (eGFR) was recorded preoperatively and at 1 day, 1 month, and 6 months postoperatively.

Results: Two hundred females and 131 males were evaluated with median BMI 26.4 kg/m^2 (range 17.1–39.6) and median age 45 years (range 19–78). MAP_d score was 0 for 231 patients (69.8%) and > 0 for 100 patients (30.2%). MAP_{nd} score was 0 for 234 patients (70.7%) and > 0 for 97 patients (29.3%). The median preoperative eGFR was 86.6 ml/min/1.73m^2 (range 48.8–138.4). After adjusting for preoperative eGFR, BMI, ASA score, and kidney sidedness, postoperative eGFR was associated with MAP score in the non-donated kidney ($p = 0.014$) but not in the donated kidney ($p = 0.24$). Compared to donors with $MAP_{nd} = 0$, donors with a $MAP_{nd} > 0$, mean eGFR was − 2.33 ml/min/1.73m^2 lower at postoperative day 1 (95% CI − 4.24 to − 0.41, $p = 0.018$), − 3.02 ml/min/1.73m^2 lower at 1 month (95% CI − 5.11 to − 0.93, $p = 0.005$), and − 2.63 ml/min/1.73m^2 lower at 6 months postoperatively (95% CI − 5.01 to − 0.26, $p = 0.030$).

Conclusions: MAP score > 0 in the non-donated kidney is associated with worse renal function in the 6 months following HALDN.

Keywords: Donor nephrectomy, MAP score, Renal function

Background

Recent studies have evaluated the impact of various preoperative patient-specific and imaging-derived characteristics on postoperative renal function following donor nephrectomy. Examinations of large cohorts of patients suggest that age, male sex, and body mass index (BMI) are predictive of decreased postoperative renal function in patients undergoing donor nephrectomy [1–4]. However, other studies have shown that BMI has no effect on long term glomerular filtration rate (eGFR) in the donor nephrectomy population [5–8]. Lee et al. examined the effect of imaging-specific characteristics on postoperative glomerular filtration rate and demonstrated a correlation between postoperative recovery of renal function and visceral/subcutaneous adipose tissue measurements [9].

* Correspondence: Thiel.David@mayo.edu
[1]Department of Urology, Mayo Clinic, 4500 San Pablo Road, Jacksonville, FL 32224, USA
Full list of author information is available at the end of the article

Adherent perinephric fat (APF) has been associated with surgical complexity and longer operative times in patients undergoing partial nephrectomy [10]. The Mayo Adhesive Probability (MAP) score was originally designed as a simple, accurate, image-based scoring system to predict the presence of troublesome APF during partial nephrectomy [11, 12]. Higher MAP score has previously been shown to be associated with longer operative time in patients undergoing hand-assisted laparoscopic donor nephrectomy [13]. The MAP score is calculated based on image-derived measures of perinephric fat distance and severity of perinephric stranding to achieve a MAP score of 0–5 [11]. Narita et al. outlined risk factors for APF in healthy patients undergoing laparoscopic donor nephrectomy. In their study, MAP score components (perinephric fat area and stranding) were correlated with the presence of APF during donor nephrectomy [14]. Motivated by these findings, we examined the relationship between MAP score and post-donation renal function in healthy patients undergoing hand-assisted laparoscopic donor nephrectomy (HALD N).

Methods

Hand-assisted laparoscopic donor nephrectomy

Hand-assisted laparoscopic donor nephrectomy (HALD N) was performed as previously described by fellowship-trained transplant surgeons at one institution using a hand-port and two additional trocars [13, 15]. The perinephric fat was dissected and the renal hilum exposed in each case. The ureter was controlled distally with a clip and sharply divided. An endovascular stapler was used to take the renal artery and the renal vein separately.

Data collection

The data set is similar to that used in our previous manuscript evaluating the relationship between MAP score and operative time in HALDN [13]. Following approval by the Mayo Clinic Institutional Review Board, 331 consecutive patients who underwent HALDN between January 2007 and April 2017 were evaluated. Data collected include patient characteristics (age, sex, race, MAP scores for donated [MAP_d] and non-donated kidneys [MAP_{nd}]), preoperative laboratory values (estimated glomerular filtration rate [eGFR], creatinine, hemoglobin [Hgb]), American Society of Anesthesiologists [ASA] score, sidedness of donor kidney, operative time), and measurement of postoperative renal function (eGFR and creatinine at postoperative day 1 [POD1], 1 month, and 6 months, calculated according to the 2006 MDRD study equation) [16]. Patients with preoperative eGFR< 60 mL/min/1.73m^2 were still considered candidates for donor nephrectomy at our institution based on measured iothalamate or creatinine clearance greater than or equal to the lower 5th percentile when age-adjusted.

Calculation of MAP score

MAP score was calculated as described in our previous manuscripts evaluating MAP score and its relationship to adherent perinephric fat, renal cell carcinoma progression free survival, and HALDN [11, 13, 17]. An independent reviewer evaluated the preoperative imaging (CT or T1-weighted MRI) for each patient undergoing HALDN to calculate MAP scores. The MAP_d score was calculated for the patient's donated kidney and the MAP_{nd} score was calculated for the patient's non-donated kidney. MAP scores were calculated for every patient utilizing the measurement of posterior renal fat thickness and the measure of severity of perinephric stranding. Perinephric fat thickness was measured at the level of the renal vein for each kidney. Posterior renal fat was measured at this level as a direct line from the level of the renal capsule to the posterior abdominal wall [11]. This variable was measured in centimeters (< 1 cm = 0 points, 1.1–1.9 cm = 1 point, > 2.0 cm = 2 points).

Perinephric stranding was identified as soft tissue attenuation in the fat surrounding the kidney. This was graded according to severity if present (0 = no stranding, 2 = thin mild stranding, 3 = diffuse stranding). The MAP score was calculated in each scenario as the sum of the values obtained for posterior renal fat and perinephric stranding to obtain a score 0–5 [11].

Statistical analysis

Box plots were constructed to show the distribution of preoperative eGFR according to MAP score. For evaluating associations of MAP score with renal function, MAP_d and MAP_{nd} scores were categorized as either 0 or > 0 given the low number of patients with MAP scores of 1–5. All analyses were done separately for MAP_d and MAP_{nd}. For cross-sectional associations of MAP score with preoperative eGFR we used linear regression. We used mixed effects regression models with preoperative eGFR as a covariate to evaluate associations of MAP score with postoperative eGFR. Mixed effects models additionally included random patient effects for intercepts and slopes, two indicator variables to represent three postoperative time points, three indicator variables to represent MAP score (> 0 vs. 0) at each postoperative time point. All regression-based models were adjusted for body mass index, ASA score, and sidedness of the donated kidney. Supplementary Table 1 shows associations of MAP score with postoperative eGFR adjusting for one covariate at a time. Our final model included all pre-specified covariates with the exception of age, sex, and race as these are used to calculate eGFR. Likelihood ratio tests (LRT) with 3 degrees of freedom were used to evaluate the overall association of MAP score on postoperative renal function. Confidence intervals and p-values corresponding to the difference in means and difference in slopes were two-sided and based on the t-distribution. P-values less than 0.05 were considered statistically significant. Fitted values obtained from regression models refer to a hypothetical "average" donor where baseline covariates are equal to the mean value of all patients included in the model. SAS statistical software (version 9.4, SAS Institute Inc., Cary, NC) was used for all statistical analyses.

Results

A total of 331 patients who underwent HALDN were included in the analysis. Median age was 45 years (range 19 to 78 years) and BMI was 26.4 kg/m^2 (range 17.1 to 39.6 kg/m^2). A large majority of the patients underwent left-sided donor nephrectomy (89.4%). Two hundred patients were female (60.4%). Of note, patient comorbidities were minimal given the rigorous screening process at our institution prior to consideration of donor nephrectomy. Two hundred and thirty one patients had a MAP_d score of 0 (69.8%) and 100 patients had a MAP_d score of 1–5 (30.2%). Two hundred and thirty four patients had a MAP_{nd} of 0 (70.7%) and 97 patients had MAP_{nd} of 1–5 (29.3%). Table 1 summarizes additional preoperative patient characteristics, ASA scores, and MAP_d and MAP_{nd} scores of the 331 renal donors.

Among the entire cohort, the preoperative eGFR ranged from 48.8 to 138.4 ml/min/1.73m^2 (mean = 86.6 ml/min/1.73m^2, n = 331). The distribution of preoperative eGFR is presented in Fig. 1 according to MAP score (0 or > 0) and kidney type (MAP_d or MAP_{nd}). Associations of MAP score with preoperative and postoperative renal function with adjustment for preoperative covariates are shown in Table 2. Donors with a $MAP_d > 0$ had a lower mean eGFR by 5.87 ml/min/1.73m^2 lower (95% CI 2.02 to 9.71 ml/min/1.73m^2) compared to kidney donors with a $MAP_d = 0$ in the donated kidney. When comparing eGFR according to MAP_{nd} score in the non-donated kidney, mean eGFR was 4.59 ml/min/1.73m^2 lower (95% CI 0.63 to 8.54 ml/min/1.73m^2) in those with a $MAP_{nd} > 0$ compared to those with $MAP_{nd} = 0$.

We also investigated the small cohort of patients (n = 10) with a high grade MAP_{nd} score (3 to 5). This cohort had a median preoperative eGFR of 75.3 ml/min/1.73m^2 (range, 62.2–87.3 ml/min/1.73m^2) with a median preoperative creatinine of 1.0 mg/dL (range, 0.9–1.2 mg/dL). At 1 month postoperatively, the median eGFR was 41.6 ml/min/1.73m^2 (range 35.9–57.1 ml/min/1.73m^2, n = 9) with a creatinine of 1.7 mg/dL (range 1.3–1.9 mg/dL, n = 9). At 6 months postoperatively, the median eGFR was 42.9 ml/min/1.73m^2 (range 38.9–58.4 ml/min/1.73m^2, n = 7) with a median creatinine of 1.6 mg/dL (range 1.3–1.7 mg/dL). No patient from this high risk group had an eGFR greater than 60 ml/min/1.73m^2 at 1 month or 6 months postoperatively.

We used mixed effects linear regression models to evaluate the impact of MAP score on postoperative eGFR while adjusting for preoperative eGFR and baseline covariates as displayed in Table 2. The overall association of MAP score with postoperative eGFR was

Table 1 Preoperative characteristics of the full cohort of patients who had a donor nephrectomy according to Mayo Adhesive Probability Score

Baseline characteristic	MAP Score 0 (N = 209)	MAP Score 1–5 (N = 122)
Age (years)	42.3 ± 12.4	48.6 ± 9.1
Sex		
Female	159 (76.1%)	41 (33.6%)
Male	50 (23.9%)	81 (66.4%)
Black race		
No	176 (84.2%)	110 (90.2%)
Yes	33 (15.8%)	12 (9.8%)
Body mass index (kg/m^2)	25.6 ± 3.9	28.3 ± 3.9
ASA score		
1	135 (64.6%)	70 (57.4%)
2	72 (34.4%)	47 (38.5%)
3	2 (1.0%)	5 (4.1%)
Donated kidney		
Right	23 (11.0%)	12 (9.8%)
Left	186 (89.0%)	110 (90.2%)
eGFR, ml/min/1.73m^2	88.9 ± 16.8	82.7 ± 14.3

Abbreviations: *MAP* Mayo Adhesive Probability, *ASA* American Society of Anesthesiologists, *eGFR* estimated glomerular filtration rate. The sample mean ± SD is shown for continuous variables. Number (percentage of patients) is shown for categorical variables

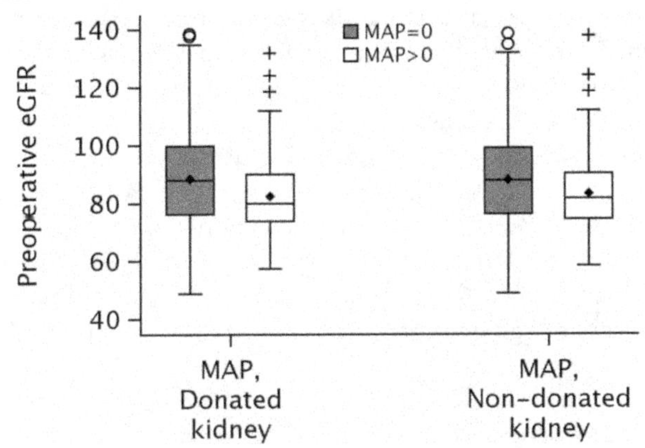

Fig. 1 Box plots of preoperative estimated glomerular filtration rate (eGFR) according to Mayo Adhesive Probability (MAP) score in the donated kidney and non-donated kidney. Units of measurement for eGFR are ml/min/1.73m^2

Table 2 Association of Mayo Adhesive Probability Score with Renal Function Before and After Donor Nephrectomy

Timing of eGFR measurement	MAP_d (> 0 vs. 0)		MAP_{nd} (> 0 vs. 0)	
	Difference in mean eGFR (95% CI), ml/min/1.73m^2	P	Difference in mean eGFR (95% CI), ml/min/1.73m^2	P
Preoperative[a]	−5.87 (−9.71 to −2.02)	0.003	−4.59 (−8.54 to −0.63)	0.023
Postoperative[b]		0.24		0.014
Day 1[c]	−0.44 (−2.33 to 1.46)	0.65	−2.33 (−4.24 to − 0.41)	0.018
1 Month [c]	−1.68 (−3.80 to 0.45)	0.12	−3.02 (−5.11 to − 0.93)	0.005
6 Month [c]	−1.99 (− 4.31 to 0.33)	0.092	−2.63 (− 5.01 to − 0.26)	0.030

MAP_d Mayo Adhesive Probability score in the donated kidney, *MAP_{nd}* Mayo Adhesive Probability score in the non-donated kidney, *eGFR* estimated glomerular filtration rate, *CI* confidence interval

[a] Associations with preoperative renal function were estimated from linear regression models with adjustment for body mass index, ASA score, and sidedness of the donated kidney

[b] The overall association of MAP score with postoperative renal function was evaluated using a likelihood ratio test with 3 degrees of freedom comparing the full mixed effects regression model to a model without the 3 MAP terms (one for each postoperative time point)

[c] Associations with renal function at each postoperative time point were estimated from mixed effects regression models with adjustment for preoperative eGFR, body mass index, ASA score, and sidedness of the donated kidney

statistically significant in the non-donated kidney (LRT $p = 0.014$, df = 3) but not in the donated kidney (LRT p value = 0.24). Compared to those with a $MAP_{nd} = 0$, donors with a $MAP_{nd} > 0$ had evidence of significantly lower eGFR at POD1 (difference in means: − 2.33 ml/min/1.73m^2; 95% CI − 4.24 to − 0.41 ml/min/1.73m^2; p = 0.018), 1 month follow-up (difference in means: − 3.02 ml/min/1.73m^2; 95% CI − 5.11 to − 0.93 ml/min/1.73m^2; p = 0.005), and 6 months follow-up (difference in means: − 2.63 ml/min/1.73m^2; 95% CI − 5.01 to − 0.26 ml/min/1.73m^2; p = 0.030). We did not find evidence of an association of MAP_{nd} with the change in eGFR from POD1 (slopes) to either 1 month (difference in slopes [$MAP_{nd} > 0$ vs. $MAP_{nd} = 0$]: − 0.67 ml/min/1.73m^2; 95% CI − 2.86 to 0.77 ml/min/1.73m^2; p = 0.53) or 6 month follow-up (difference in slopes [$MAP_{nd} > 0$ vs. $MAP_{nd} = 0$]: − 0.31 ml/min/1.73m^2; 95% CI − 2.70 to 2.08 ml/min/1.73m^2; p = 0.80). Figure 2 displays the fitted estimates of postoperative eGFR according to MAP score in the donated kidney (panel A) and MAP score in the non-donated kidney (panel B). In a separate subgroup analysis, we obtained fitted estimates of postoperative eGFR according to MAP score separately for males and females (Supplementary Figure 1).

The MDRD 2006 formula, by definition, inherently demonstrates a correlation between age, sex, and race with eGFR [15]. Six months following nephrectomy, 47% (47/100) of donors younger than 45 years, 80% (79/99) of donors 45 to 65 years, and 100% (9/9) of donors over 65 years of age presented with an eGFR less than 60 mL/min/1.73m^2.

Discussion

In preoperative examination of candidates for donor nephrectomy, assessment of patient-specific factors is crucial in preparation for surgery [18]. Part of that workup includes an analysis of the patient's BMI. There have been conflicting studies regarding the association between donor BMI and postoperative renal compromise [1–8]. Motivated by these conflicting studies, we examine the association of kidney MAP score with postoperative renal function in healthy donors.

The MAP score serves as a patient-specific and donor site-specific score that is widely applicable to the kidney donor, given that most renal donors have pre-operative cross-sectional imaging (CT scan or MRI). It has also been previously discovered to be an accurate imaged-based predictor of intraoperative APF and postoperative outcomes in patients undergoing laparoscopic and open partial nephrectomy [11, 12, 18]. Narita et al. found a correlation between MAP score variables and the identification of APF at the time of living-donor nephrectomy in their evaluation of 92 patients [14]. Lee et al. examined the correlation between CT measurement of visceral adipose tissue and postoperative renal function in their study of 75 living donors. Their study found a correlation between visceral to subcutaneous adipose tissue measurements and postoperative recovery of eGFR [9]. Studies have shown that BMI is not always a reliable measure of adipose tissue composition, especially when the visceral fat is in question [17, 19, 20]. Additionally, studies have shown that visceral fat is the most metabolically active type of fat [21, 22]. We believe the surgery specific measurement of perinephric fat and perinephric stranding may have more of an association with postoperative renal function than BMI alone due to these being inherently kidney-specific measures. Due to its proximity to the kidney and metabolically active nature, we believe an analysis of visceral fat by the MAP score may be a more effective measure than BMI when trying to understand how body fat composition affects kidney function. Results of our study indicate that MAP score in the non-donated kidney contributes to the prediction of postoperative renal function beyond the association of BMI with postoperative renal function (Likelihood ratio

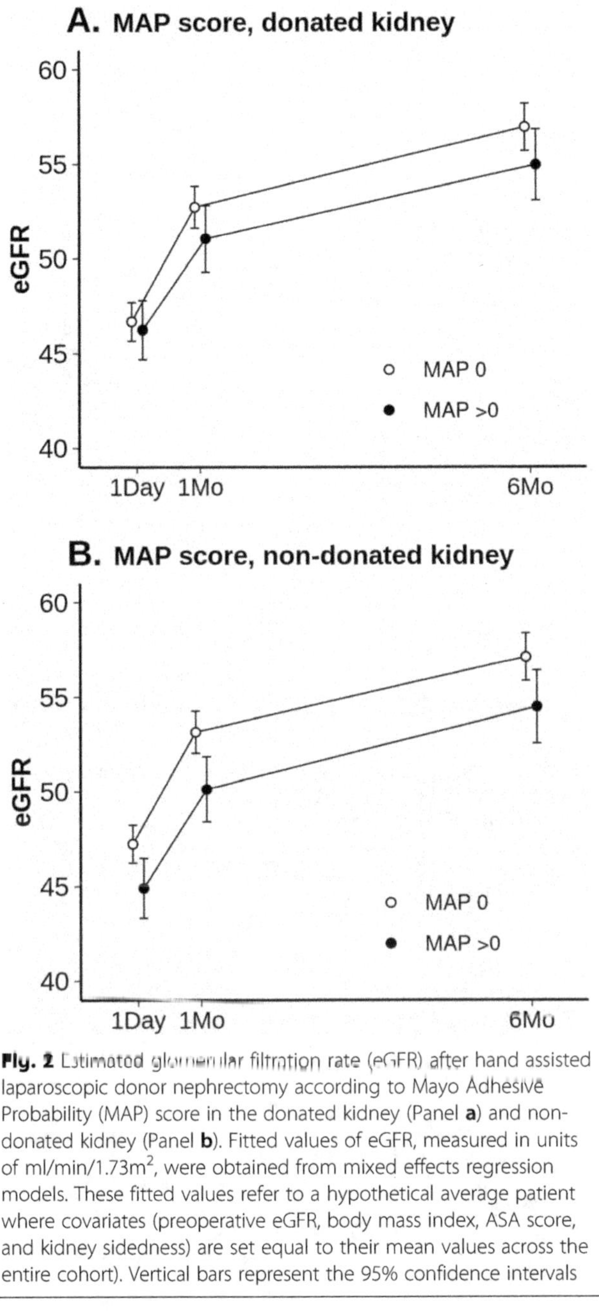

Fig. 2 Estimated glomerular filtration rate (eGFR) after hand assisted laparoscopic donor nephrectomy according to Mayo Adhesive Probability (MAP) score in the donated kidney (Panel **a**) and non-donated kidney (Panel **b**). Fitted values of eGFR, measured in units of ml/min/1.73m^2, were obtained from mixed effects regression models. These fitted values refer to a hypothetical average patient where covariates (preoperative eGFR, body mass index, ASA score, and kidney sidedness) are set equal to their mean values across the entire cohort). Vertical bars represent the 95% confidence intervals

test p = 0.014, comparing the full model to the model without MAP score, Table 2). In addition, perinephric stranding can be indicative of underlying inflammatory or metabolic processes that can also ultimately affect intraoperative dissection and renal function. This may be most relevant to renal function on POD 1 given intraoperative challenges presented by adherent perinephric fat. However, our study also incorporates these concepts in the examination of long term renal function in a cohort of patients undergoing HALDN.

Additionally, age and male sex have previously been correlated with decreased postoperative donor renal function [3, 23]. By definition, the MDRD 2006 equation correlates age, sex, and race with eGFR because these variables are included in the calculation of eGFR.

Our study findings show that patients with MAP_{nd} scores from 1 to 5 were significantly associated with worse post-donation renal function than patients with MAP_{nd} scores of 0 (p = 0.014). After donor nephrectomy, recovery of renal function is dependent upon adaptive hypertrophy and hyperfiltration of the remaining kidney. This may explain why high MAP_{nd} scores proved to be significantly associated with diminished renal function following HALDN. The MAP score enables evaluation of the thickness and quality of the fat surrounding the non-donated kidney. An evaluation by Yoon et al. demonstrated that an increased area of visceral fat is associated with decreased eGFR and renal function [24]. The use of the MAP_{nd} score quantifies the posterior perinephric fat, a quantifiable measure of visceral fat, that may be more specific in predicting remaining renal function in kidney donors compared to BMI. We believe the MAP score may be utilized as an imaged-based adjunct to aid in the evaluation of potential donor renal dysfunction; however larger studies are needed for confirmation.

We believe the results from this study may contribute to how patients are evaluated for kidney donation in the future. The information may also contribute to patient counseling. For example, a healthy 58-year-old white male included in this study had a MAP_d of 4 and MAP_{nd} of 3. His preoperative eGFR was 76.7 ml/min/1.73m^2 with a creatinine of 1 mg/dL. Postoperatively, his eGFR dropped to 41.6 ml/min/1.73m^2 at 1 month, 41.5 ml/min/1.73m^2 at 6 months, and 32.5 ml/min/1.73m^2 at 12 months. All postoperative creatinine measurements were greater than or equal to 1.7. Due to his age, this patient will likely be living with chronic renal insufficiency for many years.

When evaluating patients who presented with a high grade MAP_{nd} score (3 to 5) (n = 12), every patient had a preoperative eGFR greater than 60 ml/min. Table 2 did reveal that patients with MAP of 1–5 also had a lower mean preoperative eGFR compared to patients with MAP = 0 (adjusted difference in means: – 4.59 ml/min/1.73m^2). However, every patient with a high MAP score had a eGFR less than 60 ml/min postoperatively at 1 month or 6 months. Data available from 8 patients showed no improvement at 12 months postoperatively; no patients had an eGFR greater than 60 ml/min and none improved to within 10% of their preoperative eGFR baseline.

One limitation of our study is the low number of patients with high MAP scores. This is expected given our otherwise healthy population of kidney donors who are screened for potential diseases or malignancies that could contribute to a higher MAP score. The low number of patients with high MAP scores in this cohort precludes us from evaluating the impact of high MAP scores on postoperative renal function. However, the screening process that limits patients with a high MAP score also removes the potential confounding contribution of additional disease processes such as diabetes and hypertension on overall renal function. We did not have statistics within our dataset regarding smoking status, percentage of patients with diabetes, and other comorbidities that can affect long term renal function. This serves as a limitation to our study. Another limitation of our study is the limited number of females with a MAP score > 0. Previous studies have shown that men tend to have a greater amount of perirenal fat compared to women [25]. In a subgroup analysis we observed a similar pattern in the fitted values of postoperative eGFR in males and females, however the wide confidence intervals among females with a MAP score indicate a high level of uncertainty in those estimates (Supplementary Figure 1). Additionally, we recognize the limitation of the MDRD 2006 formula to most accurately calculate eGFR. This study was retrospective in nature therefore, only measurements considered "standard of care" were recorded and made available for analysis.

Conclusion

The MAP scoring system can be universally applied to preoperative imaging in the evaluation of patients undergoing HALDN. Our study suggests that MAP scores greater than 0 in the non-donated kidney aid in estimating postoperative renal function. It is important to note that none of the 10 patients with a MAP score > 2 recovered baseline renal function or had post-donation eGFR > 60 ml/min/1.73m^2.

Supplementary information

Additional file 1: Supplementary Figure 1. Estimated glomerular filtration rate (eGFR) after hand assisted laparoscopic donor nephrectomy according to patient sex and Mayo Adhesive Probability (MAP) score in the donated kidney and non-donated kidney. Fitted values of eGFR, measured in units of ml/min/1.73m^2, were obtained from mixed effects regression models separately for males and females. These fitted values refer to a hypothetical average patient where covariates (preoperative eGFR, body mass index, ASA score, and kidney sidedness) are set equal to their mean values, separately for males and females). Vertical bars represent the 95% confidence intervals.

Additional file 2: Supplementary Table 1. Exploration of the impact of preoperative characteristics on the association of Mayo Adhesive Probability score with postoperative renal function.

Abbreviations

eGFR: Estimated glomerular filtration rate; APF: Adherent perinephric fat; MAP: Mayo Adhesive Probability score; HALDN: Hand-assisted laparoscopic donor nephrectomy; MAP$_d$: MAP scores for donated; MAP$_{nd}$: Non-donated kidneys; BMI: Body mass index; Hgb: Hemoglobin; WBC: White blood cell count; ASA: American Society of Anesthesiologists score; POD1: Postoperative day 1

Acknowledgements

None.

Authors' contributions

KJC contributed to manuscript writing and review. AEK contributed to manuscript writing. SMY contributed to data collection. CTB contributed to statistical analysis. MLM, CTB, and DKP contributed with content expertise. DDT contributed to project conception, conduction and design as well as manuscript writing and review. All authors read and approved the manuscript.

Author details

[1]Department of Urology, Mayo Clinic, 4500 San Pablo Road, Jacksonville, FL 32224, USA. [2]Department of Health Sciences Research, Mayo Clinic, Jacksonville, FL, USA. [3]Division of Biomedical Statistics and Informatics, Mayo Clinic, Jacksonville, FL, USA. [4]Department of Transplantation, Mayo Clinic, Jacksonville, FL, USA.

References

1. Lim J, Kong YG, Kim YK, et al. Risk factors associated with decreased renal function after hand-assisted laparoscopic donor nephrectomy: a multivariate analysis of a single surgeon experience. Int J Med Sci. 2017;14:159–66. https://doi.org/10.7150/ijms.17585 eCollection 2017. PubMed PMID: 28260992; PubMed Central PMCID: PMC5332845.
2. Mjøen G, Oyen O, Midtvedt K, et al. Age, gender, and body mass index are associated with renal function after kidney donation. Clin Transplant. 2011; 25:E579–83. https://doi.org/10.1111/j.1399-0012.2011.01503.x.Epub 2011 Sep 9. PubMed PMID: 21906171.
3. Unger LW, Feka J, Sabler P, et al. High BMI and male sex as risk factor for increased short-term renal impairment in living kidney donors - retrospective analysis of 289 consecutive cases. Int J Surg. 2017;46:172–7. https://doi.org/10.1016/j.ijsu.2017.09.007 Epub 2017 Sep 11. PubMed PMID: 28912105.
4. Locke JE, Reed RD, Massie A, et al. Obesity increases the risk of end-stage renal disease among living kidney donors. Kidney Int. 2017;91:699–703. https://doi.org/10.1016/j.kint.2016.10.014 Epub 2016 Dec 29. PubMed PMID: 28041626; PubMed Central PMCID: PMC5313335.
5. Kerkeni W, Rebai MH, Bouzouita A, et al. The effect of body mass index at the time of donation on postoperative and remote consequences of nephrectomy in 189 living-related kidney donors. Arab J Urol. 2015;13:221–4. https://doi.org/10.1016/j.aju.2015.06.002 Epub 2015 Jul 9. PubMed PMID: 26413352; PubMed Central PMCID: PMC4563005.
6. Tavakol MM, Vincenti FG, Assadi H, et al. Long-term renal function and cardiovascular disease risk in obese kidney donors. Clin J Am Soc Nephrol. 2009;4:1230–8. https://doi.org/10.2215/CJN.01350209 Epub 2009 May 14. PubMed PMID: 19443625; PubMed Central PMCID: PMC2709512.
7. Heimbach JK, Taler SJ, Prieto M, et al. Obesity in living kidney donors: clinical characteristics and outcomes in the era of laparoscopic donor nephrectomy. Am J Transplant. 2005;5:1057–64 PubMed PMID: 15816886.
8. O'Brien B, Mastoridis S, Sabharwal A, et al. Expanding the donor pool: living donor nephrectomy in the elderly and the overweight. Transplantation. 2012;93:1158–65. https://doi.org/10.1097/TP.0b013e31824ef1ae PubMed PMID: 22495495.
9. Lee HH, Kang SK, Yoon YE, et al. Impact of the ratio of visceral to subcutaneous adipose tissue in donor nephrectomy patients. Transplant Proc. 2017;49:940–3. https://doi.org/10.1016/j.transproceed.2017.03.039 PubMed PMID: 28583563.
10. Kocher NJ, Kunchala S, Reynolds C, et al. Adherent perinephric fat at minimally invasive partial nephrectomy is associated with adverse peri-operative outcomes and malignant renal histology. BJU Int. 2016;117:636–41. https://doi.org/10.1111/bju.13378 Epub 2015 Dec 13. PubMed PMID: 26573951.
11. Davidiuk AJ, Parker AS, Thomas CS, et al. Mayo adhesive probability score:

an accurate image-based scoring system to predict adherent perinephric fat in partial nephrectomy. Eur Urol. 2014;66:1165–71. https://doi.org/10.1016/j.eururo.2014.08.054 Epub 2014 Sep 2. PubMed PMID: 25192968.

12. Martin L, Rouviere O, Bezza R, et al. Mayo adhesive probability score is an independent computed tomography scan predictor of adherent Perinephric fat in open partial nephrectomy. Urology. 2017;103:124–8. https://doi.org/10.1016/j.urology.2016.11.043 Epub 2017 Feb 1. PubMed PMID: 28161321.
13. Cockerill KJ, Young S, T Ball C, Custer K, Taner CB, Perry DK, Thiel DD. The Association of the Mayo Adhesive Probability (MAP) Score With Total Operative Time in Patients Undergoing Hand-assisted Laparoscopic Donor Nephrectomy. Urology. 2019;124:142–147. doi: https://doi.org/10.1016/j.urology.2018.10.041. Epub 2018 Nov 8. PubMed PMID: 30414890.
14. Narita S, Kumazawa T, Tsuchiya N, et al. Host-related risk factors for adherent Perinephric fat in healthy individuals undergoing laparoscopic living-donor nephrectomy. Surg Laparosc Endosc Percutan Tech. 2017;27:e69–73. https://doi.org/10.1097/SLE.0000000000000433 PubMed PMID: 28644262; PubMed Central PMCID: PMC5542780.
15. Wolf JS, Tchetgen MB, Merion RM. Hand-assisted laparoscopic live donor nephrectomy. Urol. 1998;52(5):885–7.
16. Stevens LA, Coresh J, Greene T, et al. Assessing kidney function--measured and estimated glomerular filtration rate. N Engl J Med. 2006;354:2473–83 PubMed PMID: 16760447.
17. Thiel DD, Davidiuk AJ, Meschia C, et al. Mayo adhesive probability score is associated with localized renal cell carcinoma progression-free survival. Urology. 2016;89:54–60. https://doi.org/10.1016/j.urology.2015.10.034.
18. Raman JD, Reynolds C, Hannon M. An increasing proportion of perinephric to subcutaneous fat is associated with adverse perioperative outcomes of robotic partial nephrectomy. J Robot Surg. 2016;10:255–9. https://doi.org/10.1007/s11701-016-0593-9 Epub 2016 May 9. PubMed PMID: 27160676.
19. Ji C, Tang S, Yang K, et al. Analysis of factors influencing Mayo adhesive probability score in partial nephrectomy. Med Sci Monit. 2017;23:6026–32.
20. Macleod LC, Hsi RS, Gore JL, et al. Perinephric fat thickness is an independent predictor of operative complexity during robot-assisted partial nephrectomy. J Endourol. 2014;28:587–91.
21. Okhunov Z, Mues AC, Kline M, et al. Evaluation of perirenal fat as a predictor of cT 1a renal cortical neoplasm histopathology and surgical outcomes. J Endourol. 2012;26:911–6.
22. Ibrahim MM. Subcutaneous and visceral adipose tissue: structure and functional differences. Obes Rev. 2010;11:11–8. https://doi.org/10.1111/j.1467-789X.2009.00623.
23. Hourmant M, Lerat L, Karam G. Donation from old living donors: how safe is it? Nephrol Dial Transplant. 2013;28:2010–4. https://doi.org/10.1093/ndt/gft069 Epub 2013 Mar 29. Review. PubMed PMID: 23543591.
24. Yoon HE, Choi SS, Kim Y, et al. The clinical usefulness of measurement of visceral fat area using multi-frequency bioimpedance: the association with cardiac and renal function in general population with relatively Normal renal function. Int J Med Sci. 2017;14:1375–81. https://doi.org/10.7150/ijms.21393.
25. Anderson KM, Lindler TU, Lamberton GR, et al. Laparoscopic donor nephrectomy: effect of perirenal fat upon donor operativetime. J Endourol. 2008;22(10):2269–74. https://doi.org/10.1089/end.2008.9725 PubMedPMID: 18831674.

6

Comparison of clinicopathologic parameters and oncologic outcomes between type 1 and type 2 papillary renal cell carcinoma

Xiang Le[1†], Xiang-Bo Wang[2†], Hao Zhao[1], Ren-Fu Chen[1*] and Peng Ge[1*]

Abstract

Background: To compare the clinicopathologic parameters and oncologic outcomes between type 1 and type 2 papillary renal cell carcinoma (PRCC).

Methods: This study was approved by the review board (NO.XYFY2019-KL032–01). Between 2007 and 2018, 52 consecutive patients who underwent surgery at a single tertiary referral hospital were included. Clinicopathologic and survival data were collected and entered into a database. The Kaplan-Meier method, and univariate and multivariate Cox proportional hazard regression analyses were performed to estimate progression-free survival (PFS) and cancer-specific survival (CSS).

Results: Of the 52 patients, 24 (46.2%) were diagnosed with type 1 PRCC, and 28 (53.8%) had type 2 PRCC. The mean tumor size was 4.8 ± 2.5 cm. The two subtypes displayed different morphological features: foamy macrophages were more common in type 1 PRCC, while eosinophils and microvascular angiolymphatic invasion were more frequent in type 2 PRCC. Type 2 cases showed higher tumor stage and World Health Organization/International Society of Urological Pathology (WHO/ISUP) grade than type 1 cases (T3-T4: 43% vs 17%, $P = 0.041$; G3-G4: 43% vs 8%, $P = 0.005$). In univariate analysis, type 2 PRCC had a lower probability for PFS and CSS than patients with type 1 PRCC ($P = 0.016$, $P = 0.049$, log-rank test, respectively). In multivariate analysis, only WHO/ISUP grade (HR 11.289, 95% CI 2.303–55.329, $P = 0.003$) and tumor size (HR 1.244, 95% CI 1.034–1.496, $P = 0.021$) were significantly associated with PFS.

Conclusions: PRCC subtype displayed different morphological features: foamy macrophages, eosinophils and microvascular angiolymphatic invasion are pathologic features that may aid in the distinction of the two subtypes. Histologic subtype of PRCC is not an independent prognostic factor and only WHO/ISUP grade and tumor size were independent predictors for PFS.

Keywords: Papillary renal cell carcinoma, WHO/ISUP grade, Prognosis, Subtype

* Correspondence: Renfu_chen@aliyun.com; gepengyzu@126.com
[†]Xiang Le and Xiang-Bo Wang contributed equally to this work.
[1]Department of Urology, the Affiliated Hospital of Xuzhou Medical University, Xuzhou, Jiangsu, China
Full list of author information is available at the end of the article

Background

Papillary renal cell carcinoma (PRCC), the second most common renal cell carcinoma (RCC) following clear cell RCC, accounts for 6 to 18% of all RCC cases [1]. It is a markedly heterogeneous entity characterized by different histologic subtypes, disease progression and clinical outcomes [2, 3]. Delahunt and Eble initially subclassified the PRCC into type 1 and type 2 based on morphological and immunohistochemical features in 1997 [4]. Typically, type 1 demonstrates the papillae covered by a single layer of simple cuboidal epithelia with scant cytoplasm, while type 2 is characterized by the presence of nuclear pseudostratifcation [5].

Recently, Magers et al. showed that type 1 PRCC was more likely to have clear cytoplasm and nuclear grooves, whereas type 2 PRCC had more abundant, granular cytoplasm and a higher nuclear grade [6]. Leroy et al. suggested that MUC1 immunostaining was usually positive in type 1 PRCC, which might be helpful in classifying such tumors [7]. However, due to the overlaps in morphologic, immunohistochemical and molecular features, it is difficult to classify all PRCCs into subtypes absolutely with current controversial criteria [2, 6, 8].

The issue whether the histologic subtypes affect oncological outcomes remains in debate. Some studies suggested type 1 PRCC was associated with a lower nuclear grade, lower tumor stage, and better prognosis than type 2 PRCC [9]. However, some other studies showed almost similar prognosis across the two subtypes [10, 11].

Herein, we performed the present study in an attempt to compare the clinicopathologic parameters and oncologic outcomes between type 1 and type 2 PRCC using a homogeneous pathological entity.

Table 1 Clinical characteristics between type 1 and type 2 papillary renal cell carcinoma

	Type 1 PRCC	Type 2 PRCC	P
Gender			
Male	18 (75.0%)	20 (71.4%)	0.772
Female	6 (25.0%)	8 (28.6%)	
Age (years)	53.4 ± 12.6	55.8 ± 15.5	0.552
Tumor size (cm)	4.6 ± 2.26	4.9 ± 2.76	0.683
Cell-based immunotherapy[a]			
Yes	3 (12.5%)	5 (17.9%)	0.882
No	21 (87.5%)	23 (82.1%)	
WHO/ISUP grade			
G1/G2	22 (91.7%)	16 (57.1%)	0.005
G3/G4	2 (8.3%)	12 (42.9%)	
Tumor stage (T)			
T1/T2	20 (83.3%)	16 (57.1%)	0.041
T3/T4	4 (16.7%)	12 (42.9%)	
Type of surgery			
Radical nephrectomy	8 (33.3%)	17 (60.7%)	0.049
Partial nephrectomy	16 (66.7%)	11 (39.3%)	
Surgical approach			
Open surgery	3 (12.5%)	9 (32.1%)	0.094
Laparoscopic surgery	21 (87.5%)	19 (67.9%)	
Disease progression			
Yes	1 (4.0%)	9 (33.3%)	0.028
No	22 (96.0%)	18 (66.7%)	
Death from tumor			
Yes	0 (0.0%)	6 (22.2%)	0.048
No	23 (100.0%)	21 (77.8%)	

Abbreviations: *WHO/ISUP* World Health Organization/International Society of Urological Pathology, *PRCC* Papillary renal cell carcinoma
[a]Cell-based immunotherapy refers to cytokine-induced killer cells therapy

Methods

Patient population and pathologic evaluation

This was a retrospective, single-institution study approved by the Affiliated Hospital of Xuzhou Medical University review board (NO.XYFY2019-KL032–01). A total of 56 tumors initially diagnosed as PRCC between 2007 and 2018 at a single tertiary hospital were evaluated. All hematoxylin and eosin–stained slides available were reviewed by the same pathologist (author Xiang-Bo Wang). Histologic subtypes were recorded according to the WHO classification of kidney tumors [12]. Four cases were excluded from the study after review. The remaining 52 patients were included in the present study.

Because of the difficulties in validation, reproducibility, and interpretation of the Fuhrman system [13], all samples were re-graded according to the four-tiered World Health Organization/International Society of Urological Pathology (WHO/ISUP) grading system [14, 15]. Pathological stage was assigned according to the American Joint of Committee on Cancer staging manual [10]. More morphological parameters were also recorded, including foamy macrophages, hemosiderin laden macrophages, necrosis, sarcomatoid differentiation, eosinophils, hyaline cells, classic papillary architecture, solid architecture, tubular architecture, perinephric/renal sinus fat invasion, and microvascular angiolymphatic invasion [6, 16].

Patient's clinicopathologic characteristics were entered into a database. Postoperative follow-up was not standardized. Generally, patients were evaluated every 3 months during the first year, every 6 months during the next 2 years, and then annually. Follow-up included physical examinations, laboratory measurements and imaging studies unless otherwise clinically indicated. The last follow-up was performed in May 2019. The outcomes of interest were progression-free survival (PFS) and cancer-specific survival (CSS). PFS was defined as the time from the date of surgery to local recurrence or distant metastasis and CSS was defined as the time from the date of surgery to a kidney cancer-related death. Surviving patients were censored at the last follow-up.

Statistical analysis

The continuous variables were compared using the independent-sample t test and the categorical variables were compared using the χ^2 - test. The Kaplan-Meier method was used to estimate the impacts of the subclassification and clinicopathologic parameters of PRCC on PFS and CSS, and the comparison was made with log-rank test. Univariate and multivariate (stepwise selection with enter and remove limits of $P = 0.05$ and $P = 0.05$, respectively) Cox proportional hazards regression analyses were performed to evaluate independency of prognostic factors for PFS and CSS. Nine variables (gender, age, WHO/ISUP grade, cell-based immunotherapy, type of surgery, surgical approach, pathological stage, PRCC subtypes and tumor size) were used in the stepwise selection analysis. Two-sided $P < 0.050$ was considered to indicate a statistically significant difference. Statistical analysis was performed using the Statistical Analysis System version 9.4 (SAS Institute, Cary, NC, USA) or Statistical Package for the Social Sciences 25.0 software (SPSS Inc., Chicago, IL, USA).

Results

Association with clinicopathologic characteristics

After histopathological review, the diagnosis of PRCC was confirmed in a total of 52 patients, including 38 males and 14 females (Table 1). The mean tumor size was 4.8 ± 2.5 cm. There were 24 (46.2%) patients with type 1 PRCC and 28 (53.8%) patients with type 2 PRCC. The age at surgery ranged from 17 to 86 years old (mean: 55.1). According to Table 1, patients with type 2 PRCC were more likely to have a higher WHO/ISUP grade (G3–4 in type 2 vs type 1: 43% vs 8%, $P = 0.005$) and an advanced tumor stage (T3–4 in type 2 vs type 1: 43% vs 17%, $P = 0.041$, Fig. 1). Moreover, patients with type 2 PRCC were more likely to receive radical nephrectomy (61% vs 33%; $P = 0.049$). Other clinical characteristics (including gender distribution, age, tumor size, and cell-based immunotherapy) demonstrated no statistically significant differences across the two groups.

Table 2 displays the pathologic characteristics of the patients. Presence of foamy macrophages was more frequent in type 1 (83%) than in type 2 (57%) ($P = 0.041$). In contrast, eosinophils and microvascular angiolymphatic invasion were more frequent in type 2 PRCC ($P = 0.012$ and $P = 0.028$, respectively). There were no statistically significant differences across the two groups in terms of hemosiderin laden macrophages, necrosis, sarcomatoid differentiation,

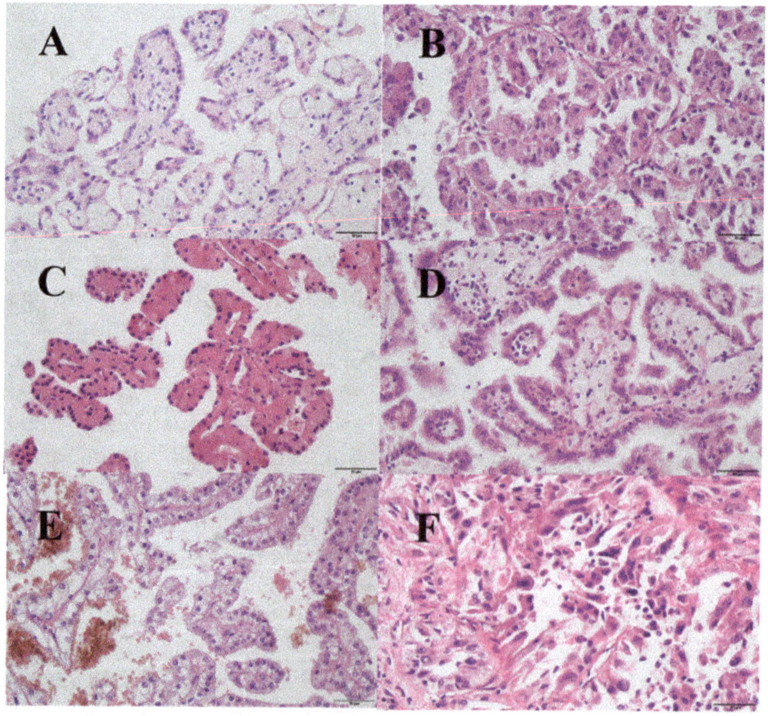

Fig. 1 Papillary renal cell carcinoma grading and types. **a**, type 1; **b**, type 2; Papillary renal cell carcinoma graded as nucleolar grade 1(**c**), 2(**d**), 3(**e**), 4(**f**). Hematoxylin and eosin stains, original magnification × 400

Table 2 Pathologic characteristics between type 1 and type 2 papillary renal cell carcinoma

	Type 1	Type 2	P
Foamy macrophages			
Yes	20 (83.3%)	16 (57.1%)	0.041
No	4 (16.7%)	12 (42.9%)	
Hemosiderin laden macrophages			
Yes	20 (83.3%)	27 (96.4%)	0.261
No	4 (16.7%)	1 (3.6%)	
Necrosis			
Yes	11 (45.8%)	18 (64.3%)	0.182
No	13 (54.2%)	10 (35.7%)	
Sarcomatoid differentiation			
Yes	0 (0.0%)	2 (7.1%)	0.493
No	24 (100.0%)	26 (92.9%)	
Eosinophils			
Yes	7 (29.2%)	18 (64.3%)	0.012
No	17 (70.8%)	10 (35.7%)	
Hyaline cells			
Yes	12 (50.0%)	18 (64.3%)	0.299
No	12 (50.0%)	10 (35.7%)	
Classic papillary architecture			
Yes	23 (95.8%)	28 (100.0%)	0.462
No	1 (4.2%)	0 (0.0%)	
Solid architecture			
Yes	4 (16.7%)	10 (35.7%)	0.123
No	20 (83.3%)	18 (64.3%)	
Tubular architecture			
Yes	15 (62.5%)	16 (57.1%)	0.695
No	9 (37.5%)	12 (42.9%)	
Perinephric/renal sinus fat invasion			
Yes	3 (12.5%)	8 (28.6%)	0.157
No	21 (87.5%)	20 (71.4%)	
Microvascular angiolymphatic invasion			
Yes	1 (4.2%)	9 (32.1%)	0.028
No	23 (95.8%)	19 (67.9%)	

hyaline cells, classic papillary architecture, solid architecture, tubular architecture, and perinephric/renal sinus fat invasion.

Association with survival

Two patients were lost to follow-up after surgery. Thus, the remaining 50 patients were included in survival analysis. The mean follow-up duration was 38 months (standard error, 4.7). Overall, 9 (33%) and 1 (4%) patients with type 2 PRCC and type 1 PRCC underwent disease progression, respectively ($P = 0.028$, Table 1). A total of 6 patients died of PRCC. The most common recurrence or metastatic sites were retroperitoneal /distant lymph node, lung, liver, and retroperitoneal cavity (Table 3).

Figure 2a exhibits the Kaplan–Meier plots for PFS estimates stratified by type 1 PRCC versus type 2. Type 2 PRCC patients had a lower probability for PFS than patients with type 1 ($P = 0.016$, log-rank test, Fig. 2a; $P = 0.045$, univariate Cox analysis, Table 4). Similarly, patients with type 2 PRCC were at significantly higher risk for cancer specific mortality than patients with type 1 PRCC ($P = 0.049$, Fig. 2b).

Multivariate analysis was performed using a Cox regression with stepwise selection of covariates. Among the nine variables (gender, age, WHO/ISUP grade, cell-based immunotherapy, type of surgery, surgical approach, pathological stage, PRCC subtypes and tumor size), only WHO/ISUP grade (HR 11.289, 95% CI 2.303–55.329, $P = 0.003$) and tumor size (HR 1.244, 95% CI 1.034–1.496, $P = 0.021$) entered the model. The histologic subtype of PRCC was not an independent predictor for PFS. In view of the fact that the statistical power was weakened by very few death events, multivariate Cox proportional hazards regression analyses were not performed for CSS.

Discussion

PRCC represents the largest subset of non-clear cell RCC [17]. It is traditionally subdivided into 2 subtypes on the basis of histomorphologic features. More recently, new PRCC subtype has been recognized [6]. In this current series, several morphological aspects of PRCC architecture and cytological features were investigated. We found that aggregates of foamy macrophages in the background stroma were common (69.2% of cases) and presence of foamy macrophages was less frequent in type 2 PRCC (57.1%) than type 1 PRCC (83.3%). Similar to our findings, Polifka et al. demonstrated that 70.9% of type 1 PRCC and 49.0% type 2 PRCC presented foamy macrophages and presence of foamy macrophages was linked with a better overall survival [18]. Unlike foamy macrophages, eosinophils and microvascular angiolymphatic invasion were more common in type 2 PRCC. Taken together, these findings in the present study may assist to discriminate between type 1 PRCC and type 2 PRCC.

The issue whether type 2 PRCC predicts poorer prognosis than type 1 PRCC remains controversial. Some claimed that type 2 has a more aggressive behavior than type 1, whereas others reported similar clinical course [9, 17–19]. From our perspectives, several points should be noted when we take the prior findings into consideration. Firstly, some studies investigated the prognosis of the subtypes after the data were adjusted against the

Table 3 Recurrence and/or metastatic site in disease progression patients

Patient ID	Recurrence and/or metastatic site
1	bone
2	distant lymph node
3	liver
4	retroperitoneal lymph node, bone
5	retroperitoneal lymph node, liver, bone
6	retroperitoneal lymph node, rectum, retroperitoneal cavity
7	lung,bone, brain
8	retroperitoneal lymph node, lung, spleen, retroperitoneal cavity, abdominopelvic cavity, abdominal wall
9	lung
10	retroperitoneal cavity, adrenal gland, liver

effects of Fuhrman grade [10, 20]. Delahunt et al. indicated that Fuhrman grading was inappropriate for PRCC and recommended WHO/ISUP grading system [21]. Secondly, some investigations were based on multicenter database, thus without a centralized pathologic review, differing criteria and nomenclature likely resulted in under- or over-reporting of PRCC [10].

The present study was designed to investigate the outcomes of PRCC using a homogeneous pathological entity by minimizing potential confounding effects associated with different diagnosis criteria. We found that type 2 PRCC showed a higher tumor stage and a higher WHO/ISUP grade than type 1 PRCC. It indicates that type 2 PRCC tends to have a more aggressive course than type 1 PRCC, which is in accordance with the results of previous studies [9]. Regarding the prognostic factors, we found differences in terms of PFS and CSS between type 1 and type 2 in univariate analysis. However, multivariate analysis failed to draw a conclusion that histologic subtype was an independent predictor of PFS. Several explanations are possible for these somewhat contradictory results. Firstly, type 2 PRCC tends to run parallel with high WHO/ISUP grade and high tumor stage and is less strongly related to outcomes than pathologic features. Besides, our study was limited by an overall short follow-up time and a small sample size. The statistical power was weakened by very few events.

Recently, a novel grading system for clear cell RCC and PRCC was proposed by ISUP and then endorsed by the WHO [14, 21]. The applicability of WHO/ISUP grading system to PRCC has been validated and recommended widely [14, 18]. Cornejo et al. reported that WHO/ISUP grade was statistically superior to Fuhrman grade in predicting survival in both univariate and multivariate analyses [16]. In this study, all samples were regraded according to the four-tiered WHO/ISPU grading system. In accordance with previous studies, we found that WHO/ISUP grade was an independent prognostic factor for PFS.

It is generally recognized that clear cell RCC conveys superior outcome than PRCC. However, different PRCC

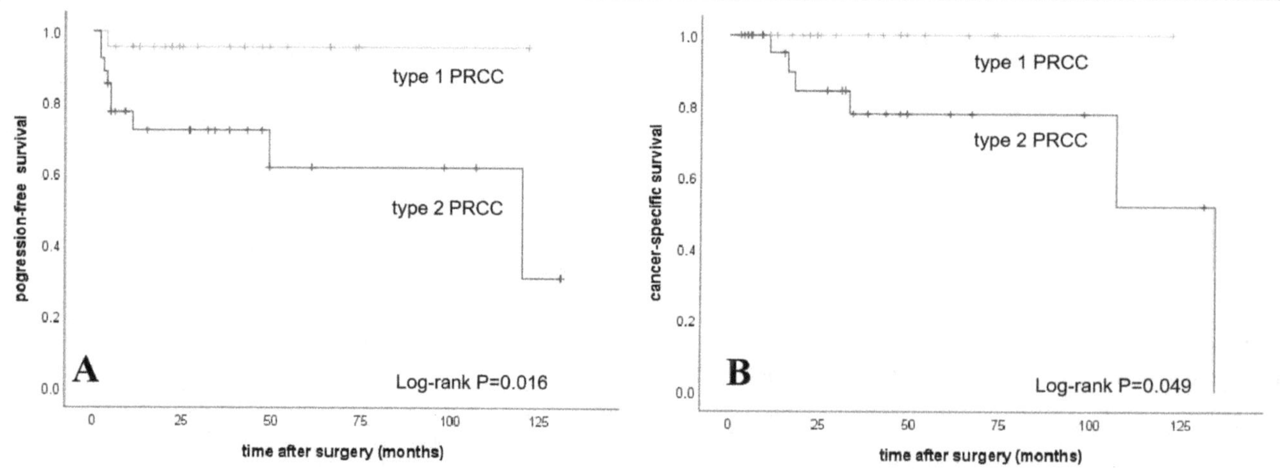

Fig. 2 Kaplan-meier curves. **a**, progression-free survival. **b**, cancer-specific survival. *P*-values are based on log-rank test. PRCC, papillary renal cell carcinoma

Table 4 Univariate Cox analysis on progression-free survival in papillary renal cell carcinoma patients

	HR	95%CI	P
Gender			
Female	1		
Male	0.364	0.095–1.389	0.139
Age			
≤ 60	1		
>60	0.885	0.248–3.156	0.851
Surgical approach			
Open surgery	1		
Laparoscopic surgery	0.323	0.086–1.205	0.092
Type of surgery			
Partial nephrectomy	1		
Radical nephrectomy	0.092	0.012–0.726	0.024
Cell-based immunotherapy			
No	1		
Yes	1.132	0.236–5.425	0.877
Tumor stage			
T1/T2	1		
T3/T4	12.136	2.557–57.599	0.002
WHO/ISUP grade			
G1/G2	1		
G3/G4	13.692	2.890–64.874	0.001
PRCC subtype			
type 1	1		
type 2	8.326	1.050–66.024	0.045
Tumor size	1.340	1.117–1.608	0.002

Abbreviations: *HR* Hazard ratio, *CI* Confidence interval, *WHO/ISUP* World Health Organization/International Society of Urological Pathology, *PRCC* Papillary renal cell carcinoma

risk subgroups may not predict the same prognosis. Steffens and colleagues [3] indicated that PRCC could apparently be differentiated into organ-confined/localised and advanced/metastatic subgroup. Compared to clear cell RCC, the former subgroup had a significantly better prognosis, while the latter subgroup had a worse prognosis. Previous studies have shown that PRCC, especially type 2 PRCC, is an heterogeneous entity with divergent spectra [18]. Hence, our understanding of PRCC should not be limited to histologic subtypes. More information about genome profiles and cell signaling of tumor induction, promotion, and progression is required.

Although our study offers new information in answering the question of prognostic differences between patients with type 1 PRCC and patients with type 2 PRCC, it is not devoid of potential limitations that need to be acknowledged. First and foremost are the limitations inherent to its retrospective nature. In addition, in order to make a homogeneous pathological entity, we only chose those patients between 2007 and 2018, thus the follow-up time and sample size were the limitations of the present study.

Conclusions

This study compared clinicopathologic parameters and oncologic outcomes between type 1 PRCC and type 2 PRCC in a homogeneous pathological entity. We found that foamy macrophages were more common in type 1 PRCC, while eosinophils and microvascular angiolymphatic invasion were more frequent in type 2 PRCC. Although type 2 PRCC tended to have a higher tumor stage and WHO/ISUP grade, histologic subtype was not an independent prognostic factor. In multivariate analysis, only WHO/ISUP grade and tumor size were significantly associated with PFS.

Abbreviations

PRCC: Papillary renal cell carcinoma; RCC: Renal cell carcinoma; WHO/ISUP: World Health Organization/International Society of Urological Pathology; PFS: Progression-free survival; CSS: Cancer-specific survival

Acknowledgements

None.

Authors' contributions

XL and XW contributed equally to this work and they designed the study, obtained data, performed the statistical analysis, wrote the manuscript and interpreted the data. HZ participated in the conception and design of the study and acquisition of data. RC and PG participated in the conception and design of the study and interpretation of the data and reviewed and edited the manuscript. All authors read and approved the final manuscript.

Author details

[1]Department of Urology, the Affiliated Hospital of Xuzhou Medical University, Xuzhou, Jiangsu, China. [2]Department of Pathology, the Affiliated Hospital of Xuzhou Medical University, Xuzhou, Jiangsu, China.

References

1. Srigley JR, Delahunt B, Eble JN, Egevad L, Epstein JI, Grignon D, Hes O, Moch H, Montironi R, Tickoo SK, et al. The International Society of Urological Pathology (ISUP) Vancouver classification of renal Neoplasia. Am J Surg Pathol. 2013;37(10):1469–89.
2. Linehan WM, Spellman PT, Ricketts CJ, Creighton CJ, Fei SS, Davis C, Wheeler DA, Murray BA, Schmidt L, Vocke CD, et al. Comprehensive molecular characterization of papillary renal-cell carcinoma. N Engl J Med. 2016;374(2):135–45.
3. Steffens S, Janssen M, Roos FC, Becker F, Schumacher S, Seidel C, Wegener G, Thuroff JW, Hofmann R, Stockle M, et al. Incidence and long-term prognosis of papillary compared to clear cell renal cell carcinoma--a multicentre study. Eur J Cancer. 2012;48(15):2347–52.
4. Delahunt B, Eble JN. Papillary renal cell carcinoma: a clinicopathologic and immunohistochemical study of 105 tumors. Mod Pathol. 1997;10(6):537–44.
5. Jiang F, Richter J, Schraml P, Bubendorf L, Gasser T, Sauter G, Mihatsch MJ, Moch H. Chromosomal imbalances in papillary renal cell carcinoma: genetic differences between histological subtypes. Am J Pathol. 1998;153(5):1467–73.
6. Magers MJ, Perrino CM, Cramer HM, Wu HH. Cytomorphologic comparison of type 1 and type 2 papillary renal cell carcinoma: a retrospective analysis of 28 cases. Cancer Cytopathol. 2019;127(6):370–6.

7. Leroy X, Zini L, Leteurtre E, Zerimech F, Porchet N, Aubert JP, Gosselin B, Copin MC. Morphologic subtyping of papillary renal cell carcinoma: correlation with prognosis and differential expression of MUC1 between the two subtypes. Mod Pathol. 2002;15(11):1126–30.
8. Akhtar M, Al-Bozom IA, Al HT. Papillary Renal Cell Carcinoma (PRCC): An Update. Adv Anat Pathol. 2019;26(2):124–32.
9. Pignot G, Elie C, Conquy S, Vieillefond A, Flam T, Zerbib M, Debre B, Amsellem-Ouazana D. Survival analysis of 130 patients with papillary renal cell carcinoma: prognostic utility of type 1 and type 2 subclassification. UROLOGY. 2007;69(2):230–5.
10. Bigot P, Bernhard JC, Gill IS, Vuong NS, Verhoest G, Flamand V, Reix B, Suer E, Gokce I, Beauval JB, et al. The subclassification of papillary renal cell carcinoma does not affect oncological outcomes after nephron sparing surgery. World J Urol. 2016;34(3):347–52.
11. Yamanaka K, Miyake H, Hara I, Inoue TA, Hanioka K, Fujisawa M. Papillary renal cell carcinoma: a clinicopathological study of 35 cases. Int J Urol. 2006; 13(8):1049–52.
12. Lopez-Beltran A, Scarpelli M, Montironi R, Kirkali Z. 2004 WHO classification of the renal tumors of the adults. Eur Urol. 2006;49(5):798–805.
13. Sika-Paotonu D, Bethwaite PB, McCredie MR, William JT, Delahunt B. Nucleolar grade but not Fuhrman grade is applicable to papillary renal cell carcinoma. Am J Surg Pathol. 2006;30(9):1091–6.
14. Moch H, Cubilla AL, Humphrey PA, Reuter VE, Ulbright TM. The 2016 WHO classification of tumours of the urinary system and male genital organs-part a: renal, penile, and testicular tumours. Eur Urol. 2016;70(1):93–105.
15. Delahunt B, Cheville JC, Martignoni G, Humphrey PA, Magi-Galluzzi C, McKenney J, Egevad L, Algaba F, Moch H, Grignon DJ, et al. The International Society of Urological Pathology (ISUP) grading system for renal cell carcinoma and other prognostic parameters. Am J Surg Pathol. 2013;37(10):1490–504.
16. Cornejo KM, Dong F, Zhou AG, Wu CL, Young RH, Braaten K, Sadow PM, Nielsen GP, Oliva E. Papillary renal cell carcinoma: correlation of tumor grade and histologic characteristics with clinical outcome. Hum Pathol. 2015;46(10):1411–7.
17. Schrader AJ, Rauer-Bruening S, Olbert PJ, Hegele A, Rustemeier J, Timmesfeld N, Varga Z, Hofmann R. Incidence and long-term prognosis of papillary renal cell carcinoma. J Cancer Res Clin Oncol. 2009;135(6):799–805.
18. Polifka I, Agaimy A, Herrmann E, Spath V, Trojan L, Stockle M, Becker F, Strobel P, Wulfing C, Schrader AJ, et al. High proliferation rate and TNM stage but not histomorphological subtype are independent prognostic markers for overall survival in papillary renal cell carcinoma. Hum Pathol. 2019;83:212–23.
19. Ha YS, Chung JW, Choi SH, Lee JN, Kim HT, Kim TH, Chung SK, Byun SS, Hwang EC, Kang SH, et al. Clinical significance of subclassification of papillary renal cell carcinoma: comparison of Clinicopathologic parameters and oncologic outcomes between papillary histologic subtypes 1 and 2 using the Korean renal cell carcinoma database. Clin Genitourin Cancer. 2017;15(2):e181–6.
20. Borgmann H, Musquera M, Haferkamp A, Vilaseca A, Klatte T, Shariat SF, Scavuzzo A, Jimenez RM, Wolff I, Capitanio U, et al. Prognostic significance of Fuhrman grade and age for cancer-specific and overall survival in patients with papillary renal cell carcinoma: results of an international multi-institutional study on 2189 patients. World J Urol. 2017;35(12):1891–7.
21. Delahunt B, Egevad L, Srigley JR, Samaratunga H. Fuhrman grading is inappropriate for papillary renal cell carcinoma. World J Urol. 2018;36(8):1335–6.

7

Limited utility of qPCR-based detection of tumor-specific circulating mRNAs in whole blood from clear cell renal cell carcinoma patients

Sinisa Simonovic[1,2,3*], Christian Hinze[3], Kai M. Schmidt-Ott[3,4], Jonas Busch[1], Monika Jung[1], Klaus Jung[1,2] and Anja Rabien[1,2]

Abstract

Background: RNA sequencing data is providing abundant information about the levels of dysregulation of genes in various tumors. These data, as well as data based on older microarray technologies have enabled the identification of many genes which are upregulated in clear cell renal cell carcinoma (ccRCC) compared to matched normal tissue. Here we use RNA sequencing data in order to construct a panel of highly overexpressed genes in ccRCC so as to evaluate their RNA levels in whole blood and determine any diagnostic potential of these levels for renal cell carcinoma patients.

Methods: A bioinformatics analysis with Python was performed using TCGA, GEO and other databases to identify genes which are upregulated in ccRCC while being absent in the blood of healthy individuals. Quantitative Real Time PCR (RT-qPCR) was subsequently used to measure the levels of candidate genes in whole blood (PAX gene) of 16 ccRCC patients versus 11 healthy individuals. PCR results were processed in qBase and GraphPadPrism and statistics was done with Mann-Whitney U test.

Results: While most analyzed genes were either undetectable or did not show any dysregulated expression, two genes, CDK18 and CCND1, were paradoxically downregulated in the blood of ccRCC patients compared to healthy controls. Furthermore, LOX showed a tendency towards upregulation in metastatic ccRCC samples compared to non metastatic.

Conclusions: This analysis illustrates the difficulty of detecting tumor regulated genes in blood and the possible influence of interference from expression in blood cells even for genes conditionally absent in normal blood. Testing in plasma samples indicated that tumor specific mRNAs were not detectable. While CDK18, CCND1 and LOX mRNAs might carry biomarker potential, this would require validation in an independent, larger patient cohort.

Keywords: Renal cell carcinoma, CDK18, CCND1, Biomarker, Blood, PAXgene

* Correspondence: sinisha555@yahoo.com
[1]Department of Urology, Charité - Universitätsmedizin Berlin, corporate member of Freie Universität Berlin, Humboldt-Universität zu Berlin, and Berlin Institute of Health, Berlin, Germany
[2]Berlin Institute for Urologic Research, Berlin, Germany
Full list of author information is available at the end of the article

Background

In the United States, it is estimated that 65,340 new cases and 14,970 deaths from kidney cancer will occur in 2018 [1]. ccRCC is the most common renal malignancy, accounting for around 80% of the cases [2]. Together with papillary and chromophobe carcinoma, it comprises 2% of all cancers worldwide [3]. Renal cell carcinoma (RCC) incidence increases markedly with age, peaking at 50–70 years, with males being affected twice more frequently than females [4]. The major risk factors for RCC include excess body weight, hypertension and cigarette smoking [5] and associations have also been made with different lifestyle, dietary, occupational and environmental factors [6]. Primary RCC displays no early clinical symptoms as most renal masses remain asymptomatic until the late stages of the disease, with over 50% of all cases of RCC being discovered by chance during imaging studies for other comorbidities [7, 8]. Only 10% of patients have the classical triad of symptoms: hematuria, flank pain and weight loss. Around 25% of RCCs have already metastasized by the time of diagnosis [9]. RCC is mostly unresponsive to conventional chemotherapy and radiation, which is the main reason for treatment failures [10, 11]. The gold standard for the management of renal masses is nephrectomy, in spite of which approximately 30% of patients develop recurrence or metastases [12, 13], which require systemic therapies and are associated with high mortality.

As current prognostic models based on conventional clinicopathological and imaging data have limited accuracy, new biomarkers are needed for early detection, improved diagnostics and the prediction of the clinical outcome of patients with RCC [14–17]. The ideal biomarker or biomarker panel should have high specificity, sensitivity, and reproducibility. Plasma, serum, and urine have recently gained interest in the field of cancer biomarker discovery. They represent potential sources of valuable biomarkers, containing proteins, DNA, and various RNA species, with blood being especially suitable in terms of kidney disease and low invasiveness. Steady progress in the field is being made, however to date, none of the identified ccRCC biomarkers have been clinically validated [18].

RNA circulating in blood is highly degraded (usually less than 100 bp in length [19]) and even after the introduction of systems that enable the stabilization and storage of whole blood mRNA (e.g. the PAXgene platform) studies tend to be limited to shorter RNA subspecies, or those protected from degradation due to their specific structure or association with proteins or membranous vesicular structures such as exosomes. Analyzing ccRCC biomarkers in urine would be particularly convenient, however this field is far less fruitful compared to blood studies. Similarly as for blood, urine is problematic in terms of RNA detection because of the presence of RNAses, but also because of PCR inhibition [20], which is steering the focus into the analysis of shorter RNA subspecies. Especially in the case of microRNA (miRNA), liquid biopsy has expanded from use in plasma to other bodily fluids in an increasing number of malignancies, making rapid progress since 2008 [21]. Along with miRNA, the use of Circulating Tumor Cells (CTCs), cell free DNA (cfDNA), and more recently circular RNA (circRNA) and long non-coding RNAs (lncRNA), are proving to be far more viable strategies, as for most tumors there is somewhat sporadic progress in detecting tumor-derived mRNA in blood and associating it with cancer prognosis, for example as described here [22–24]. A further issue that complicates tumor-derived RNA detection in blood is the uncertainty regarding the exact RNA origin, i.e. whether it is derived from solid tumor or CTCs, and what percentage of source cells are living and actively secreting RNA as opposed to undergoing apoptosis [25].

The first of the five proposed stages in biomarker development is the comparison of tumor with nontumor tissue [26]. Here techniques such as microarrays and more recently RNAseq are used to assess gene expression, while protein expression profiles are based on immunohistochemistry and mass spectroscopy, with the goal of discovering genes displaying dysregulation (usually overexpression in tumor compared to normal tissue). This phase is followed by the development of a clinical assay utilizing blood for non-invasive screening. Of course, the blood levels of selected genes do not have to precicely mirror the expression in tissue, as a result of e.g. the specific rate of mRNA release from cancer tissue into blood. The approach of using mRNA expression of tumor tissue as a starting point and analyzing the levels od respective transcripts in blood by RT-qPCR has been previously used with success, resulting in promising assays deserving of clinical validation. A recent study showed the validation of an RT-PCR assay based on prostate-specific RNA in whole blood from patients with metastatic castration-resistant prostate cancer (mCRPC) [27]. Several databases were consulted to select a panel of genes that were overexpressed in prostate tissue but showed no detection in peripheral blood mononuclear cells (PBMC). This was followed by RT-PCR analysis of blood samples of cancer patients and volunteers, resulting in the establishment of a 5-gene panel that enhances and complements the previously established CTC enumeraration assay. Similarly, in another study focusing on early detection of colorectal cancer [28], meta-analysis of microarray data was used to identify RNAs with highest diffeential expression between cancer tissue and normal blood samples. Subsequent RT-qPCR analysis revealed that blood expression of 3 specific genes shows promising sensitivity and specificity with respect to detection of this cancer.

In this study, TCGA database was used as a starting point to identify genes which are most highly overexpressed in the tissue of ccRCC patients, after which a subset containing genes that according to other databases have no blood expression was evaluated by qPCR in whole blood samples from ccRCC patients and healthy individuals. While RNA transcripts of some of these genes had good detectability in blood, none of the genes were significantly up-regulated in blood from ccRCC patients and two genes paradoxically displayed downregulation.

Methods

Patients and samples

The staging and grading of the tumor samples were done according to the 2002 TNM classification and the Fuhrman grading system [29, 30]. The ccRCC tissue samples were obtained during partial or radical nephrectomy at the University Hospital Charité in Berlin in 2011 and blood samples in the period between 2010 and 2016. Tissue samples were frozen in liquid nitrogen directly after surgical resection and stored at − 80 °C until RNA extraction. They came from tumor and matched normal tissue of 3 male patients without diagnosed metastasis (ages: 47–71; tumor stages: 2 x pT1, and pT3; grading: G1, G2, G3). PAXgene blood samples were obtained from 27 individuals and included 16 ccRCC samples, out of which 10 were non-metastatic (8 male and 2 female patients; median age 70, range 47–84 years; tumor staging: 1x pT1, 2x pT2, 7x pT3; grading: 2x G1, 7x G2, 1x G3) and 6 metastatic: (5 male and 1 female patients; median age 67, range 47–72 years; tumor staging: 6x pT3; grading: 5x G2, 1x G3). In total there were 11 samples without diagnosed cancer, 4 from patients suffering from non-cancer kidney illnesses, and 7 healthy volunteers (7 male and 4 female; median age 47, range 29–80 years).

Bioinformatics analysis

The first stage in gene selection was the analysis of ccRCC expression in TCGA database, followed by the use of GEO and GTEx databases to remove genes present in blood (Fig. 1). Subsequently, in order to evaluate candidate genes with respect to their suitability to serve as blood biomarkers by distinguishing ccRCC vs. normal patients, their expression was first tested by RT-qPCR in ccRCC and normal tissues, and secondly in blood samples of cancer patients versus non-cancer patients and healthy donors. According to the bioinformatics analysis, the higher expression in ccRCC tissue would be expected to be confirmed as compared to normal tissue, and subsequently, when PAXgene blood

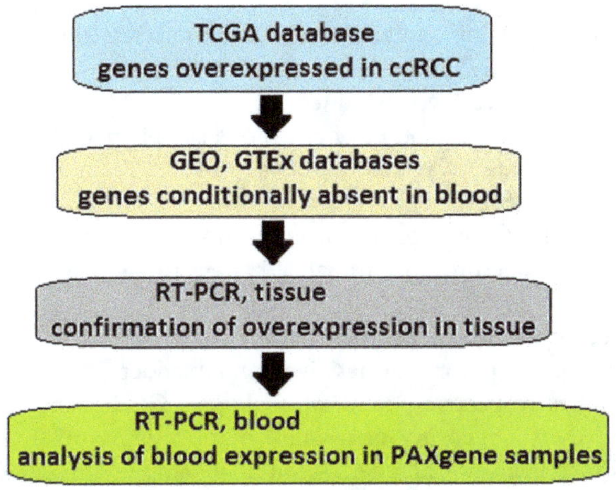

Fig. 1 Workflow diagram

samples are tested, the higher expression of at least some of the candidate genes would hopefully be determined in PAX blood from cancer patients compared to healthy. In order to obtain RNA seq based expression profiles in ccRCC and compare them to normal tissue as well as blood, the Cancer Genome Atlas database (TCGA, [31]) was used. The TCGA data portal is the largest and most commonly used public resource providing somatic and germline mutation, gene expression, gene methylation and copy number variation (CNV) data sets, amongst others, for several thousands of tumor samples. Data was obtained for 470 ccRCC patients, including 68 samples from matched normal tissue. In cases where multiple samples corresponded to a single patient, average expression values were calculated. Out of 20,533 TCGA genes in total, blood expression data from sources described below was found for 20,466 genes. Ideally candidate genes should not have wide expression domains; so as to provide a measure of kidney specificity for a gene, Tissue-specific Gene Expression and Regulation database (TiGER, [32]) was consulted, which is based on the analysis of the NCBI EST database [33] for 30 human tissues and contains tissue-specific expression profiles for 20,000 UniGenes. From 458 enriched in kidney, genes also expressed in blood, liver, prostate and bladder were deducted, leaving a list of 95 conditionally named 'kidney specific' genes.

In order to obtain blood expression profiles, a comprehensive search for RNA seq expression data from healthy individuals was made in literature and online databases. Gene Expression Omnibus database (GEO, [34]) archives and freely distributes microarray, next-generation sequencing, and other forms of high-throughput functional genomics data. This database was searched by variations of 'blood [Sample Source] AND *Homo sapiens* [Organism]

AND high throughput sequencing [Platform Technology Type]' providing a total of seven usable datasets altogether comprising 91 individual blood samples. Further 376 blood samples were obtained from GTEx database [35] and an additional source of one blood sample pooled from five individuals was kindly provided by Dr. Zhao and Dr. Zhang of Pfizer.

In order for expression profiles in important organs or organs related to the urological system to be given some relevance, RNA seq data from normal tissue was also considered in the analysis. From TCGA database, data was obtained for normal liver and bladder (9 and 11 samples respectively) and an analogous GEO search resulted in a recovery of a small number of samples for kidney, liver and bladder. Additional samples for kidney and liver (pooled from multiple donors) were included from RNA seq Atlas [36] (Table 1).

Processing of data downloaded from TiGER database, RNA seq expression data, calculation of rpkm values (reads per kilobase million) where necessary, translation of gene names and statistics were done in Python. Rpkm values were calculated according to the formula: raw count × 1,000,000/(gene length x library size). Translation of gene names was done using BioMart [38]. Mann-Whitey U test was used to discern between cancer and matched normal samples from TCGA with statistical significance defined as $p < 0.05$. In cases of gene expression entries with multiple isoforms, replicate samples, duplicate gene names, absolute highest values were taken, so as not to underestimate the possible presence in blood.

Table 1 Sources of expression profile datasets

Database	Tissue	Sample number	Source
GEO/GSE53655	blood	6	whole blood/PAXgene
GEO/GSE72509	blood	18	whole blood/PAXgene
GEO/GSE51799	blood	6	whole blood/PAXgene
GEO/GSE51799	blood	16	peripheral blood mononuclear cells
GEO/GSM833103	blood	16	whole blood/ PAXgene
GEO/GSM1647922, Personal correspondence	blood	12	whole blood/EDTA, Tempus
Personal correspondence, Pfizer [37]	blood	1, pooled from 5	whole blood/PAXgene
GTEx	blood	376	whole blood
TCGA	liver, normal matched	9	cancer patients
TCGA	bladder, normal matched	11	cancer patients
GEO/GSE69360	kidney	2	adult normal tissue
GEO/GSE69360	liver	2	adult normal tissue
RNA seq Atlas	kidney	1, pooled	normal tissue
RNA seq Atlas	liver	1, pooled	normal tissue
GEO/GSE35178	bladder	1	adult normal tissue

RNA isolation and RT-qPCR analysis

Total tissue RNA (1 μg) was purified using miRNeasy Kit (Qiagen, Hilden, Germany) following homogenization using TissueLyser II (Qiagen). Total RNA from PAXgene blood tubes was purified using the PAXgene Blood miRNA Kit (Qiagen). Total RNA concentration was determined by NanoDrop 1000 Spectrometer (Thermo Fisher Scientific Inc., Wilmington, DE, USA) by measuring the absorbance at 260 nm and RNA purity by measuring A260/280 ratios. The integrity and size distribution of the tissue and blood derived RNA was analyzed using Bioanalyzer (Agilent RNA 6000 Nano Kit). Only samples with RNA integrity number values equal or above 7 were included. RNA samples from normal tissues were pooled together and the same was done with the ones from cancer, producing one normal pool (NN) and one cancer pool (NC). Complementary DNA synthesis was performed using the Transcriptor First Strand cDNA Synthesis Kit (Roche Applied Science, Mannheim, Germany) with a mix of random hexamer and anchored-oligo(dT) primers. RNA was also isolated and transcribed from the renal cell carcinoma cell line 786–0 to assess the quality of all newly made cDNA from tissue and PAXgene blood samples. Normalization of the RT-qPCR data was done using the kidney reference gene peptidylproline isomerase A (PPIA) [39].

Primers were designed for SYBR Green using NCBI's PrimerBlast and Primer3 (see Additional file 1), so as to cover the maximum number of isoforms. The criteria for primer design were: amplicon length 60–150 nt, primer length 18–30 nt, intron spanning (intron length > 1000 nt), GC content 40–60%. For certain genes UPL probes were used in which case primers were automatically suggested with a given probe by the online tool (Universal Probe Library, Roche [40]), and common assays were selected for genes with multiple isoforms.

The relative quantification of transcripts was done on the Light Cycler 480 (Roche) using the QuantiTec SYBR Green PCR Kit (Qiagen) as previously described [37]. In case of UPL probes LightCycler 480 Probes Master Kit (Roche) was used. PCR was done on 96-well plates, with kidney cancer cell line 786–0 and ccRCC tissues as positive controls. PCR conditions were optimized where necessary and the size of PCR products was confirmed by electrophoresis using Bioanalyzer (Agilent DNA 1000 Kit). PCR data were analyzed by qBasePLUS software (Biogazelle NV, Gent, Belgium). With respect to the qBasePLUS processing, the samples were divided in 2 or

3 groups: normal vs. all cancer samples, i.e. cancer and metastatic cancer in a single group, as shown in the table 'qBasePLUS results: normal vs. all cancer samples' (see Additional file 2), normal vs. non-metastatic cancer, normal vs. metastatic cancer, and non-metastatic cancer vs. metastatic, as shown in the table 'qBasePLUS results: non-metastatic cancer vs. metastatic samples' (see Additional file 3). Results were calculated for 100% PCR efficiency and ′unpaired′ experimental design.

Statistics

Statistical analysis was done with GraphPad Prism 6.07 (GraphPad Software, San Diego, CA, USA) and qBasePLUS, using the Mann-Whitney U-test. *P* values < 0.05 were considered statistically significant. Graphs were *generated in GraphPad Prism using the* Mann-Whitney U-test.

Results

Candidate gene selection

In order to obtain a list of genes potentially useful as biomarkers, only genes with supposedly no blood expression, favorable statistical distance between distributions of cancer and normal values and high expression in cancer were taken into account. Regarding blood expression, values below 1 rpkm were considered low enough as to signify possible non expression, with respect to the sensitivity of detection. As a measure of distance of cancer and matched normal tissue distributions, the ratio of 5th percentile of cancer distribution with 95th percentile from normal was taken, and values above 0.5 considered favorable. Another measure of distance was calculated where the score represents the multiplication of probabilities of patients from each distribution falling within the overlap interval (score = Xprob x Yprob). Individual probabilities are calculated as the number of patients whose rpkm values fall within the overlap interval, divided by the total number of patients in the distribution (Xprob = patients within the overlap interval/total number of patients). Score is assigned 0 if the distributions do not overlap, and 1 for identical distributions. In cases when one distribution is within the other, but there are no patients from the larger one which fall into the overlap interval (they are distributed on both sides of it) score is assigned 1 as those genes are not valuable for further analysis. This method of calculating statistical distance is generally stricter then the percentile ratio, with favorable distance represented by values less than 0.3.

For genes of interest, the expression levels in liver, bladder, prostate and kidney in healthy individuals were also taken into account, giving preferential ranking to genes with lower rpkm values. Literature, the Human Protein Atlas [41], and OMIM [42] were consulted to gather information regarding gene function and expression domains of selected genes. Gene functions related to metabolic pathways in kidney or implicated in cancer (especially genes linked to ccRCC and hypoxia-inducible factors HIF1α and HIF2α) together with absence of expression in bone marrow and immune system, low or no expression in most tissues, and enrichment in kidney were considered favorable with respect to gene ranking.

A group of 20 genes were found to strictly fulfill expression criteria (defined as: blood expression GEO sources 95th percentile <1rpkm, GTEx 95th percentile <=1; fold change TCGA cancer median/matched normal tissue median > 1; distribution distance 5th percentile TCGA cancer/95th percentile matched normal tissue > 0.5, TCGA cancer median > 5rpkm) (Table 2, first 20 genes). The first 13 genes have median cancer values above 10. In addition, when it is considered that the rate of release of RNA from ccRCC into blood may be much higher than from normal kidney, as well as the presence of circulating tumor cells, the fold change median cancer/matched normal tissue, as well as the percentile ratio distribution distance measure become less relevant and may be relaxed in terms of gene selection. A similar argument follows for blood expression considering that individual blood sources may not be fully reliable and false outliers may be present. This enables the inclusion of certain genes which do not satisfy all the criteria fully, but may excel in some (last 11 genes in the table).

Many of these genes have previously been implicated in ccRCC, largely in micro-array studies [43–50]. This analysis identified this group of genes as having zero or low RNA blood presence, suggesting their potential use as ccRCC biomarkers in blood.

Analysis of the expression of candidate genes

To obtain an approximate overview of the levels in tissue, the expression was analyzed in cancer versus normal tissue for 15 genes of highest interest and the bioinformatics analysis was confirmed, as all these genes showed increased levels in cancer, notably so CA9 and NDUFA4L2 (Fig. 2). Certain genes were excluded from the analysis because of detection issues (multiple isoforms, etc.).

Blood testing consisted of two stages: in the first stage 3 PAXgene cancer samples were used (Table 3), and only genes with good (Cq < 33) detectability were selected for the second stage of blood testing with 24 more PAXgene samples (13 cancer and 11 normal/healthy), in order to broadly evaluate their expression. Especially good detectability was shown for following genes: CDK18 (Cq = 27), EGLN3 (Cq = 26), TMEM45A (Cq = 28), CAV2 (Cq = 26). A larger number of genes was undetectable or with extremely high Cq values. The genes with the supposedly highest potential based on

Table 2 Candidate genes

GENE	MEDIAN RPKM in ccRCC (based on expression data from TCGA consortium, [31])	FOLD DIFFERENCE, median rpkm in ccRCC vs. median rpkm in normal kidney (based on expression data from TCGA consortium, [31])	RPKM DISTRIBUTION DISTANCE, 5th percentile ccRCC/ 95th percentile normal kidney (based on expression data from TCGA consortium, [31])	BLOOD RPKM value of 95th percentile (based on GEO database [34])	BLOOD RPKM value of 95th percentile (based on GTEx database [35])
NDUFA4L2	701	145	1.06	0.16	0.15
EGLN3	174	23.2	0.93	0.72	0.62
CA9	117	1218	3.74	1	0.13
CCND1	138	4.34	0.58	0.58	0.37
CAV2	110	3.98	0.69	0.43	0.43
ESM1	92.5	12.4	0.6	0.77	0.2
PPP1R3C	20.1	3.66	0.54	0.03	0.67
STC2	19.1	22.3	1.33	0	0.07
NPTX2	18.4	150	1.48	0.07	0.13
ANGPT2	17.1	10.4	0.54	0.11	0.08
DGCR5	15.2	25.9	0.99	0.3	0.17
DOCK6	13.2	2.08	0.51	0.26	0.68
FABP6	11.9	91.3	1.18	0.62	0.85
TMEM133	8.9	2.67	0.52	0.60	0.24
LZTS1	8.81	5.54	0.52	0.26	0.25
COX4I2	6.85	4.37	0.52	0.06	0.15
KIAA1274	6.71	4.11	0.58	0.78	0.41
LPIN3	6.14	2.29	0.54	0.12	0.17
FKBP9L	6.11	1.32	0.51	0.71	0.14
RAB42	5.90	5.47	1.02	0.17	0.49
MET	112	2.08	0.36	0.07	0.1
CDK18	85.4	5.29	0.28	1.21	0.85
CP	79.7	21.3	0.11	0.89	0.4
TMEM45A	62.9	2.43	0.71	0.13	2.31
LOX	51.0	10.8	0.22	0.22	0.29
GAL3ST1	49.4	8.14	0.3	0.15	0.11
CYP2J2	49	39.3	0.27	0.65	0.2
NOL3	44.1	10.6	1.36	1.98	2.47
FBXO17	38.7	2.77	0.5	2	0.12
FABP7	19.9	974	0.22	0	0.05
BARX2	19.1	6.01	0.27	0.42	0.04

bioinformatics and tissue PCR analysis (NDUFA4L2 and CA9) had low detectability with very high Cq values (around 34). Nevertheless, NDUFA4L2 was tested on all 27 samples and was confirmed to be undetectable. In summary, 9 genes were finally selected for the second stage of testing (CAV2a, FABP7, ESM1, NOL3, LOX, CDK18, EGLN3, TMEM45A, CCND1). In the second stage, the expression levels turned out to be similar in cancer versus normal blood for most genes, except for CDK18 and CCND1 which paradoxically turned out to be downregulated in cancer blood (Table 4). Additional testing with 10 plasma samples indicated non-measurable expression. There was no correlation between the expression levels in blood for CDK18, CCND1, and LOX, and patient data such as age, tumor grade and stage.

The downregulation of CDK18 RNA in cancer blood (metastatic and non-metastatic grouped together) compared to normal was significant with p value = 0.001,

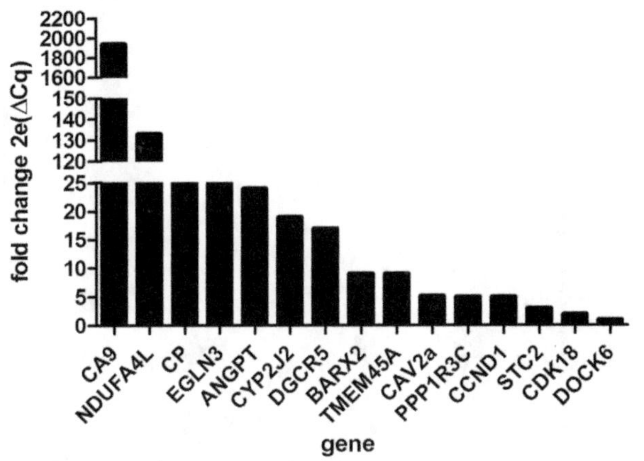

Fig. 2 Confirmation of TCGA data by RT-qPCR: Candidate genes were overexpressed in ccRcc compared to normal tissue (all values are above 1). Fold change is calculated as 2exp (Cqnormal-Cqcancer)

Table 3 Evaluation of candidate genes by RT-qPCR in tissue and 3 blood samples

Candidate genes	Confirmed Higher Expression In Ccrcc Vs Normal Tissue; fold change cancer/normal	Detectability In 3 PAX blood ccRCC SAMPLES, mean Cq value
NDUFA4L2	yes; 133	> 33
EGLN3	yes; 25	26.1
CA9	yes; 1938	> 33
CCND1	yes; 5	31.5
CAV2	not tested	26.1
ESM1	not tested	30.6
PPP1R3C	yes; 5	> 33
STC2	yes; 3	> 33
NPTX2	yes; 24	> 33
ANGPT2	yes; 24	> 33
DOCK6	yes; 1	> 33
FABP6	not tested	> 33
MET	not tested	> 33
CDK18	yes; 2	27.6
CP	yes; 40	> 33
TMEM45A	yes; 9	28.8
LOX	not tested	30.7
GAL3ST1	not tested	> 33
CYP2J2	yes; 19	> 33
NOL3	not tested	29.8
FABP7	not tested	32.5
BARX2	yes; 9	> 33

Table 4 Evaluation of expression in the second stage of blood testing with 27 samples

Candidate genes	Fold change cancer/normal	*P* value	Significantly different expression of ccRCC vs. normal in 27 pax blood samples
EGLN3	−1.26	0.215	No
CCND1	−1.55	0.039	Downregulated in ccRCC
CAV2	1.16	0.497	No
ESM1	−1.21	0.668	No
CDK18	−2.10	0.001	Downregulated in ccRCC
TMEM45A	−1.04	0.734	No
LOX	−1.31	0.668	No, tendency towards upregulation in metastatic ccRCC
NOL3	−1.05	0.641	No
FABP7	−1.13	0.671	No

whereas CCND1 was downregulated with $p = 0.039$ (Fig. 3). For both genes, there was no significant difference in levels when non-metastatic and metastatic samples were compared with each other. The results also showed a tendency towards upregulation for LOX when non-metastatic were compared to metastatic cancer samples, with the p value very close to significant ($p = 0.058$) (Fig. 3).

Discussion

In this study, a gene panel was made comprising the most highly overexpressed genes in ccRCC tissue whose mRNA also had the potential of being absent in the blood of healthy individuals. The first stage in the construction of this panel was the TCGA database- to select a panel of the most overexpressed genes in ccRCC, followed by the GEO and GTEx databases- to deduct from this panel genes showing measurable expression in the blood of healthy individuals. After confirming the tissue overexpression on samples from ccRCC patients in the next step, RT-qPCR analysis was done to evaluate mRNA levels in whole blood of ccRCC patients vs. patients without ccRCC and healthy donors. Measurable genes did not show overexpression in normal blood while two genes exhibited downregulation.

Whole blood analysis of selected genes does not show increased mRNA levels

The genes that had highest potential based on the bioinformatics analysis were NDUFA4L2 and CA9. According to the TCGA, the former has very high median expression in ccRCC tissue (701 rpkm) whereas the latter has the highest overexpression in ccRCC compared to normal tissue (1218). However, we found both to be undetectable in whole blood by qPCR. Several other

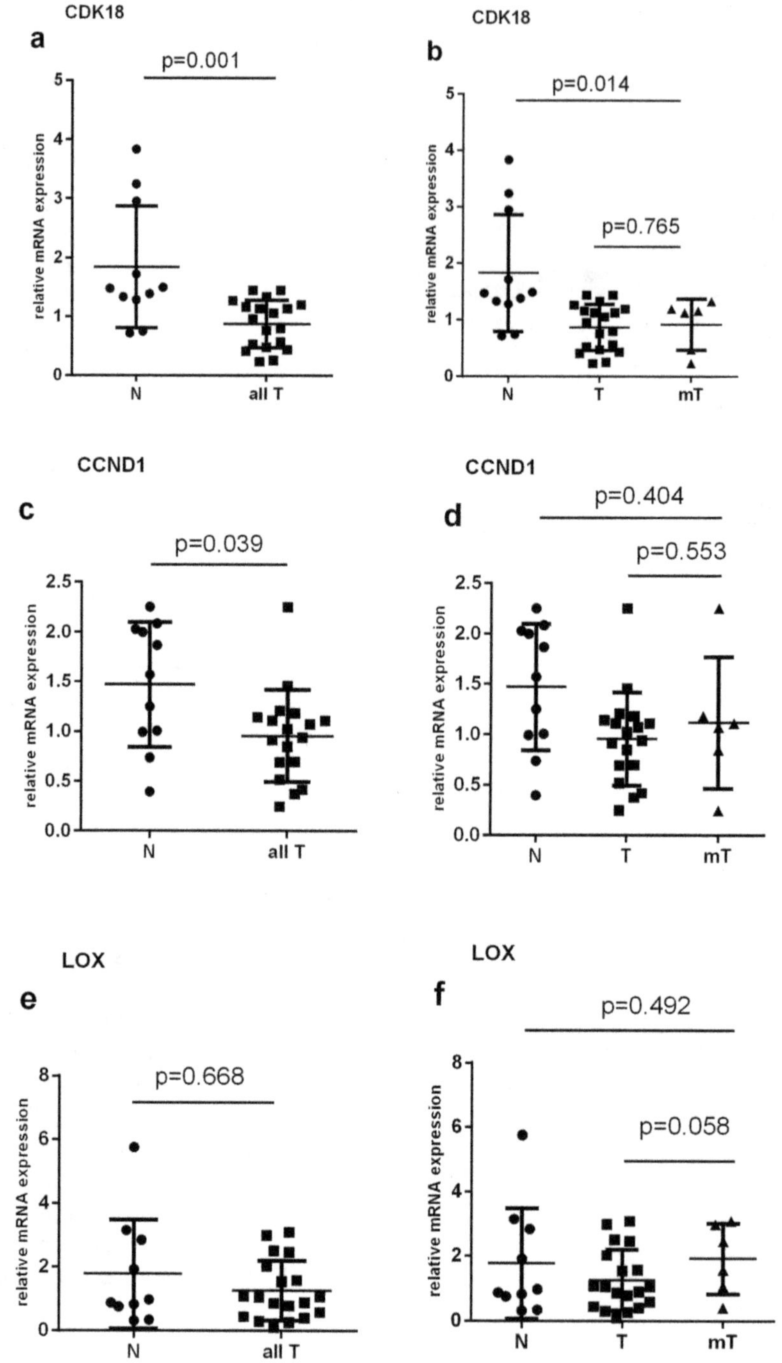

Fig. 3 Blood relative mRNA expression of CDK18, CCND1, and LOX based on the qBase exported relative quantity (RQ) values, calculated from Cq values, according to the formula: $RQ = 2^{(meanCq\text{-}Cq)}$; results from qBase (RQ values) were processed in *GraphPad Prism in order to generate graphs using the* Mann-Whitney U-test. N- normal patient samples; T- tumor patient samples; mT- metastatic. **a** CDK18 was underexpressed in PAX blood tumor samples compared to normal PAX blood. **b** There is no significant difference in expression of CDK18 between tumor and metastatic tumor PAX blood samples. **c** CCND1 was underexpressed in PAX blood tumor samples compared to normal PAX blood. **d** There is no significant difference in expression of CCND1 between tumor and metastatic tumor PAX blood samples. **e** There is no significant difference in expression of LOX in PAX blood tumor samples compared to normal PAX blood. **f** Lox shows a tendency towards upregulation in metastatic compared to non-metastatic tumor PAX blood samples

candidate genes were found to be undetectable in whole blood, while most of the genes that were detectable (EGLN3, CAV2, ESM1, TMEM45A, NOL3, FABP7) did not exhibit significant dysregulation in expression between cancer and healthy PAXgene samples. A plausible path to overcoming this outcome was to examine these genes in plasma, as the mRNA levels (supposedly originating from the expression in blood cells) could significantly drop in healthy samples compared to cancer ones once the blood cells are removed, revealing the effect of the tumor derived RNA. However, after testing 10 plasma samples, our conclusion was that gene expression in the plasma was not measurable. The PAXgene system is used for stabilization and isolation of mRNA and other classes of nucleic acids (such as genomic DNA and miRNA). Blood specimens are collected in tubes containing a stabilization reagent preventing nuclease degradation and transcriptional changes in antic oagulated whole blood, and stabilizing RNA for up to 3 days at room temperature, for the purpose of expression profiling [51]. All handling of RNA was done with special care, and although it is reasonable to assume that for many or all of the candidate genes RNA was degraded by blood RNAses, the RNA integrity of whole PAXgene samples was indeed satisfactory, reflected by their high RIN values. Apart from the issues regarding RNA stability and concerning expression interference from blood cells, possible limitations of this work design may stem from the bioinformatics phase. Acquired GEO datasets, which were used to screen for genes absent from blood (with supposedly no blood expression) may not be 100% reliable; they came from many different sources and were not in a perfect mutual accordance. A separate issue is the cutoff value of < 1 rpkm to signify absence of blood presence for a gene. Most authors somewhat arbitrarily define the expression threshold as 1 rpkm (more generally anywhere between 0.3 rpkm and 1 rpkm), below which the sensitivity of RNA sequencing is insufficient to confirm expression and distinguish it from the background [52, 53]. Our cutoff potentially may have enabled genes with minute expression in blood cells to be included in the wet lab analysis.

CDK18, CCND1, lox

The study also revealed the downregulation of two genes, CDK18 and CCND1, in ccRCC blood compared to healthy samples, as well as a tendency towards upregulation for LOX in metastatic compared to non-metastatic ccRCC. These results may be suitable for additional analysis in a larger patient cohort.

Cyclin-dependent kinase 18 (CDK18, PCTK3, PCTAIRE, PCTAIRE3) belongs to the PCTAIRE protein kinases, which are a subfamily of cdc2-related serine/threonine protein kinases named for a cysteine-for-serine substitution in the PCTAIRE motif conserved in the initially characterized CDK proteins (PCTAIRE sequence instead of the PSTAIRE sequence). They have unique N and C-terminal domains that extend forth from a serine/threonine kinase domain that is highly homologous to cdc2 [54]. PCTAIRE kinase subfamily includes three members, PCTK1/CDK16, PCTK2/CDK17, and PCTK3/CDK18 which are poorly researched. Insights into the activation of CDK18 have recently been obtained- it binds cyclin A2 and cyclin E1 (pulldown experiment with HEK293T cells) and is activated by cyclin A2 and PKA (cAMP-dependent protein kinase) [55]. CDK18 has recently been shown to regulate cell migration and adhesion in HEK293T cells by negatively modulating FAK (focal adhesion kinase) activity and reorganizing actin and associated skeletal/adhesion proteins such as cofilin, and has also been implicated in vesicular transport via interaction with Sec23Ap [56]. Overexpression of CDK18 also led to the formation of filopodia during the early stages of cell adhesion in HeLa cells [57]. Interestingly, it has also been recently found to play a role in replication stress and positively regulate genome stability, by associating with RAD proteins [58]. Lastly, PCTAIRE-3 as well as PCTAIRE-2 have been implicated in Alzheimer's disease [59, 60]. CDK18 was induced by CTS-1 (Chimeric tumor suppressor-1, p53-derived synthetic tumor suppressor) and mediated growth arrest and death in glioma cells [61]. Apart from its activation by cyclin A2, in the same study CDK18 was shown to phosphorylate retinoblastoma tumorsupressor protein (Rb) in vitro [55]. *Although PCTAIRE1 has been found to be upregulated in many cancers, so far there is no such data for CDK18.*

Cyclin D1 (CCND1) regulates CDK4 or CDK6, whose activity is necessary for G1/S transition of the cell cycle. CCND1 is more frequently dysregulated in human cancers and therefore more studied than cyclin D2 or D3. Its overexpression leads to aberrant CDK activation resulting in rapid growth and division and is correlated with tumor stage, increased metastasis and poor prognosis in various cancers [62]. It is also involved in processes such as DNA repair and the control of mitochondrial activity and cell migration; it may assume CDK-independent functions as well [63]. CCND1 was investigated by microarray and TMA in ccRCC, and found to be upregulated and a potential therapeutic target [64]. In another study, CCND1 was found to be a useful immunohistochemical marker to discriminate between chromophobe renal cell carcinoma and renal oncocytoma [65].

Lysyl oxidase (LOX) performs covalent cross linking in elastin and collagen by oxidizing lysine residues, and therefore is important for the integrity of extracellular matrix [66]. It has both intracellular and extracellular functions and is involved in a number of pathological processes that affect the connective tissue [67]. It is up-regulated in many cancers and involved in tumor progression, although it has been reported to function as a tumor-suppressor as well. Its concrete roles in various aspects of tumorigenesis have been reviewed recently [68]. LOX is a HIF target [69] and in ccRCC, LOX has been shown to be strongly overexpressed compared to normal tissue; it is one of the genes postranscriptionally regulated by miR-141-3p and miR-145-5p; and has prognostic relevance for the overall survival of ccRCC patients [70]. In ccRCC cell cultures, it has been found to function in a positive-regulative loop with HIF-1α, and to influence ccRCC progression by modifying cellular adhesion, migration, and the rigidity of the collagen matrix [71].

Conclusions

In summary, with the goal of finding potential blood-based biomarkers for ccRCC, this study investigated the blood presence of genes highly overexpressed in ccRCC tissue and compared their blood mRNA levels between healthy and ccRCC patient samples. The overexpression in tissue was not reflected in the increase in the levels of mRNAs circulating in the blood of ccRCC patients. The analysis revealed the transcripts of CDK18 and CCND1 as underexpressed in the blood of ccRCC patients, and LOX as showing a tendency towards upregulation in metastatic ccRCC compared to non-metastatic. Further analysis of the selected gene panel by using a larger patient cohort may prove useful.

Supplementary information

Additional file 1:. A subset of genes were detected using UPL probes in which case probe numbers are given.

Additional file 2: All cancer samples (metastatic and non-metastatic) were included in a single group and compared with normal samples.

Additional file 3: Metastatic cancer samples were taken as a separate group and compared to non-metastatic.

Abbreviations

CCND1: Cyclin d1; ccRCC: Clear cell renal cell carcinoma; CDK18: Cyclin-dependent kinase 18; CEA: Carcinoembryonic antigen; cfDNA: Circulating cell-free dna; circRNA: Circular rna; CNV: Copy number variation; CTCs: Circulating tumor cells; GEO: Gene expression omnibus database; HCC: Hepatocellular carcinoma; HIF: Hypoxia inducible factor; lncRNA: Long non-coding rnas; LOX: Lysyl oxidase; miRNAs: Micrornas; PSA: Prostate-specific antigen; RCC: Renal cell carcinoma; RT-qPCR: Quantitative real time pcr; TCGA: Cancer Genome Atlas database; TiGER: Tissue-specific Gene Expression and Regulation database

Acknowledgements

We are grateful to Silke Rabenhorst for excellent technical assistance.

Authors' contributions

Study design: KMS, KJ, AR, SS; bioinformatics: CH, SS; acquisition of data: JB, MJ, SS; interpretation of data: KMS, KJ, AR, SS; manuscript preparation: SS; substantial revision: JB, KJ, KMS, AR. We confirm that all authors read and approved the final manuscript.

Author details

[1]Department of Urology, Charité - Universitätsmedizin Berlin, corporate member of Freie Universität Berlin, Humboldt-Universität zu Berlin, and Berlin Institute of Health, Berlin, Germany. [2]Berlin Institute for Urologic Research, Berlin, Germany. [3]Max-Delbrück-Center for Molecular Medicine (MDC), Berlin, Germany. [4]Department of Nephrology and Medical Intensive Care, Charité - Universitätsmedizin Berlin, Berlin, Germany.

References

1. Siegel RL, Miller KD, Jemal A. Cancer statistics, 2018. CA Cancer J Clin. 2018; 68:7–30.
2. Srigley JR, Delahunt B, Eble JN, Egevad L, Epstein JI, Grignon D, et al. The International Society of Urological Pathology (ISUP) Vancouver classification of renal neoplasia. Am J Surg Pathol. 2013;37:1469–89.
3. Rydzanicz M, Wrzesiński T, Bluyssen HA, Wesoły J. Genomics and epigenomics of clear cell renal cell carcinoma: recent developments and potential applications. Cancer Lett. 2013;341:111–26.
4. Martel CL, Lara PN. Renal cell carcinoma: current status and future directions. Crit Rev Oncol Hematol. 2003;45(2):177–90.
5. McLaughlin J, Lipworth L, Tarone R, Blot W. Cancer Epidemiology and Prevention. Oxford Univ. Press; 2006. p. 1087–100.
6. Chow WH, Dong LM, Devesa SS. Epidemiology and risk factors for kidney cancer. Nat Rev Urol. 2010;7:245–57.
7. Gospodarowicz MK, Miller D, Groome PA, Greene FL, Logan PA, Sobln LH. The process for continuous improvement of the TNM classification. Cancer. 2004;100(1):1–5.
8. Powles T, Staehler M, Ljungberg B, Bensalah K, Canfield SE, Dabestani S, et al. European Association of Urology guidelines for clear cell renal cancers that are resistant to vascular endothelial growth factor receptor-targeted therapy. Eur Urol. 2016;70(5):705–6.
9. Jonasch E, Gao J, Rathmell WK. Renal cell carcinoma. BMJ. 2014;349:4797.
10. Ljungberg B, Bensalah K, Bex A, Canfield S, Dabestani S, Hofmann F, et al. Guidelines on renal cell carcinoma: 2014 update. Eur Assoc Urol. 2015;67: 913–24.
11. Singer EA, Gupta GN, Srinivasan R. Update on targeted therapies for clear cell renal cell carcinoma. Curr Opin Oncol. 2011;23(3):283–9.
12. MacLennan S, et al. Systematic review of oncological outcomes following surgical management of localised renal cancer. Eur Urol. 2012;61:972–93.
13. Janzen NK, Kim HL, Figlin RA, Belldegrun AS. Surveillance after radical or partial nephrectomy for localized renal cell carcinoma and management of recurrent disease. Urol Clin North Am. 2003;30:843–52.
14. Sun M, Shariat SF, Cheng C, et al. Prognostic factors and predictive models in renal cell carcinoma: a contemporary review. Eur Urol. 2011;60:644–61.
15. Atzpodien J, Royston P, Wandert T, et al. Metastatic renal carcinoma comprehensive prognostic system. Br J Cancer. 2003;88:348–53.
16. Kim HL, Seligson D, Liu X, et al. Using tumor markers to predict the survival of patients with metastatic renal cell carcinoma. J Urol. 2005;173:1496–501.
17. Adashek JJ, Salgia MM, Posadas EM, Figlin RA, Gong J. Role of Biomarkers in Prediction of Response to Therapeutics in Metastatic Renal-Cell Carcinoma. Clin Genitourin Cancer. 2019;17(3):e454–e460. Review.
18. Majer W, Kluzek K, Bluyssen H, Wesoły J. Potential approaches and recent advances in biomarker discovery in clear-cell renal cell carcinoma. J Cancer. 2015;6(11):1105–13.
19. Reddi KK, Holland JF. Elevated serum ribonuclease in patients with pancreatic cancer. Proc Natl Acad Sci U S A. 1976;73:2308–10.
20. Huggett JF, Novak T, Garson JA, Green C, Morris-Jones SD, Miller RF, et al. Differential susceptibility of PCR reactions to inhibitors: an important and unrecognised phenomenon. BMC Res Notes. 2008;1:70.
21. Connolly ID, et al. The "liquid biopsy": the role of circulating DNA and RNA in central nervous system tumors. Curr Neurol Neurosci Rep. 2016;16(3):25.
22. Yörüker EE, Holdenrieder S, Gezer U. Blood-based biomarkers for

diagnosis, prognosis and treatment of colorectal cancer. Clin Chim Acta. 2016;455:26–32.
23. Zane K, et al. Emerging blood-based biomarkers for detection of gastric cancer. World J Gastroenterol. 2015;21(41):11636–53.
24. Nandagopal L, Sonpavde G. Circulating biomarkers in bladder cancer. Bladder Cancer. 2016;2(4):369–79.
25. Stroun M, Lyautey J, Lederrey C, et al. About the possible origin and mechanism of circulating DNA apoptosis and active DNA release. Clin Chim Acta. 2001;313(1–2):139–42.
26. Pepe MS, Etzioni R, Feng Z, Potter JD, Thompson ML, Thornquist M, et al. Phases of biomarker development for early detection of cancer. J Natl Cancer Inst. 2001;93(14):1054–61.
27. Danila DC, Anand A, Schultz N, et al. Analytic and clinical validation of a prostate cancer-enhanced messenger RNA detection assay in whole blood as a prognostic biomarker for survival. Eur Urol. 2014;65(6):1191–7.
28. Rodia MT, et al. Systematic large-scale meta-analysis identifies a panel of two mRNAs as blood biomarkers for colorectal cancer detection. Oncotarget. 2016;7(21):30295–306.
29. Fuhrman SA, Lasky LC, Limas C. Prognostic significance of morphologic parameters in renal cell carcinoma. Am J Surg Pathol. 1982;6:655–63.
30. Sobin LH, Wittekind C. TNM classification of malignant tumours. New York: Wiley-Liss; 2002. p. 193–5.
31. Cancer Genome Atlas Research Network. Comprehensive molecular characterization of clear cell renal cell carcinoma. Nature. 2013;499:43–9.
32. Liu X, Yu X, Zack DJ, Zhu H, Qian J. TIGER: a database for tissue-specific gene expression and regulation. BMC Bioinformatics. 2008;9:271.
33. Boguski MS, Lowe TM, Tolstoshev CM. dbEST--database for "expressed sequence tags". Nat Genet. 1993;4:332–3.
34. Edgar R, Domrachev M, Lash AE. Gene expression omnibus: NCBI gene expression and hybridization array data repository. Nucleic Acids Res. 2002;30:207–10.
35. Lonsdale J, et al. The genotype-tissue expression (GTEx) project. Nat Genet. 2013;45:580–5.
36. Krupp M, Marquardt JU, Sahin U, Galle PR, Castle J, Teufel A. RNA-Seq atlas-a reference database for gene expression profiling in normal tissue by next-generation sequencing. Bioinformatics. 2012;28(8):1184–5.
37. Zhao S, et al. Comparison of stranded and non-stranded RNA-seq transcriptome profiling and investigation of gene overlap. BMC Genomics. 2015;16:675.
38. BioMart. http://www.ensembl.org. Accessed 20 Apr 2016.
39. Jung M, Ramankulov A, Roigas J, Johannsen M, Ringsdorf M, Kristiansen G, et al. In search of suitable reference genes for gene expression studies of human renal cell carcinoma by real-time PCR. BMC Mol Biol. 2007;8:47.
40. Universal Probe Library. www.universalprobelibrary.com. Accessed 5 May 2016.
41. Uhlen M, et al. A human protein atlas for normal and cancer tissues based on antibody proteomics. Mol Cell Proteomics. 2005;4(12):1920–32.
42. Hamosh A, et al. Online Mendelian inheritance in man (OMIM), a knowledgebase of human genes and genetic disorders. Nucleic Acids Res. 2002;30(1):52–5.
43. Meyer HA, Tolle A, Jung M, Fritzsche FR, Haendler B, Kristiansen I, et al. Identification of stanniocalcin 2 as prognostic marker in renal cell carcinoma. Eur Urol. 2009;55:669–78.
44. Thibodeau BJ, Fulton M, Fortier LE, Geddes TJ, Pruetz BL, Ahmed S, et al. Characterization of clear cell renal cell carcinoma by gene expression profiling. Urol Oncol. 2016;34(4):168.
45. Feng JY, Diao XW, Fan MQ, Wang PX, Xiao Y, Zhong X, et al. Screening of feature genes of the renal cell carcinoma with DNA microarray. Eur Rev Med Pharmacol Sci. 2013;17(22):2994–3001.
46. Fu L, Minton DR, Zhang T, Nanus DM, Gudas LJ. Genome-wide profiling of track kidneys shows similarity to the human ccRCC transcriptome. Mol Cancer Res. 2015;13(5):870–8.
47. Schrödter S, Braun M, Syring I, Klümper N, Deng M, Schmidt D, et al. Identification of the dopamine transporter SLC6A3 as a biomarker for patients with renal cell carcinoma. Mol Cancer. 2016;15:10.
48. Minton DR, Fu L, Mongan NP, Shevchuk MM, Nanus DM, Gudas LJ. Role of NADH dehydrogenase (ubiquinone) 1 alpha subcomplex 4-like 2 in clear cell renal cell carcinoma. Clin Cancer Res. 2016;22(11):2791–801.
49. Klatte T, Kabbinavar F, Zomordian N, Belldegrun AS, Pantuck AJ. Prospective evaluation of carbonic anhydrase IX (CAIX) as a molecular marker in metastatic renal cell carcinoma: interim results. J Urol. 2007;177:164.
50. Bruick RK, McKnight SL. A conserved family of prolyl-4-hydroxylases that modify HIF. Science. 2001;294:1337–40.
51. Rainen L, Oelmueller U, Jurgensen S, et al. Stabilization of mRNA expression in whole blood samples. Clin Chem. 2002;48:1883–90.
52. Ramsköld D, Wang ET, Burge CB, Sandberg R. An abundance of ubiquitously expressed genes revealed by tissue transcriptome sequence data. PLoS Comput Biol. 2009;5(12):e1000598.
53. Magee R, Loher P, Londin E, Rigoutsos I. Threshold-seq: a tool for determining the threshold in short RNA-seq datasets. Bioinformatics. 2017;33(13):2034–6.
54. Meyerson M, Enders GH, Wu CL, et al. A family of human cdc2-related protein kinases. EMBO J. 1992;11:2909–17.
55. Matsuda S, Kominato K, Koide-Yoshida S, et al. PCTAIRE kinase 3/cyclin-dependent kinase 18 is activated through association with cyclin a and/or phosphorylation by protein kinase a. J Biol Chem. 2014;289(26):18387–400.
56. Palmer KJ, Konkel JE, Stephens DJ. PCTAIRE protein kinases interact directly with the COPII complex and modulate secretory cargo transport. J Cell Sci. 2005;118:3839–47.
57. Matsuda S, Kawamoto K, Miyamoto K, Tsuji A, Yuasa K. PCTK3/CDK18 regulates cell migration and adhesion by negatively modulating FAK activity. Sci Rep. 2017;7:45545.
58. Barone G, Staples CJ, Ganesh A, Patterson KW, Bryne DP, Myers KN, et al. Human CDK18 promotes replication stress signaling and genome stability. Nucleic Acids Res. 2016;44(18):8772–85.
59. Herskovits AZ, Davies P. The regulation of tau phosphorylation by PCTAIRE 3: implications for the pathogenesis of Alzheimer's disease. Neurobiol Dis. 2006;23(2):398–408.
60. Chaput D, Kirouac L, Stevens SM Jr, Padmanabhan J. Potential role of PCTAIRE-2, PCTAIRE-3 and P-histone H4 in amyloid precursor protein-dependent Alzheimer pathology. Oncotarget. 2016;7(8):8481–97.
61. Naumann U, Huang H, Wolburg H, Wischhusen J, Weit S, Ohgaki H, et al. PCTAIRE3: a putative mediator of growth arrest and death induced by CTS-1, a dominant-positive p53-derived synthetic tumor suppressor, in human malignant glioma cells. Cancer Gene Ther. 2006;5:469–78.
62. Qie S, Diehl JA. Cyclin D1, cancer progression, and opportunities in cancer treatment. J Mol Med (Berl). 2016;94(12):1313–26.
63. Zwijsen RM, Wientjens E, Klompmaker R, van der Sman J, Bernards R, Michalides RJ. CDK-independent activation of estrogen receptor by cyclin D1. Cell. 1997;88(3):405–15.
64. Karim S, Al-Maghrabi JA, Farsi HM, Al-Sayyad AJ, Schulten HJ, Buhmeida A, et al. Cyclin D1 as a therapeutic target of renal cell carcinoma- a combined transcriptomics, tissue microarray and molecular docking study from the Kingdom of Saudi Arabia. BMC Cancer. 2016;16(Suppl 2):741.
65. Zhao W, Tian B, Wu C, Peng Y, Wang H, Gu WL, et al. DOG1, cyclin D1, CK7, CD117 and vimentin are useful immunohistochemical markers in distinguishing chromophobe renal cell carcinoma from clear cell renal cell carcinoma and renal oncocytoma. Pathol Res Pract. 2015;211(4):303–7.
66. Kumari S, Panda TK, Pradhan T. Lysyl oxidase: its diversity in health and diseases. Indian J Clin Biochem. 2017;32(2):134–41.
67. Zheng W, et al. Low extracellular lysyl oxidase expression is associated with poor prognosis in patients with prostate cancer. Oncol Lett. 2016;12(5):3161–6.
68. Wang TH, Hsia SM, Shieh TM. Lysyl oxidase and the tumor microenvironment. Int J Mol Sci. 2017;8(1):62.
69. Tanaka T, et al. Anthracycline inhibits recruitment of hypoxia-inducible transcription factors and suppresses tumor cell migration and cardiac Angiogenic response in the host. J Biol Chem. 2012;287(42):34866–82.
70. Liep J, Kilic E, Meyer HA, Busch J, Jung K, Rabien A. Cooperative effect of miR-141-3p and miR-145-5p in the regulation of targets in clear cell renal cell carcinoma. PLoS One. 2016;11(6):e0157801.
71. Di Stefano V, Torsello B, Bianchi C, Cifola I, Mangano E, Bovo G, et al. Major action of endogenous Lysyl oxidase in clear cell renal cell carcinoma progression and collagen stiffness revealed by primary cell cultures. Am J Pathol. 2016;186(9):2473–85.

8

Impact of sarcomatoid differentiation and rhabdoid differentiation on prognosis for renal cell carcinoma with vena caval tumour thrombus treated surgically

Bin Yang[1†], Haizhui Xia[1†], Chuxiao Xu[1], Min Lu[2], Shudong Zhang[1], Guoliang Wang[1*] and Lulin Ma[1*]

Abstract

Background: Sarcomatoid differentiation in renal cell carcinoma (RCC) with vena caval tumour thrombus has been shown to be associated with aggressive behaviours and poor prognosis; however, evidence of the impact of rhabdoid differentiation on prognosis is lacking. This study evaluated the impact of sarcomatoid differentiation and rhabdoid differentiation on oncological outcomes for RCC with vena caval tumour thrombus treated surgically.

Methods: We retrospectively analysed patients treated surgically for RCC with vena caval tumour thrombus at our institute from Jan 2015 to Nov 2018. Prognostic variables were evaluated for associations with progression-free survival (PFS) and cancer-specific survival (CSS) by Kaplan–Meier survival analysis and log-rank test. Univariate and multivariate analyses were performed to determine independent prognostic variables.

Results: We identified 125 patients with RCC and vena caval tumour thrombus, including 17 (13.6%) with sarcomatoid differentiation alone, 8 (6.4%) with rhabdoid differentiation alone and 3 (2.4%) with both sarcomatoid and rhabdoid differentiation. Compared to pure RCC, patients with sarcomatoid differentiation but not rhabdoid differentiation have worse PFS ($p = 0.018$ and $p = 0.095$, respectively). The univariate and multivariate analyses both showed sarcomatoid differentiation as a significant predictor of PFS. Compared to pure RCC, patients with sarcomatoid differentiation ($p = 0.002$) and rhabdoid differentiation ($p = 0.001$) both had significantly worse CSS. The univariate analysis showed sarcomatoid differentiation, rhabdoid differentiation, metastasis and blood transfusion as significant predictors of CSS (All, $p < 0.05$). In the multivariate analysis, sarcomatoid differentiation (HR 3.90, $p = 0.008$), rhabdoid differentiation (HR 3.01, $p = 0.042$), metastasis (HR 3.87, $p = 0.004$) and blood transfusion (HR 1.34, $p = 0.041$) all remained independent predictors of CSS.

Conclusions: Sarcomatoid differentiation and rhabdoid differentiation are both independent predictors of poor prognosis in RCC with vena caval tumour thrombus treated surgically.

Keywords: Sarcomatoid, Rhabdoid, Renal cell carcinoma, Vena cava, Thrombus, Prognosis

* Correspondence: wangguoliang@medmail.com.cn; malulin@bjmu.edu.cn
[†]Bin Yang and Haizhui Xia contributed equally to this work.
[1]Department of Urology, Peking University Third Hospital, 49 North Garden Road, Haidian District, Beijing 100191, People's Republic of China
Full list of author information is available at the end of the article

Background

Renal cell carcinoma (RCC) is the most common kidney tumour, comprising an estimated 2.2% of all new cancer diagnoses with 403,262 new cases and 175,098 deaths in 2018 [1]. Overall 4–10% of patients with RCC present with venous tumour thrombus [2]. Sarcomatoid differentiation in RCC is characterized histologically by a dedifferentiated growth pattern of epithelial neoplasm into malignant spindle-shaped mesenchymal cells [3]. Sarcomatoid differentiation can arise in any histologic subtype of RCC; thus, it is no longer considered a distinct histologic subtype [4]. Approximately 5% of all RCCs and up to 15% of stage IV cases contain sarcomatoid differentiation [5, 6]. Previous studies suggested that sarcomatoid differentiation is associated with aggressive behaviours, poor response to targeted therapy and worse prognosis [6–8]. However, the impact of sarcomatoid differentiation on prognosis for RCC with vena caval tumour thrombus treated surgically has not been studied extensively.

Rhabdoid differentiation in RCC is characterized by "sheets and clusters of variably cohesive, large epithelioid cells with vesicular nuclei, prominent nucleoli and large paranuclear intracytoplasmic inclusions" [9]. It is present in approximately 5% of all RCCs and 27% of grade 4 RCCs [9, 10]. Rhabdoid differentiation in RCC is considered a predictor of poor prognosis, similar to sarcomatoid differentiation. Therefore, the World Health Organization International Society of Urological Pathology (WHO/ISUP) grading system formally classifies RCC with either sarcomatoid differentiation or rhabdoid differentiation as grade 4 [11]. The impact of rhabdoid differentiation in RCC on prognosis has been studied to some extent, but the available reports have inconsistent conclusions. Furthermore, there is little evidence on the prognostic role of rhabdoid differentiation in RCC with vena caval tumour thrombus treated surgically.

Therefore, this report describes the survival outcomes of a consecutive series of patients treated surgically for RCC with vena caval tumour thrombus and our evaluation of the impact of sarcomatoid differentiation and rhabdoid differentiation on survival outcomes.

Methods

Patients

After receiving approval from the Peking University Third Hospital Medical Science Research Ethics Committee, we retrospectively analysed the data of patients treated with nephrectomy and thrombectomy for RCC with vena caval tumour thrombus at our institute from Jan 2015 to Nov 2018. Among the 131 patients pathologically diagnosed with RCC with vena caval tumour thrombus, 6 were excluded from the study: 1 with metachronous vena caval tumour thrombus, 2 with two-stage operation for RCC with vena caval tumour thrombus and 3 with incomplete follow-up data. Thus, 125 patients were included in our study. None of the patients underwent neoadjuvant therapy before surgery. Comprehensive clinical and pathological data was collected for each patient, including age, gender, tumour size, thrombus level, blood transfusion, TNM stage, histologic subtype, Fuhrman grade, tumour necrosis, sarcomatoid differentiation, rhabdoid differentiation and adjuvant target therapy of tyrosine kinase inhibitors.

Clinical and pathological evaluation

Tumour size was collected as the largest diameter reported in computed tomography or magnetic resonance imaging examination. The level of tumour thrombus was assigned using the Mayo classification [12]. TNM stage was determined according to the 8th edition American Joint Committee on Cancer TNM classification [13]. Histologic subtype was assigned based on the 2016 WHO classification of renal tumour [14]. The tumour grade was determined following the Fuhrman system. A commonly accepted definition of sarcomatoid differentiation and rhabdoid differentiation morphology was used [3, 9]. One urological pathologist reviewed the pathologic specimens.

Surgical procedures

First, nephrectomy was performed following routine procedures, and lymph node dissection was performed for patients suspected to have lymph node metastasis based on enhanced CT or PET/CT results. Second, the inferior vena cava (IVC) and contralateral renal vein were isolated and blocked as follows: (a) For Mayo I tumour thrombus, the IVC tumour thrombus was squeezed back into the renal vein using the milking technique, and the IVC was partially blocked with vessel forceps. (b) For Mayo II tumour thrombus, several short hepatic veins and lumbar veins were ligated to expose the retrohepatic segment of the IVC, and the contralateral renal vein and distal and proximal IVC were blocked with rubber bands. (c) For Mayo III tumour thrombus, the liver was mobilized to expose the hepatic portal vein before blocking the IVC. (d) For Mayo IV tumour thrombus without entrance to the atrium, the milking technique and Foley catheter-assisted technique could be used to downgrade the tumour thrombus to level III. (e) For Mayo IV tumour thrombus into the atrium, thoracoabdominal midline incision and cardiopulmonary bypass were commonly necessary. Next, the junction of the renal vein and IVC was curvilinearly incised, and the tumour thrombus was pulled out once confirmed to be completely isolated. Finally, the IVC was sutured continuously after flushing the lumen with heparin saline.

Follow-up

Follow-up was executed every 3 months for the first 2 years and semi-annually thereafter and included physical examination, laboratory tests and chest and abdomen-pelvis scans. Follow-up information was obtained through review of outpatient records and telephone calls. Progression-free survival (PFS) was calculated from the date of surgery to radiological evidence of tumour progression, death from any cause or the last follow-up. Cancer specific survival (CSS) was calculated from the date of surgery to death from RCC or the last follow-up.

Statistical analysis

Normally distributed continuous variables were reported as means and standard deviations. Non-normally distributed continuous variables were reported as medians and interquartile ranges. The Student's t test and Mann–Whitney U test were applied to compare continuous variables. The Chi-square test was applied to compare categorical variables. The Kaplan–Meier method with log-rank test was used for survival analysis and comparisons. Univariate and multivariate Cox proportional hazard models were performed to identify independent predictors associated with PFS and CSS. All statistical analyses were conducted with SPSS Statistics 22.0 (IBM Corp, Armonk, NY, USA). Two-tailed tests were used for all comparisons, and $p < 0.05$ was considered statistically significant.

Results

Baseline characteristics

A total of 125 patients treated surgically for RCC with vena caval tumour thrombus were included in our study. Thrombus levels were Mayo I, II, III, and IV in 38, 49, 25 and 13 patients, respectively. Among those patients, 17 (13.6%) had sarcomatoid differentiation alone, 8 (6.4%) had rhabdoid differentiation alone and 3 (2.4%) had both sarcomatoid and rhabdoid differentiation. The patients' clinicopathological demographics are outlined in Table 1 and are stratified by the presence of sarcomatoid and/or rhabdoid differentiation. There was no significant difference in gender, age, thrombus level, histological subtype, T stage, nodal status or adjuvant target therapy between the patients with sarcomatoid and/or rhabdoid differentiation and the patients with pure RCC. RCC with sarcomatoid and/or rhabdoid differentiation tended to have a higher incidence of synchronous metastasis than pure RCC, but this difference was not significant (39.3 vs 21.6%, $p = 0.060$). However, RCC with sarcomatoid and/or rhabdoid differentiation more frequently had larger tumour size (median 8.5 vs 10.4 cm, $p = 0.012$) and higher blood transfusion (median 1600 vs 400 cc, $p = 0.038$) than pure RCC. Similarly, RCC with sarcomatoid and/or rhabdoid differentiation more frequently displayed high-grade disease (84.6 vs 59.6%, $p = 0.018$) and tumour necrosis (71.4 vs 45.4%, $p = 0.015$).

Impact of sarcomatoid and rhabdoid differentiation

The mean follow-up was 13.6 ± 10.1 months. At the last follow-up, 55 (44.0%) patients had reported disease progression with a mean PFS of 22.7 ± 1.9 months and 22 (17.6%) had died as a consequence of RCC, with a mean CSS of 33.1 ± 1.8 months. The perioperative mortality within 90 days was 10.4% (13/125). One of them died of intraoperative pulmonary embolism. Based on the Kaplan–Meier survival analysis, non-clear cell RCC (mean 10.1 vs 26.3 months, $p < 0.001$) and metastasis (mean 14.2 vs 26.3 months, $p = 0.001$) were significantly associated with PFS (Fig. 1). Compared to pure RCC, RCC with sarcomatoid differentiation (mean 11.9 vs 25.2 months, $p = 0.018$), but not RCC with rhabdoid differentiation (mean 12.1 vs 25.2 months, $p = 0.095$), had significantly worse PFS (Fig. 2). In the univariate analysis, metastasis (HR 2.48, $p = 0.001$), non-clear cell RCC (HR 2.73, $p = 0.001$) and sarcomatoid differentiation (HR 1.99, $p = 0.037$) were significant predictors of PFS (Additional file 1: Table S1). In the multivariate analysis, metastasis (HR 2.64, $p = 0.001$), non-clear cell RCC (HR 3.23, $p < 0.001$) and sarcomatoid differentiation (HR 2.08, $p = 0.029$) all remained independent predictors of PFS (Additional file 1: Table S1). We did not include T stage in the model due to the important collinearity between T stage and thrombus level.

Based on the Kaplan–Meier survival analysis, RCC with sarcomatoid differentiation (mean 19.8 vs 35.3 months, $p = 0.002$) and rhabdoid differentiation (mean 16.0 vs 35.7 months, $p = 0.001$) had significantly worse CSS than pure RCC (Fig. 3). Metastasis was also significantly associated with CSS (mean 26.1 vs 35.9 months, $p = 0.010$). Thrombus level and histologic subtype were not associated with CSS. In the univariate analysis, sarcomatoid differentiation (HR 3.54, $p = 0.011$), rhabdoid differentiation (HR 3.82, $p = 0.009$), metastasis (HR 2.88, $p = 0.014$) and blood transfusion (HR 1.36, $p = 0.017$) were significant predictors of CSS (Table 2). In the multivariate analysis, sarcomatoid differentiation (HR 3.90, $p = 0.008$), rhabdoid differentiation (HR 3.01, $p = 0.042$), metastasis (HR 3.87, $p = 0.004$) and blood transfusion (HR 1.34, $p = 0.041$) all remained significant independent predictors of CSS (Table 2). In the univariate and multivariate analysis only blood transfusion was both significant predictor of perioperative mortality within 90 days (Additional file 1: Table S2).

Discussion

RCC with sarcomatoid differentiation was first reported as a distinct histologic subtype termed sarcomatoid RCC

Table 1 Clinicopathological demographics of patients treated surgically for RCC with vena caval tumour thrombus

Characteristics	Pure RCC ($n = 97$)	RCC with sarcomatoid and/or rhabdoid differentiation ($n = 28$)	p
Age (years), median (IQR)	60 (53–67)	55 (52–63)	0.205
Gender, n (%)			0.614
Male	68 (70.1)	21 (75.0)	
Female	29 (29.9)	7 (25.0)	
Tumour side, n (%)			0.510
Left	25 (25.8)	9 (32.1)	
Right	72 (74.2)	19 (67.9)	
Tumour size (cm), mean ± SD	8.5 ± 3.2	10.4 ± 4.1	0.012
Thrombus level (Mayo), n (%)			0.790 0.038 0.319
I	29 (29.9)	9 (32.1)	
II	40 (41.2)	9 (32.1)	
III	19 (19.6)	6 (21.4)	
IV	9 (9.3)	4 (14.3)	
Blood transfusion (cc), median (IQR)	400 (0–2000)	1600 (400–3200)	
Tumour stage, n (%)			
T3b	84 (86.6)	21 (75.0)	
T3c	9 (9.3)	4 (14.3)	
T4	4 (4.1)	3 (10.7)	
Nodal status, n (%)			1.000
N0/Nx	88 (90.7)	26 (92.9)	
N+	9 (9.3)	2 (7.1)	
Metastatic status, n (%)			0.060
M0	76 (78.4)	17 (60.7)	
M1	21 (21.6)	11 (39.3)	
Metastatic sites, n (%)			0.701
Lung	16 (64.0)	8 (57.1)	
Bone	6 (24.0)	5 (35.7)	
Liver	3 (12.0)	1 (7.1)	
Histologic subtype, n (%)			0.454
Clear cell RCC	77 (79.4)	24 (85.7)	
Non-clear cell RCC	20 (20.6)	4 (14.3)	
Fuhrman grade, n (%) ($n = 120$)			0.018
1–2	38 (40.4)	4 (15.4)	
3–4	56 (59.6)	22 (84.6)	
Tumour necrosis, n (%)			0.015
Absent	53 (54.6)	8 (28.6)	
Present	44 (45.4)	20 (71.4)	
Adjuvant target therapy	38(39.2)	11(39.3)	0.992

RCC renal cell carcinoma, *IQR* interquartile range, *SD* standard deviation

in 1968 [15]. Subsequent studies confirmed that sarcomatoid RCC can occur in all subtypes of RCC, but it does have a higher incidence in clear cell RCC [4, 6, 16]. Sarcomatoid differentiation is currently considered a rare histologic variant that predicts aggressive behaviour and poor prognosis. According to previous studies, RCC with sarcomatoid differentiation more frequently has larger tumour size, higher risk of necrosis and higher tumour stage and grade [6, 7, 16], which is consistent with the results of our study. In our cohort of RCC with vena caval tumour thrombus treated surgically, the presence of sarcomatoid differentiation in RCC was found to be an independent predictor for PFS and CSS after adjusting for other known prognostic factors. The association between sarcomatoid differentiation with poor oncologic outcomes has been consistently confirmed by many previous studies [5, 6, 16, 17]. Using the Surveillance, Epidemiology, and End Results–Medicare database, Trudeau et al. [7] identified one of the largest RCC cohorts including 234 RCCs with sarcomatoid differentiation. The results of that study showed that RCC with sarcomatoid differentiation has a worse 5-year CSS compared to pure clear cell RCC (67% vs 14%).

RCC with sarcomatoid differentiation is classified as grade 4 by the WHO/ISUP grading system [11]. However, grade 4 RCC with sarcomatoid differentiation has significantly worse CSS than grade 4 RCC without differentiation [10, 18]. We believe that the equivalence of sarcomatoid differentiation and grade 4 classification in RCC may underestimate the prognostic value of sarcomatoid differentiation. Furthermore, Adibi et al. [19] found that the percentage of sarcomatoid differentiation (PSD) was a prognostic factor for overall survival in RCC. Zhang et al. [20] suggested that PSD was an independent predictor of prognosis. However, the prognostic value of PSD in patients with RCC is still under debate [21, 22]. Our study failed to include PSD in the multivariate analysis model due to insufficient data. Insufficient pathologic material can result in incomplete and inaccurate assessment of PSD in retrospective studies. This may be one explanation for the conflicting conclusions of the above studies.

Rhabdoid differentiation, which can arise in any histologic subtype of RCC, including clear cell, papillary, chromophobe and unclassified RCC, may be a prognostic variation of RCC, similar to sarcomatoid differentiation. However, rhabdoid differentiation has not been studied as thoroughly as sarcomatoid differentiation. Gökden et al. [9] reported an incidence of rhabdoid differentiation of 4.7% and revealed associations between rhabdoid differentiation and increased grade and stage for the first time. Delahunt et al. [11] reviewed previous studies that reported survivals ranging from 8 to 31 months. In a more recent study of grade 4 RCC, 45

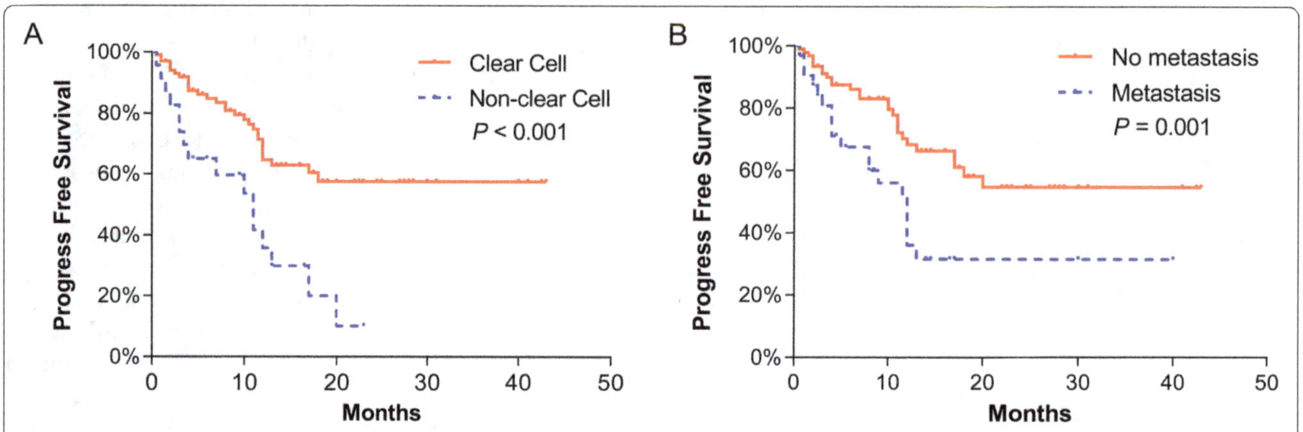

Fig. 1 Kaplan–Meier curves of progression-free survival stratified by histologic subtype (**a**) and metastatic status (**b**)

(28.3%) cases had rhabdoid differentiation, with a median CSS of 3.8 years [18]. To our knowledge, our study is the first to evaluate the prognostic impact of sarcomatoid differentiation and rhabdoid differentiation in RCC with vena caval tumour thrombus. We identified an incidence of rhabdoid differentiation of 8.8%, and our results supported the above hypothesis that rhabdoid differentiation in RCC is associated with adverse prognostic factors. Furthermore, we confirmed that rhabdoid differentiation in RCC is a predictor of CSS independent from sarcomatoid differentiation, thrombus level and other prognostic variables. In a prior cohort of 49 clear cell RCCs with rhabdoid differentiation, the presence of rhabdoid differentiation was shown to be an independent predictor of poor prognosis, which is consistent with the results of our study [23].

In contrast, a study of grade 4 RCC showed that rhabdoid differentiation alone was not associated with worse CSS [18]. To our knowledge, the study by Zhang et al. [10] with 111 cases and a 2-year survival of 46% is the largest reported to date; it demonstrated that RCC with rhabdoid differentiation confers an increased risk of death compared to grade 3 RCC. However, the multivariate subgroup analysis of grade 4 RCC revealed that rhabdoid differentiation was not associated with CSS. The existing studies have consistently supported the incorporation of sarcomatoid differentiation and/or rhabdoid differentiation into grade 4 RCC to improve outcome prediction. However, we suggest that it is inappropriate to treat sarcomatoid differentiation and rhabdoid differentiation equally when evaluating the prognosis of RCC.

Furthermore, we found histologic subtype to be a significant predictor of PFS and CSS, in keeping with previous studies [24, 25]. However, studies of grade 4 RCC accounting for sarcomatoid differentiation and/or rhabdoid differentiation failed to show an independent association between histologic subtype and prognosis [18, 20]. Since the cohorts only included grade 4 RCC, some non-clear cell RCCs that could not be graded using the existing Fuhrman classification system may have been excluded generating selection bias. The small

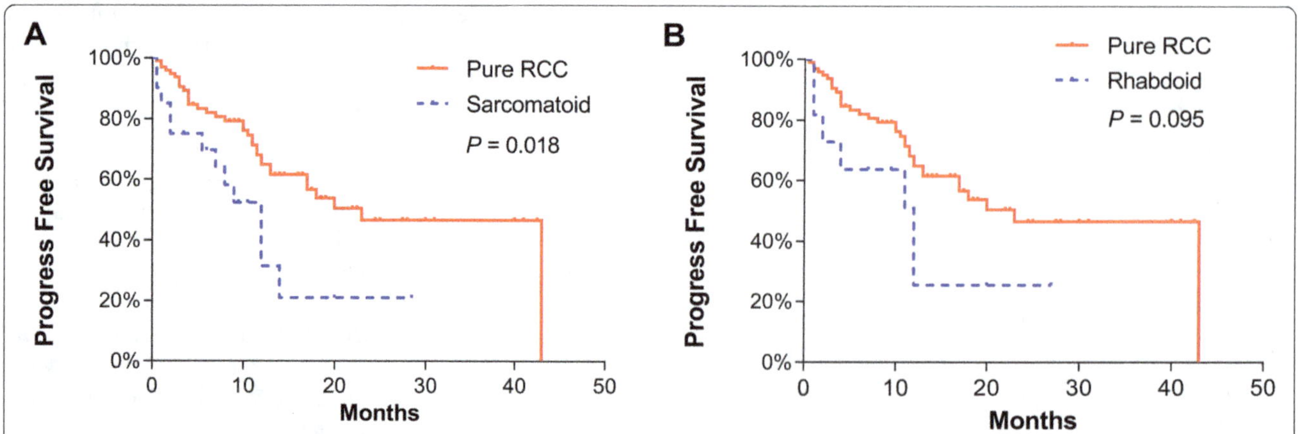

Fig. 2 Kaplan–Meier curves of progression-free survival for patients with pure renal cell carcinoma (RCC) vs RCC with sarcomatoid differentiation (**a**) and pure RCC vs RCC with rhabdoid differentiation (**b**)

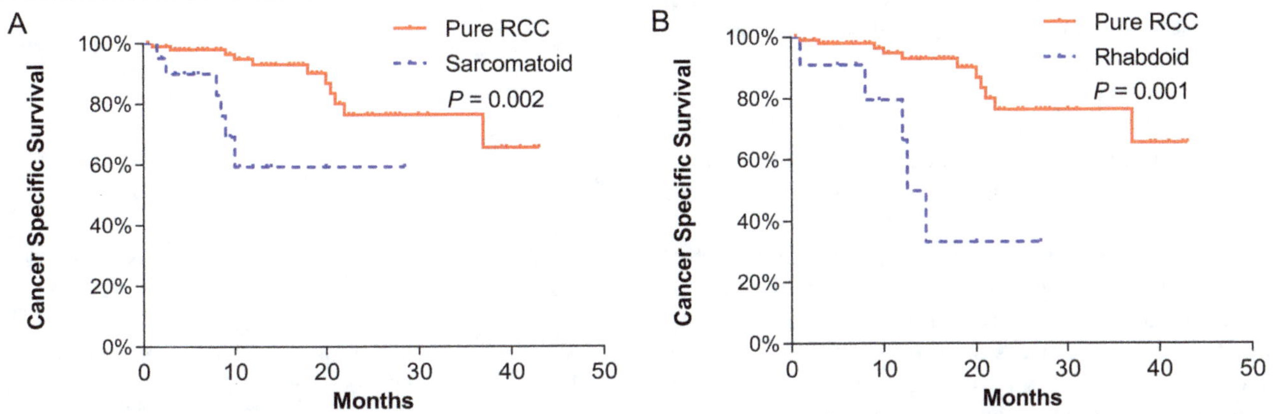

Fig. 3 Kaplan–Meier curves of cancer-specific survival for patients with pure renal cell carcinoma (RCC) vs RCC with sarcomatoid differentiation (**a**) and pure RCC vs RCC with rhabdoid differentiation (**b**)

sample for the sarcomatoid differentiation and rhabdoid differentiation cohorts may have been insufficient to detect differences in prognosis between the histologic subtypes. In our study, potential predictors, such as thrombus level and tumour necrosis, were not significantly associated with PFS or CSS. In contrast, most recent studies have supported the impact of thrombus level on oncologic outcomes in RCC with vena caval tumour thrombus [17, 24, 26], although some results are conflicting [27]. Currently, the prognostic significance of tumour necrosis is less certain. A study based on 3017 cases of clear cell RCC showed that the WHO/ISUP grading system achieves a better predictive ability for prognosis when the presence of tumour necrosis is

Table 2 Univariate and multivariate Cox proportional hazard regression analyses of CSS

	Univariate		Multivariate	
	HR (95% CI)	*p*	HR (95% CI)	*p*
Gender, female	1.07 (0.43–2.66)	0.878		
Age (years)	0.99 (0.95–1.03)	0.620		
Tumour size (cm)	1.06 (0.95–1.18)	0.323		
Thrombus level				
I	Ref.			
II	1.09 (0.37–3.15)	0.881		
III	1.83 (0.61–5.46)	0.280		
IV	0.57 (0.07–4.73)	0.601		
Blood transfusion (10^3 cc)	1.36 (1.06–1.76)	0.017	1.34 (1.01–1.77)	0.041
Lymph node involvement	1.96 (0.58–6.67)	0.279		
Metastasis	2.88 (1.24–6.70)	0.014	3.87 (1.56–9.61)	0.004
Histologic subtype				
Clear cell RCC	Ref.			
Non-clear cell RCC	1.87 (0.72–4.85)	0.196		
Sarcomatoid differentiation	3.54 (1.34–9.38)	0.011	3.90 (1.42–10.71)	0.008
Rhabdoid differentiation	3.82 (1.39–10.51)	0.009	3.01 (1.04–8.74)	0.042
Fuhrman grade				
1–2	Ref.			
3–4	1.47 (0.57–3.76)	0.423		
Tumour necrosis	1.78 (0.75–4.24)	0.191		
Adjuvant target therapy	0.55 (0.23–1.36)	0.199		

CSS cancer specific survival, *RCC* renal cell carcinoma

incorporated [28]. However, in several studies, tumour necrosis was not shown to be an independent predictor of oncologic outcomes [18, 23, 26]. Compared to the cytokine therapy era, the targeted therapy era has achieved significant improvement in survival in RCC. However, RCC with sarcomatoid differentiation has been shown to have a poor response to targeted therapy [4, 29], and this may influence prognosis and survival.

Our study has some limitations, including its retrospective nature, single-centre experience and relatively shorter follow-up compared to previous studies. Although multivariate analyses were used to identify independent predictors of PFS and CSS, it is possible that unmeasured differences existed considering the small sample of our study. In addition, we did not perform lymph node dissection routinely for all patients which may have reduced the reliability of our results regarding the prognostic impact of lymph node involvement. Finally, there was some heterogeneity in treatment after surgery which can result in different oncologic outcomes.

Conclusion

Our study shows that sarcomatoid differentiation and rhabdoid differentiation are associated with worse CSS in patients with RCC and vena caval tumour thrombus treated surgically. Furthermore, RCC with sarcomatoid differentiation was an independent predictor for worse PFS. Blood transfusion was an important predictor of early perioperative mortality.

Supplementary information

Additional file 1: Table S1. Univariate and multivariate Cox proportional hazard regression analyses of PFS. **Table S2.** Univariate and multivariate logistic regression analyses of perioperative mortality within 90 days.

Abbreviations

CSS: Cancer-specific survival; ISUP: International Society of Urological Pathology; IVC: Inferior vena cava; PFS: Progression-free survival; PSD: Percentage of sarcomatoid differentiation; RCC: Renal cell carcinoma; WHO: World Health Organization

Acknowledgements

Not applicable.

Authors' contributions

LLM, GLW proposed the protocol. BY, HZX, CXX, ML were involved in data collection and management. BY, HZX, SDZ analysed the data. BY, HZX contributed to statistical analysis. BY contributed to manuscript writing. LLM, GLW critically revised the manuscript. All authors read and approved the final manuscript.

Author details

[1]Department of Urology, Peking University Third Hospital, 49 North Garden Road, Haidian District, Beijing 100191, People's Republic of China. [2]Department of Pathology, Peking University Health Science Center, Beijing, China.

References

1. Bray F, Ferlay J, Soerjomataram I, Siegel RL, Torre LA, Jemal A. Global cancer statistics 2018: GLOBOCAN estimates of incidence and mortality worldwide for 36 cancers in 185 countries. CA Cancer J Clin. 2018;68(6):394–424.
2. Lardas M, Stewart F, Scrimgeour D, Hofmann F, Marconi L, Dabestani S, Bex A, Volpe A, Canfield SE, Staehler M, et al. Systematic review of surgical management of nonmetastatic renal cell carcinoma with vena caval thrombus. Eur Urol. 2016;70(2):265–80.
3. Delahunt B. Sarcomatoid renal carcinoma: the final common dedifferentiation pathway of renal epithelial malignancies. Pathology. 1999;31(3):185–90.
4. Bergerot P, Agarwal N, Pal SK, Jones J. Sarcomatoid renal cell carcinoma: the apple Doesn't fall far from the tree. Clin Cancer Res. 2017;23(21):6381–3.
5. Shuch B, Bratslavsky G, Shih J, Vourganti S, Finley D, Castor B, Treat E, Linehan WM, Pantuck AJ, Said JW, Belldegrun AS. Impact of pathological tumour characteristics in patients with sarcomatoid renal cell carcinoma. BJU Int. 2012;109(11):1600–6.
6. Gu L, Li H, Wang H, Ma X, Wang L, Chen L, Zhao W, Zhang Y, Zhang X. Presence of sarcomatoid differentiation as a prognostic indicator for survival in surgically treated metastatic renal cell carcinoma. J Cancer Res Clin Oncol. 2017;143(3):499–508.
7. Trudeau V, Larcher A, Sun M, Boehm K, Dell Oglio P, Sosa J, Tian Z, Fossati N, Briganti A, Shariat SF, Karakiewicz PI. Comparison of oncologic outcomes between sarcomatoid and clear cell renal cell carcinoma. World J Urol. 2016;34(10):1429–36.
8. Mouallem NE, Smith SC, Paul AK. Sarcomatoid renal cell carcinoma: Biology and treatment advances. Urol Oncol. 2018;36(6):265–71.
9. Gökden N, Nappi O, Swanson PE, Pfeifer JD, Vollmer RT, Wick MR, Humphrey PA. Renal cell carcinoma with Rhabdoid features. Am J Surg Pathol. 2000;24(10):1329–38.
10. Zhang BY, Cheville JC, Thompson RH, Lohse CM, Boorjian SA, Leibovich BC, Costello BA. Impact of Rhabdoid differentiation on prognosis for patients with grade 4 renal cell carcinoma. Eur Urol. 2015;68(1):5–7.
11. Delahunt B, Eble JN, Egevad L, Samaratunga H. Grading of renal cell carcinoma. Histopathology. 2019;74(1):4–17.
12. Blute ML, Leibovich BC, Lohse CM, Cheville JC, Zincke H. The Mayo Clinic experience with surgical management, complications and outcome for patients with renal cell carcinoma and venous tumour thrombus. BJU Int. 2004;94(1):33–41.
13. Paner GP, Stadler WM, Hansel DE, Montironi R, Lin DW, Amin MB. Updates in the eighth edition of the tumor-node-metastasis staging classification for urologic cancers. Eur Urol. 2018;73(4):560–9.
14. Moch H, Cubilla AL, Humphrey PA, Reuter VE, Ulbright TM. The 2016 WHO classification of Tumours of the urinary system and male genital organs—part a: renal, penile, and testicular Tumours. Eur Urol. 2016; 70(1):93–105.
15. Farrow GM, Harrison EG Jr, Utz DC. Sarcomas and sarcomatoid and mixed malignant tumors of the kidney in adults. 3. Cancer. 1968;22(3):556–63.
16. Cheville JC, Lohse CM, Zincke H, Weaver AL, Leibovich BC, Frank I, Blute ML. Sarcomatoid renal cell carcinoma: an examination of underlying histologic subtype and an analysis of associations with patient outcome. Am J Surg Pathol. 2004;28(4):435–41.
17. Abel EJ, Spiess PE, Margulis V, Master VA, Mann M, et al. Cytoreductive nephrectomy for renal cell carcinoma with venous tumor Thrombus. J Urol. 2017;198(2):281–8.
18. Kara O, Maurice MJ, Zargar H, Malkoc E, Akca O, Andrade HS, Ramirez D, Caputo PA, Nelson RJ, Rini B, Kaouk JH. Prognostic implications of sarcomatoid and rhabdoid differentiation in patients with grade 4 renal cell carcinoma. Int Urol Nephrol. 2016;48(8):1253–60.
19. Adibi M, Thomas AZ, Borregales LD, Merrill MM, Slack RS, et al. Percentage of sarcomatoid component as a prognostic indicator for survival in renal cell carcinoma with sarcomatoid dedifferentiation. Urol Oncol. 2015;33(10):427 e17–23.

20. Zhang BY, Thompson RH, Lohse CM, Leibovich BC, Boorjian SA, Cheville JC, Costello BA. A novel prognostic model for patients with sarcomatoid renal cell carcinoma. BJU Int. 2015;115(3):405–11.
21. Merrill MM, Wood CG, Tannir NM, Slack RS, Babaian KN, et al. Clinically nonmetastatic renal cell carcinoma with sarcomatoid dedifferentiation: Natural history and outcomes after surgical resection with curative intent. Urol Oncol. 2015;33(4):166 e21–9.
22. Korenbaum C, Pierard L, Thiery A, Story F, Lindner V, Lang H, Kurtz JE, Barthelemy P. Treatments, outcomes, and validity of prognostic scores in patients with Sarcomatoid renal cell carcinoma: a 20-year single-institution experience. Clin Genitourin Cancer. 2018;16(3):e577–86.
23. Przybycin CG, McKenney JK, Reynolds JP, Campbell S, Zhou M, Karafa MT, Magi-Galluzzi C. Rhabdoid differentiation is associated with aggressive behavior in renal cell carcinoma: a Clinicopathologic analysis of 76 cases with clinical follow-up. Am J Surg Pathol. 2014;38(9):1260–5.
24. Tilki D, Nguyen HG, Dall Era MA, Bertini R, Carballido JA, et al. Impact of histologic subtype on Cancer-specific survival in patients with renal cell carcinoma and tumor Thrombus. Eur Urol. 2014;66(3):577–83.
25. Nguyen DP, Vilaseca A, Vertosick EA, Corradi RB, Touijer KA, Benfante NE, Sjoberg DD, Russo P. Histologic subtype impacts cancer-specific survival in patients with sarcomatoid-variant renal cell carcinoma treated surgically. World J Urol. 2016;34(4):539–44.
26. Rodriguez Faba O, Linares E, Tilki D, Capitanio U, Evans CP, Montorsi F, Martínez-Salamanca JI, Libertino J, Gontero P, Palou J. Impact of Microscopic Wall invasion of the renal vein or inferior vena cava on Cancer-specific survival in patients with renal cell carcinoma and tumor Thrombus: a multi-institutional analysis from the international renal cell carcinoma-venous Thrombus consortium. Eur Urol Focus. 2018;4(3):435–41.
27. Wagner B, Patard J, Méjean A, Bensalah K, Verhoest G, et al. Prognostic value of renal vein and inferior vena cava involvement in renal cell carcinoma. Eur Urol. 2009;55(2):452–9.
28. Delahunt B, McKenney JK, Lohse CM, Leibovich BC, Thompson RH, Boorjian SA, Cheville JC. A novel grading system for clear cell renal cell carcinoma incorporating tumor necrosis. Am J Surg Pathol. 2013;37(3):311–22.
29. Keskin SK, Msaouel P, Hess KR, Yu K, Matin SF, et al. Outcomes of patients with renal cell carcinoma and Sarcomatoid dedifferentiation treated with nephrectomy and systemic therapies: comparison between the cytokine and targeted therapy eras. J Urol. 2017;198(3):530–7.

9

Metatarsal metastasis from clear cell renal cell carcinoma

Hongzeng Wu[1], Ruoqi Han[2], Qianqian Zhang[3], Yi Zhao[1] and Helin Feng[1*]

Abstract

Background: Bone metastasis is known to occur in some patients with cancer, usually in the spine, pelvis or ribs, and less than 0.01% of patients have metastases in the foot bone, so metatarsal metastasis is quite rare. The initial symptoms of osseous metastases are swelling, pain, or both.

Case presentation: We report a 68-year-old man with solitary metatarsal metastasis 26 months after a diagnosis of renal clear cell carcinoma. The patient suffered intermittent swelling of his right foot and pain for one year due to trauma and was not treated. The doctor attributed the symptoms to trauma, administering massage therapy and a plaster cast to the patient at the local clinic. After reviewing the medical records, we found that this patient had a history of clear cell renal cell carcinoma. The patient underwent radiological examination and open biopsy of the first metatarsal bone of the right foot. These findings confirmed that the patient had a metatarsal metastasis from clear cell renal cell carcinoma. The patient subsequently underwent right foot amputation. No local recurrence or distant metastasis was found after a 6-month follow-up.

Conclusion: Clinicians should be aware of a history of renal cell carcinoma (RCC) and fully understand the patient's past medical history. When treating patients with clear cell renal cell carcinoma who have unresolving bony pain or swelling, clinicians should always keep in mind the possibility of bone metastasis of RCC.

Keywords: Metatarsal metastasis, Renal cell carcinoma (RCC), Foot bone

Background

Metastatic disease of the skeleton often occurs in patients with malignancy, with bone damage and pain as the main manifestations. Malignant tumours prone to bone metastasis are breast cancer, lung cancer, kidney cancer, and other common primary cancers, including prostate cancer [1]. The sites of bone metastases are frequently localized in the axial skeleton, such as the spine and pelvis. Metastatic diseases of the distal knee and elbow joints are unusual. Bone metastasis of the foot is rare, occurring in approximately 0.01% of all metastatic bone diseases and is usually a late manifestation of disseminated disease [2, 3]. We report metatarsal metastasis from clear cell renal cell carcinoma in a 68-year-old man and review the related literature.

Case presentation

A 68-year-old male with intermittent swelling of his right foot and pain for one year was admitted in July 2019. The patient had a history of a mild right foot sprain that caused pain a year prior. Initially, the pain was relieved after rest but progressed with worsening pain and swelling after daily activities. At the local clinic, the doctor attributed the symptoms to trauma, administering massage therapy and a plaster cast to the patient, and the symptoms were alleviated. Two months before hospitalization, the patient's right foot was continuously swollen with worsening, severe pain that limited ambulation. For further treatment, the patient came to our outpatient clinic and underwent X-ray examination of the right foot. The physical examination demonstrated that the soft tissue was mildly swollen. There was pain on

* Correspondence: helinfeng0311@163.com
[1]Department of Orthopedics, The Fourth Hospital of Hebei Medical University, 12 Health Road, Shijiazhuang, Hebei 050011, People's Republic of China
Full list of author information is available at the end of the article

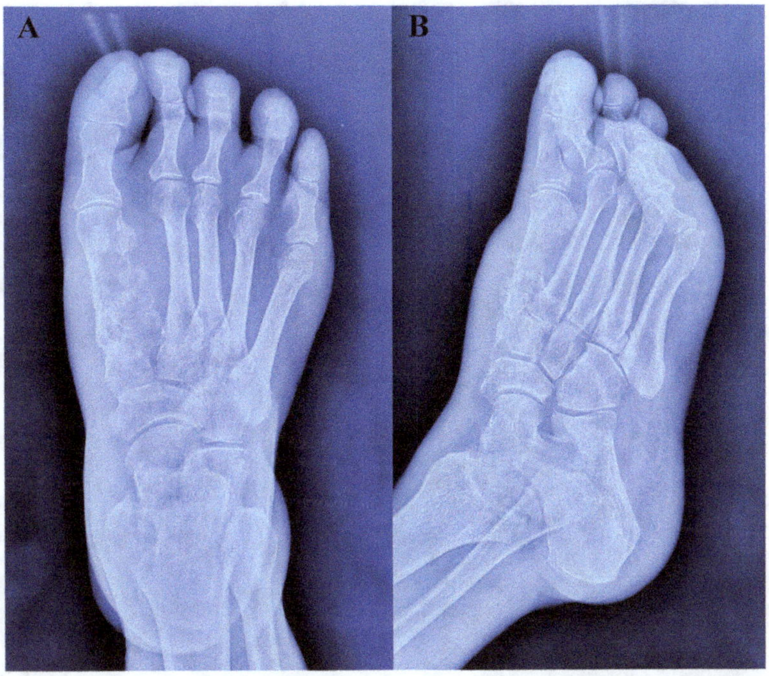

Fig. 1 X-ray scan of the patient. **a** Posteroanterior radiograph. **b** Lateral radiograph

palpation in the first metatarsus of the right foot. There was no paresthesia of the surrounding skin. The results of radiographs confirmed bone destruction of the first metatarsus of the right foot, which suggested underlying malignancy (Fig. 1a and b).

After reviewing the medical history, we discovered that the patient had a history of a large left renal mass discovered in April 2017 (Fig. 2). Computed tomography (CT) showed a round low-density shadow in the left inferior kidney, approximately 13*10 cm in size, with uneven density. There were flaky low-density shadows and point-like high-density shadows. Subsequently, the work-up was negative for metastatic disease, and radical nephrectomy was performed. Postoperative pathological results demonstrated stage II (T2N0M0) clear cell renal cell carcinoma (Fuhrman nuclear grade 2). After discharge, the patient was reviewed regularly in a polyclinic and received Chinese herbal treatment. Therefore, in the context of a known primary RCC, a metatarsal metastasis was suspected. The patient was admitted to the orthopaedic department for further treatment.

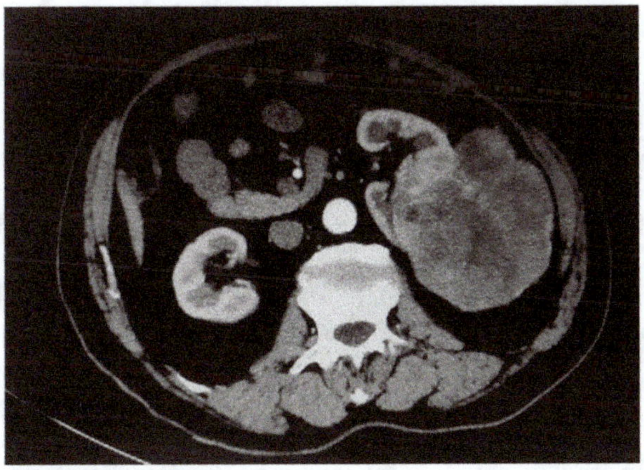

Fig. 2 Abdominal CT showing a tumour in the left kidney

After admission, the patient underwent magnetic resonance imaging (MRI), revealing a mass on the right first metatarsal bone with a less clear margin, approximately 5.19 cm in diameter, which had an isointense signal on T1-weighted images (Fig. 3a) and a mixed slightly high signal on T2-weighted images (Fig. 3b), with bone destruction, which was considered to be a malignant tumour. The results of the CT scan were consistent with those of MRI. After thorough examination and evaluation, no other distant metastatic lesions were found in the patient. Next, the patient underwent open biopsy of the first metatarsal bone of the right foot. Histological examination revealed clear cell carcinoma with nephrogenic implications (Fig. 4). Therefore, metatarsal metastasis from clear cell renal cell carcinoma was confirmed. The patient subsequently underwent right foot amputation (Fig. 5a and b). Six months after surgery, the patient walked with crutches and was re-examined at the orthopaedic clinic of our hospital. No local recurrence or distant metastasis was found.

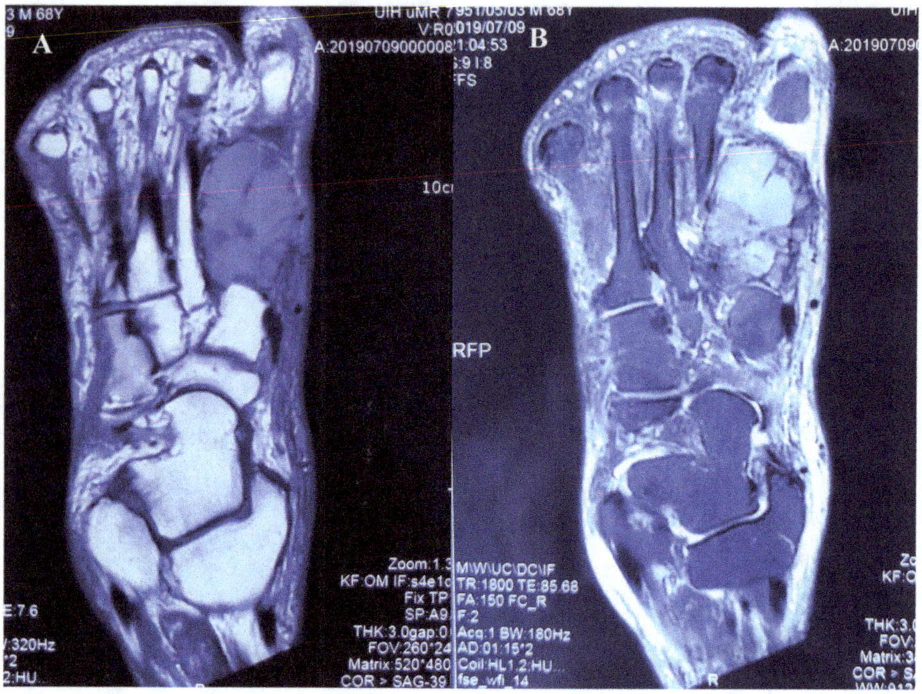

Fig. 3 Foot magnetic resonance imaging scans of the patient. **a** T1-weighted images. **b** T2-weighted images

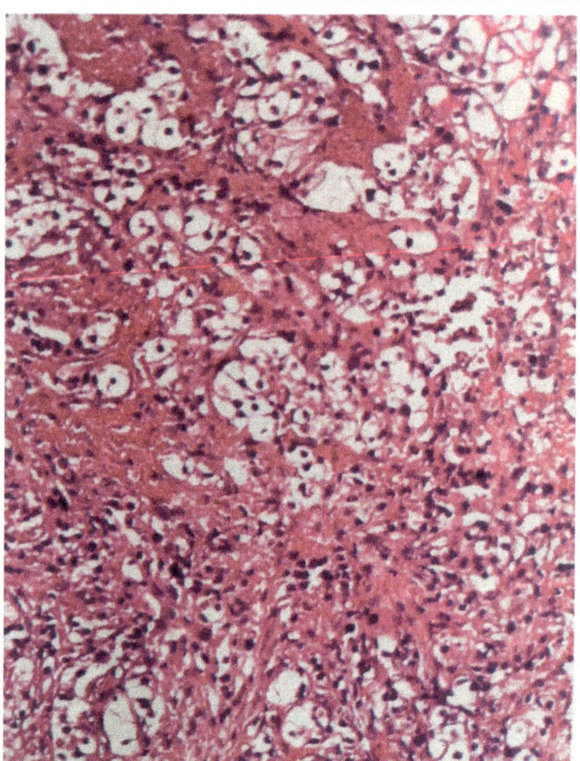

Fig. 4 Postoperative pathology of the metatarsal bone

Discussion and conclusion

RCC is commonly known to metastasize to the lungs, bone, and brain, but RCC can metastasize to some atypical sites as well, such as skeletal muscle [4], scalp [5] and uvula [6], as described in the literature. This report describes the metastasis of clear cell renal cell carcinoma to the metatarsus. Previously reported malignant tumours that metastasized to the foot skeleton are listed in Tables 1 and 2. The most common primary cancer of foot bone metastasis is lung cancer, followed by renal and intestinal tumours [7, 50, 51]. In metastatic RCC, bone metastases occur in almost 30% of patients [52]. Bone metastases are a common site of relapse in many types of solid cancers. Most bone metastases occur in the spine, followed by the pelvis and long bones. Acrometastasis (defined as metastasis to the hand or foot) is quite rare [2]. The metastatic sites of foot bones are summarized in Table 3 according to previous case reports. The calcaneus is the foot bone most commonly involved [18, 35].

In this case report, the clinician did not inquire about the patient's previous medical history, nor did he perform any image examination for the foot for the patient upon first presentation. During the 1-year period, the patient developed intermittent swelling of the right foot with mild pain and an inability to walk without receiving definite diagnosis and timely treatment. Diagnostic delay may lead to pathological fractures; therefore, metastatic bone disease of the foot may affect the quality of life of

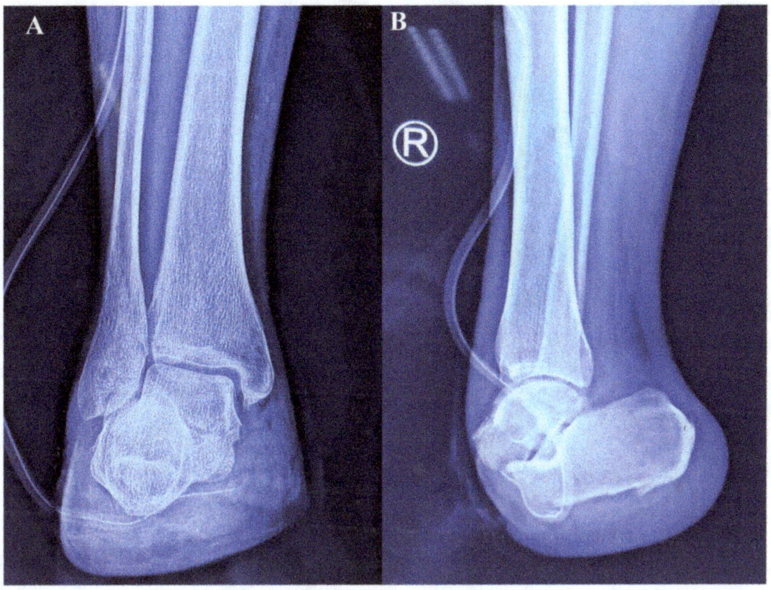

Fig. 5 Postoperative X-ray scan of the patient. **a** Positive radiograph. **b** Lateral radiograph

Table 1 Malignant tumors metastasized to the foot skeleton

Primary carcinoma	Number	(Refs.)
Lung cancer	11	[2, 7–16]
Cervical carcinoma	2	[16, 17]
Endometrial cancer	5	[18–20]
Prostatic cancer	5	[23–25]
Breast cancer	3	[3, 28, 29]
Intestinal tumor	7	[30, 31]
Bladder cancer	2	[3, 34]
Kidney cancer	7	[35–39]
Gastric adenocarcinoma	2	[42, 43]

patients, particularly as they are ambulating. However, the combination of medical history and imaging examination usually reveals the underlying diagnosis and provides a reference for treatment. For that reason, we report metatarsal metastasis from clear cell renal cell carcinoma in a 68-year-old man and review cases of foot bone metastasis of renal cancer reported in previous literature (Table 4). In these cases, the most common pathological type of foot bone metastasis was clear cell renal cell carcinoma, which represents the most common histology of renal carcinoma and has a worse prognosis than other RCCs [54–56]. All patients in Table 4 were male. Studies have reported a 4:1 male predominance in clear cell renal cell carcinoma with bone metastasis [57]. Almost all the patients received surgical treatment.

Table 2 Malignant tumors metastasized to the foot skeleton

Others	Urothelial carcinoma of the urete [44], Submandibular gland carcinoma [45], Hypopharyngeal epidermoid carcinoma [9], Melanoma [46], Multiple myeloma [3],Humeral osteogenic sarcoma [30], Non-Hodgkin Lymphoma [47], Nasopharyngeal carcinoma [48], Esophagus carcinoma [49], Hypernephroma [30]

As no therapeutic standard or guideline currently exists for RCC with bone metastasis. The median survival time of RCC with bone metastasis is usually below 24 months [57]. Acrometastases are often associated with extensive metastasis in other sites, so the prognosis is poor. The treatment is usually palliative and needs to be adapted to each patient's individual condition. Relief of pain is often the therapeutic goal. Palliative treatment of bone metastases has always been conservative: radiotherapy, chemotherapy, immunotherapy, targeted therapy, bisphosphonates and analgesics [58]. More recently, minimally invasive techniques, including ethanol ablation, laser ablation, microwave ablation, cryoablation and radiofrequency ablation, have been used for painful

Table 3 Metastatic sites of foot bones

Location	Number	[Refs.]
Calcaneus	15	[3, 8, 16, 18, 22, 24, 26, 27, 29, 32, 38, 42]
Metatarsals	14	[2, 7, 10–12, 19, 31–35, 39, 46, 49]
Phalanges	13	[9, 17, 20, 21, 28, 36, 40, 41, 43, 45, 47, 48, 53]
Talus	1	[13]
Cuboid	4	[25, 32, 33, 47]
Navicular bones	3	[14, 23, 33]
Cuneiform bones	4	[2, 15, 33, 37]

Table 4 Review of the previously reported cases of foot bone metastasis of renal cancer

Age	FS	Sex	Metastatic sites	Pathology	Treatment	[Refs.]
72	Y	Male	Phalanges	Clear cell carcinoma	Surgery	[36]
55	Y	Male	Metatarsals	Clear cell carcinoma	–	[35]
58	Y	Male	Cuneiform bones	Clear cell carcinoma	Surgery and Medication and Radiotherapy	[37]
59	N	Male	Calcaneus	Clear cell carcinoma	Surgery	[38]
–	–	–	Metatarsals	Adenocarcinoma	Surgery	[39]
55	Y	Male	Phalanges	Adenocarcinoma	Surgery	[40]
59	Y	Male	Phalanges	Clear cell carcinoma	Surgery	[41]

FS first presentation

bone lesions [59–63]. Surgical resection of bone metastasis from RCC has been reported to improve the prognosis of patients, and the effect is further improved for solitary metastasis if feasible [64]. These conditions were all met in our case. We believe that the best treatment for a single metastasis is always surgical excision if there is a long time from nephrectomy to the detection of isolated metastasis.

In conclusion, clinicians should fully understand the patient's past medical history. Even though acrometastasis is rare, this diagnosis should be considered in any patient with a history of RCC, particularly male patients, with local pain and swelling. Appropriate clinical and radiographic evaluation of these patients is essential to offer timely local therapy that may improve prognosis and enhance patient quality of life.

Abbreviations

CT: Computed Tomography; MRI: Magnetic Resonance Imaging; RCC: Renal Cell Carcinoma

Acknowledgements

Not applicable.

Authors' contributions

HW, RH, and HF collected the patient's data. HW, QZ and YZ analysed the data and performed the reference search. HW, RH, QZ and HF drafted and revised the manuscript. All authors contributed to data analysis and drafting and revision of the manuscript, and read and approved the final manuscript.

Author details

[1]Department of Orthopedics, The Fourth Hospital of Hebei Medical University, 12 Health Road, Shijiazhuang, Hebei 050011, People's Republic of China. [2]Department of Breast Surgery, The Fourth Hospital of Hebei Medical University, 12 Health Road, Shijiazhuang, Hebei 050011, People's Republic of China. [3]Department of Gynecology, Hebei Medical University Second Affiliated Hospital, 215 Heping Road, Shijiazhuang, Hebei 050011, People's Republic of China.

References

1. Salapura V, Zupan I, Seruga B, Gasljevic G, Kavcic P. Osteoblastic bone metastases from renal cell carcinoma. Radiol Oncol. 2014;48(3):243–6.
2. Rice B, Ross J, Todd N, Caputo L, Rush S, Shrestha B. Pulmonary pleomorphic carcinoma metastasis to the midfoot. J Foot Ankle Surg. 2015; 54(3):483–6.
3. Maheshwari AV, Chiappetta G, Kugler CD, Pitcher JD Jr, Temple HT. Metastatic skeletal disease of the foot: case reports and literature review. Foot Ankle Int. 2008;29(7):699–710.
4. Salman R, Sebaaly MG, Asmar K, Nasserdine M, Bannoura S, Khoury NJ. Rare skeletal muscle metastasis from renal cell carcinoma: case report and review of the literature. CEN Case Rep. 2018;7(2):316–9.
5. Errami M, Margulis V, Huerta S. Renal cell carcinoma metastatic to the scalp. Rare Tumors. 2016;8(4):6400.
6. Khade P, Devarakonda S. Atypical metastasis of renal cell carcinoma to the uvula: case report and review of literature. Int Med Case Rep J. 2018;11:29–32.
7. Kemnitz MJ, Erdmann BB, Julsrud ME, Jacobs PM, Ringstrom JB. Adenocarcinoma of the lung with metatarsal metastasis. J Foot Ankle Surg. 1996;35(3):210–2.
8. Dai H, Qiang M, Chen Y, Zhai W, Zhang K. Lung cancer presenting as heel pain: a case report. Oncol Lett. 2014;8(2):736–8.
9. Baran R, Tosti A. Metastatic carcinoma to the terminal phalanx of the big toe: report of two cases and review of the literature. J Am Acad Dermatol. 1994;31(2 Pt 1):259–63.
10. Delgadillo LA, Nichols DE. Oat cell carcinoma metastasis to the foot. J Foot Ankle Surg. 1998;37(1):55–62.
11. Wu KK. Bronchogenic carcinoma with metastases to the foot: a report of two cases. J Foot Ankle Surg. 1995;34(3):322–6.
12. Trinidad J, Kaplansky D, Nerone V, Springer K. Metastatic adenosquamous carcinoma of the foot: a case report. J Foot Ankle Surg. 2012;51(3):345–51.
13. Gan K, Shen Y. Metastatic pulmonary adenocarcinoma of the talus: a case report. J Foot Ankle Surg. 2017;56(4):827–31.
14. Iselin LD, Symeonidis PD, Stavrou P. Solitary navicular metastasis of a pulmonary adenocarcinoma. Foot Ankle Spec. 2011;4(6):373–5.
15. Li W, Li W, Zhang R. Metastasis to the medial cuneiform bone from squamous cell carcinoma of the lung revealed by bone Scintigraphy. Clin Nucl Med. 2016;41(12):946–7.
16. Singh C, Gupta M, Singh J, Ali A. Isolated calcaneal metastasis: an unusual presentation of lung carcinoma as heel pain. Clin Nucl Med. 2016;41(3):214–6.
17. Ciccone MA, Conturie CL, Lee CM, Matsuo K. Toe metastasis: a rare pattern of cervical cancer spread. Gynecol Oncol Case Rep. 2014;8:7–9.
18. Cooper JK, Wong FL, Swenerton KD. Endometrial adenocarcinoma presenting as an isolated calcaneal metastasis. A rare entity with good prognosis. Cancer. 1994;73(11):2779–81.
19. Longo R, Gamelon-Benichou C, Elias-Matta C, Platini C, Eid N, Yacoubi M, Quetin P. An unusual solitary metatarsal metastasis from an Endometrioid endometrial adenocarcinoma. Am J Case Rep. 2015;16:473–7.
20. Ali ZA, Wimhurst JA, Ali AA, Tempest ME, Edwards DJ. Endometrial cancer metastasis presenting as a grossly swollen toe. Int J Gynecol Cancer. 2003; 13(6):909–11.
21. Amiot RA, Wilson SE, Reznicek MJ, Webb BS. Endometrial carcinoma metastasis to the distal phalanx of the hallux: a case report. J Foot Ankle Surg. 2005;44(6):462–5.
22. Manolitsas TP, Fowler JM, Gahbauer RA, Gupta N. Pain in the foot: calcaneal metastasis as the presenting feature of endometrial cancer. Obstet Gynecol. 2002;100(5 Pt 2):1067–9.
23. Reyes DK, Miller JA, Cerrato RA, Pienta KJ. Oligometastatic prostate cancer to the navicular bone: case report. Urol Case Rep. 2015;3(3):59–62.
24. Agrawal S, Irvine A, Money-Kyrle J, Ellis BW. Isolated calcaneal metastasis from prostate cancer. Ann R Coll Surg Engl. 2008;90(3):W7–9.
25. Oh WK, Loda M, Kantoff PW, Janicek M. Progressive sclerosis of isolated foot metastasis of prostate cancer. J Urol. 2002;167(3):1392.
26. McCarthy MT, Ebrahem H, Aibdeen Z, Hodnett PA, Mulcahy E, Osman N. Prostate cancer metastasis to calcaneus: a solitary lesion at an atypical site, dormant for more than 10 years. JRSM Open. 2016;7(10):2054270416660934.
27. Bibbo C, Hatfield SP, Albright JT. Treatment of metastatic prostate adenocarcinoma to the calcaneus. J Foot Ankle Surg. 2010;49(2):159): e115–20.
28. Ravind R, Prameela CG, Gurram BC, Dinesh M. Synchronous phalangeal metastases in upper and lower limbs from primary breast malignancy: a

rare case scenario with a review of the literature. BMJ Case Rep. 2015;2015.
29. Groves MJ, Stiles RG. Metastatic breast cancer presenting as heel pain. J Am Podiatr Med Assoc. 1998;88(8):400–5.
30. Wu KK, Guise ER. Metastatic tumors of the foot. South Med J. 1978;71(7): 807–8 812.
31. Wijayaratna R, Ng JW. Metatarsal metastasis as the presenting feature of occult colorectal carcinoma. BMJ Case Rep. 2013;2013:bcr2013010353.
32. Ellington JK, Kneisl JS. Acrometastasis to the foot: three case reports with primary colon cancer. Foot Ankle Spec. 2009;2(3):140–5.
33. Sworn MJ, Buchanan R, Moynihan FJ. Rectal carcinoma presenting as massive metastatic involvement of foot bones. Br Med J. 1978;2(6130):98–9.
34. Petkovic M, Muhvic D, Zamolo G, Jonjic N, Mustac E, Mrakovcic-Sutic I, Seili-Bekafigo I. Metatarsal metastasis from transitional cell cancer of the urinary bladder. Coll Antropol. 2004;28(1):337–41.
35. Yadav R, Ansari MS, Dogra PN. Renal cell carcinoma presenting as solitary foot metastasis. Int Urol Nephrol. 2004;36(3):329–30.
36. Perdona S, Autorino R, Gallo L, Des M, Marra L, Claudio L, Caraco C, Franco R, Fazzioli F, Gallo A. Renal cell carcinoma with solitary toe metastasis. Int J Urol. 2005;12(4):401–4.
37. Choufani E, Diligent J, Galois L, Mainard D. Metastatic renal cell carcinoma presenting as foot metastasis: case report and review of the literature. J Am Podiatr Med Assoc. 2011;101(3):265–8.
38. Tonogai I, Nishisho T, Miyagi R, Sairyo K. Total calcanectomy for metastasis of renal cell carcinoma in the calcaneus: a case report. Foot Ankle Surg. 2018;24(1):e7–e12.
39. Chauveaux D, Liquois F, Le Huec JC, Le Rebeller A. Metatarsal metastasis. A case treated by exeresis an reconstruction. Rev Chir Orthop Reparatrice Appar Mot. 1990;76(7):525–7.
40. Kumar PP, Kovi J. Metastases to bones of the hands and feet. J Natl Med Assoc. 1978;70(11):837–40.
41. Anderson EE, Leitner WA, Boyarsky S, Small MP, McCollum DE. Renal-cell carcinoma metastatic to great toe. J Bone Joint Surg Am. 1968;50(5):997–8.
42. Bergqvist D, Mattsson J. Solitary calcaneal metastasis as the first sign of gastric cancer. A case report. Ups J Med Sci. 1978;83(2):115–8.
43. Kakarala G, Chatha H, Ferns B, Ebizie A. Metastatic gastric adenocarcinoma mimicking osteomyelitis of second toe. Foot (Edinb). 2008;18(3):171–3.
44. Ryder JH, McGarry SV, Wang J. Calcaneal acrometastasis from urothelial carcinoma of the ureter: a case report and literature review. Clin Interv Aging. 2013;8:395–9.
45. Zhang J, Sun Y, Li Z, Feng H. Metastasis of submandibular gland carcinoma to the toe bone: a case report. Br J Oral Maxillofac Surg. 2019;57(4):368–70.
46. Friend G, Mitchell J. Metastatic melanoma of a MetatarsalA case report. J Am Podiatr Med Assoc. 2017;107(1):90–4.
47. Allman LM. Metastatic bone involvement of the hallux distal phalanx and cuboid in an elderly patient with non-Hodgkin lymphoma. Foot Ankle Spec. 2008;1(6):355–8.
48. Lee DK. Distant metastases to the hallux in nasopharyngeal carcinoma. J Am Podiatr Med Assoc. 2008;98(3):239–41.
49. Mohanty A, Dutta D, Das S, Samanta DR, Senapati S. Carcinoma esophagus with isolated metatarsal metastasis. Indian J Cancer. 2011;48(1):112–3.
50. Nakagawa R, Susa M, Nakayama R, Watanabe I, Horiuchi K, Toyama Y, Nakamura M, Matsumoto M, Morioka H. Metastasis of renal cell carcinoma to the trapezium. J Hand Surg Asian Pac Vol. 2017;22(2):262–5.
51. Malone M, Gannass A, Binahmed A, Bowling FL, Boulton AJ. An extensive primary nodular melanoma of the foot with associated distant metastases: a case report. Foot (Edinb). 2012;22(3):235–9.
52. Woodward E, Jagdev S, McParland L, Clark K, Gregory W, Newsham A, Rogerson S, Hayward K, Selby P, Brown J. Skeletal complications and survival in renal cancer patients with bone metastases. Bone. 2011;48(1): 160–6.
53. Zhang J, Li Z, Ma X, Feng H: A pathological toe fracture as the first presentation of cervical cancer: A case report. Medicine (Baltimore) 2019, 98(3):e14190.
54. Keegan KA, Schupp CW, Chamie K, Hellenthal NJ, Evans CP, Koppie TM. Histopathology of surgically treated renal cell carcinoma: survival differences by subtype and stage. J Urol. 2012;188(2):391–7.
55. Capitanio U, Cloutier V, Zini L, Isbarn H, Jeldres C, Shariat SF, Perrotte P, Antebi E, Patard JJ, Montorsi F, et al. A critical assessment of the prognostic value of clear cell, papillary and chromophobe histological subtypes in renal cell carcinoma: a population-based study. BJU Int. 2009;103(11):1496–500.
56. Leibovich BC, Lohse CM, Crispen PL, Boorjian SA, Thompson RH, Blute ML, Cheville JC. Histological subtype is an independent predictor of outcome for patients with renal cell carcinoma. J Urol. 2010;183(4):1309–15.
57. Huang Z, Du Y, Zhang X, Liu H, Liu S, Xu T. Clear cell renal cell carcinoma bone metastasis: what should be considered in prognostic evaluation. Eur J Surg Oncol. 2019;45(7):1246–52.
58. Fizazi K, Lipton A, Mariette X, Body JJ, Rahim Y, Gralow JR, Gao G, Wu L, Sohn W, Jun S. Randomized phase II trial of denosumab in patients with bone metastases from prostate cancer, breast cancer, or other neoplasms after intravenous bisphosphonates. J Clin Oncol. 2009;27(10):1564–71.
59. Gangi A, Kastler B, Klinkert A, Dietemann JL. Injection of alcohol into bone metastases under CT guidance. J Comput Assist Tomogr. 1994;18(6):932–5.
60. Groenemeyer DH, Schirp S, Gevargez A. Image-guided percutaneous thermal ablation of bone tumors. Acad Radiol. 2002;9(4):467–77.
61. Simon CJ, Dupuy DE, Mayo-Smith WW. Microwave ablation: principles and applications. Radiographics. 2005;25(Suppl 1):S69–83.
62. Callstrom MR, Atwell TD, Charboneau JW, Farrell MA, Goetz MP, Rubin J, Sloan JA, Novotny PJ, Welch TJ, Maus TP, et al. Painful metastases involving bone: percutaneous image-guided cryoablation--prospective trial interim analysis. Radiology. 2006;241(2):572–80.
63. Toyota N, Naito A, Kakizawa H, Hieda M, Hirai N, Tachikake T, Kimura T, Fukuda H, Ito K. Radiofrequency ablation therapy combined with cementoplasty for painful bone metastases: initial experience. Cardiovasc Intervent Radiol. 2005;28(5):578–83.
64. Ljungberg B, Bensalah K, Canfield S, Dabestani S, Hofmann F, Hora M, Kuczyk MA, Lam T, Marconi L, Merseburger AS, et al. EAU guidelines on renal cell carcinoma: 2014 update. Eur Urol. 2015;67(5):913–24.

10

Management of complex renal cysts in Canada: Results of a survey study

Félix Couture[1], Antonio Finelli[2], Amélie Tétu[3], Bimal Bhindi[4], Rodney H. Breau[5], Anil Kapoor[6], Wassim Kassouf[7], Luke Lavallée[5], Simon Tanguay[7], Philippe D. Violette[8] and Patrick O. Richard[1*]

Abstract

Background: Bosniak III and IV cysts have a high risk of malignancy and have traditionally been managed surgically. However, growing evidence suggests that many can be managed by active surveillance. The main objective of this study was to characterize the use of surveillance in the management of complex renal cysts.

Methods: A web-based survey was sent to all registered, active members of the Canadian Urological Association ($N = 583$) in October 2018.

Results: The survey response rate was 24.7%. Management of Bosniak III cysts varied considerably. A large proportion of respondents (33.1%) offered active surveillance in > 50% of cases. Only 13.7% of respondents reported never or rarely (< 5% of cases) offering surveillance. In contrast, for Bosniak IV cysts, 60.1% of urologists never or rarely offered surveillance, while only 10.1% offer it in > 50% of cases. A significantly greater proportion of academic urologists, compared to non-academic urologists, viewed surveillance as a management option for patients with a Bosniak III or IV cyst. The most commonly reported barriers to a greater adoption of surveillance were concerns regarding its oncologic safety, the lack of data to support surveillance in this population, and the lack of triggers for discontinuation of active surveillance and intervention.

Conclusions: Despite active surveillance being included as a management option in guidelines, many Canadian urologists are reluctant to offer surveillance to patients with Bosniak III or IV cysts. Practice patterns are heterogeneous among those offering surveillance. High-quality studies are required to better define the benefits and risks of cystic renal mass surveillance.

Keywords: Complex renal cysts, Bosniak, Active surveillance, Surgery, Management

Background

Up to one third of individuals over 60 years of age will be diagnosed with a renal cyst following abdominal imaging [1]. Renal cysts are classified according to the Bosniak classification, which categorizes the cysts according to their degree of complexity and risk of malignancy [2–4]. Cystic renal cell carcinoma represents approximately 5–10% of all renal malignancies [5]. Bosniak III and IV cysts have a high risk of malignancy (40–60% and 80–90%, respectively) and have traditionally been managed with surgical excision [6, 7]. However, similar to small non-cystic renal masses, there is growing evidence suggesting that most of these cysts are indolent and unlikely to metastasize [5, 8–15]. Thus, active surveillance has been proposed as an alternative to surgery [6, 16].

Recent observational data has provided support for the use of active surveillance among patients with complex renal cysts [17, 18]. However, the adoption of this treatment strategy for the management of complex cysts in Canada and the criteria used by urologists as triggers for discontinuation of surveillance and intervention have yet to be defined.

* Correspondence: patrick.richard@usherbrooke.ca
[1]Division of Urology, Department of Surgery, Centre Hospitalier Universitaire de Sherbrooke, 3001, 12e avenue N, Sherbrooke, Quebec J1H 5N4, Canada
Full list of author information is available at the end of the article

The objectives of this survey study were to characterize the use of active surveillance in the management of complex renal cysts in Canada and to elicit the perceived barriers to adoption. We also aimed to characterize patient and disease factors associated with use of active surveillance and triggers used as criteria for intervention.

Methods

This is a descriptive cross-sectional study using electronic surveys and conducted based on known guidelines [19, 20]. Following approval from the CIUSSS de l'Estrie - CHUS Research Ethics Board, a pilot questionnaire was developed and tested among 20 urologists in October 2018. All items were then revised according to the feedback received in the pilot survey. The survey questions were formatted as short answer, multiple choice, or Likert rating scale questions. Responses were anonymous and no personal information was collected or stored. An electronic open survey was generated on REDcap™ and distributed via email. The survey was distributed to all active members of the Canadian Urological Association (CUA) with a functional email address. Three emails (one initial and two reminders) containing a link to the English language questionnaire were sent out to all 583 members between October 30 and November 19, 2018. Questions covered practice patterns regarding complex renal cysts, criteria used to select candidates for active surveillance, triggers to intervene in patients on active surveillance, and perceived barriers to a greater adoption of active surveillance (Additional file 1). In analyses, we excluded non-practicing urologists, urologists who reported not managing complex renal cysts, and urologists who gave incomplete demographic information or who did not answer questions beyond the demographic section.

Continuous and categorical variables were reported using medians (interquartile range [IQR]) and proportions, respectively. Chi-squared tests were used to assess differences between specific groups of respondents (types of practice). Statistical analyses were conducted using SAS/STAT® software, version 9.4. All statistical tests were two-sided and p-values < 0.05 were considered statistically significant.

Results

In total, 144 urologists (24.7%) responded to the survey. From these, we excluded three urologists who were not actively in practice or did not manage complex cysts, and two urologists because they did not answer any questions other than demographics. Therefore, our study included 139 respondents, of which 88.8% (N = 122) answered every survey question.

Demographic data are presented in Table 1. Of the eligible respondents, 71 (51.1%) practiced in an academic center, while 68 (48.9%) practiced in a non-academic setting. The majority (87.0%) of respondents reported managing ≤20 new complex renal cysts on an annual basis.

Table 1 Demographic data of the included respondents (N = 139)

Variables	N (%)
Years in independent practice	
•1 to 5	56 (40.3)
•6 to 10	29 (20.9)
•11 to 15	21 (15.1)
• > 15	33 (23.7)
Fellowship training	
•Urologic oncology	46 (33.1)
•Endourology/Minimally invasive surgery	30 (21.6)
•Other fellowship	23 (16.6)
•No fellowship training	40 (28.8)
Type of practice	
•Academic hospital	71 (51.1)
•Community or rural hospital	66 (47.5)
•Office-based practice	2 (1.4)
Area of practice	
•British Columbia	10 (7.2)
•Prairies	18 (13.0)
•Ontario	59 (42.5)
•Quebec	43 (30.9)
•Atlantic Canada	9 (6.5)
Annual number of new complex renal cysts cases (Bosniak III-IV)	
•1–5	24 (17.3)
•6–10	42 (30.2)
•11–20	55 (39.6)
•21–30	10 (7.2)
• > 30	8 (5.8)

Use of active surveillance

Of the eligible respondents, 13.7% of urologists never or rarely (< 5% of cases) offered active surveillance, while 33.1% offered active surveillance in > 50% of patients with a Bosniak III cysts in whom surgical excision is considered a suitable treatment option (Fig. 1). When compared to non-academic urologists, a significantly greater proportion of academic urologists offered active surveillance as a treatment option to their patients with a Bosniak III cyst. When patients with a Bosniak III cyst were offered active surveillance as a treatment option, it was perceived by nearly half of the urologists (45.7%) that this option was accepted in a majority of cases. The likelihood of a patient accepting active surveillance for the management of a Bosniak III cyst was perceived to be significantly greater by urologists from academic centres than by urologists from non-academic centres.

Unlike for Bosniak III cyst, a majority of urologists (60.1%) never or rarely (< 5% of cases) offered active surveillance for Bosniak IV cysts, while only 10.1% offered

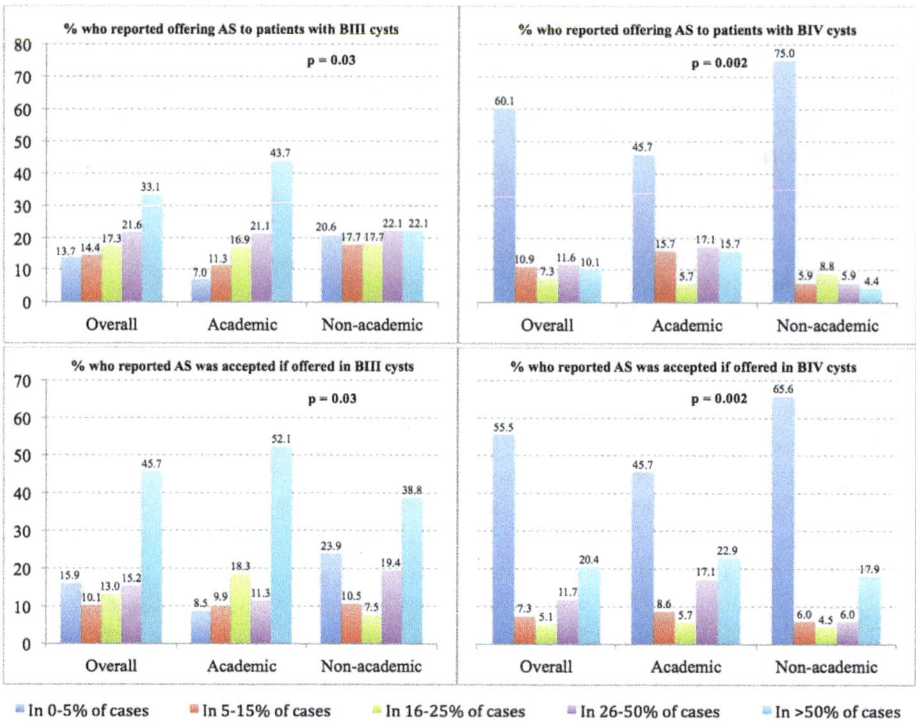

Fig. 1 Active surveillance use – Percentage of respondents who reported offering active surveillance (AS) to a certain proportion of patients and percentage of these patients they felt accept surveillance, for Bosniak III (BIII) and for Bosniak (BIV) cysts (overall and according to type of practice)

active surveillance in > 50% of cases. A significantly greater proportion of academic than non-academic urologists viewed active surveillance as a viable treatment alternative for patients with a Bosniak IV cyst. However, even when active surveillance was proposed to a patient as a treatment option, only 20.4% of urologists stated that this option was accepted by > 50% of patients.

Barriers to active surveillance adoption

Several potential barriers to a greater adoption of active surveillance were noted (Table 2). The most commonly reported ones were [1] the patient's and physician's concerns regarding the oncologic safety and/or benefits of active surveillance (89.8%), [2] the lack of data supporting active surveillance in patients with Bosniak III-IV cysts (74.2%), and

Table 2 Perceived barriers to a more widespread adoption of active surveillance for Bosniak III-IV cysts ($N = 128$)

Concerns	Disagree N (%)	Neither agree nor disagree N (%)	Agree N (%)
1) Patient and physician concerns regarding the oncologic safety and/or benefits of active surveillance.	8 (6.3)	5 (3.9)	114 (89.8)
2) The psychological burden for the physicians or patients	33 (25.8)	29 (22.7)	66 (51.6)
3) The belief that active surveillance is not an appropriate alternative since an effective surgical option already exists.	43 (33.6)	31 (24.2)	54 (42.2)
4) The lack of data to support active surveillance in patients with BIII-IV	17 (13.3)	16 (12.5)	95 (74.2)
5) The lack of specific triggers for intervention during active surveillance for cystic tumors	11 (8.6)	20 (15.6)	97 (75.8)
6) The lack of guidance/knowledge/decision-aid tool on how to best manage and follow patients on active surveillance	22 (17.2)	30 (23.4)	76 (59.4)
7) The belief that active surveillance is not an efficient trade-off to surgery because it increases the burden of care (i.e., more visits and repeated tests).	69 (53.9)	36 (28.1)	23 (18.0)
8) The reliability of patients and the possibility of patients being lost to follow-up on active surveillance.	47 (36.7)	48 (37.5)	33 (25.8)

[3] the lack of specific triggers for intervention during surveillance for complex renal cysts (75.8%).

Factors increasing likelihood of offering active surveillance

For both Bosniak III and IV cysts, age and the presence of comorbidities were perceived as having an impact on the likelihood of a patient being offered active surveillance as a treatment alternative (Table 3). The majority of urologists viewed older patients (> 75 years of age) as being ideal candidates. Nevertheless, nearly 30% of urologists thought that the lower age cut-off should be 65 years old for patients with Bosniak III cysts. Likewise, most urologists viewed that cyst size influenced their decision to offer surveillance and that cysts < 4 cm were ideal for active surveillance.

More specifically, for Bosniak III cysts, the presence of cyst wall nodularity (74.8%) and the maximal thickness of septa/calcification (44.1%) were also considered characteristics that impacted the likelihood of offering active surveillance. An upper limit threshold of 3 mm (IQR 2–5 mm) in maximal thickness of septa/calcification was perceived as being most appropriate for surveillance. For Bosniak IV cysts, the size of the nodular component was seen as important to the decision to offer active surveillance (69.9%) with a median perceived upper limit cut-off of 2 cm (IQR 1–3 cm).

Triggers for intervention during active surveillance

Several characteristics were perceived by urologists as being criteria for intervention for patients initially managed by active surveillance (Table 4). The most commonly reported criteria for Bosniak III cysts were [1] progression on imaging from Bosniak III to IV cysts, [2] worsening or change in the wall or septa enhancement, [3] progression or development of cyst wall nodularity. For Bosniak IV cysts, the two most common triggers for intervention were perceived as being [1] the growth rate of solid component (> 0.5 cm/year) and [2] the growth of solid component (> 3 cm).

Surgical management

When managed surgically, over half of respondents (57.3%) were more likely to offer a minimally invasive

Table 3 Association of patient and tumor factors with likelihood of recommending active surveillance and specific cut-offs viewed as most appropriate for active surveillance (*N* = 127 for Bosniak III; *N* = 124 for Bosniak IV)

	Significant impact on likelihood to recommend active surveillance reported N (%)	
Characteristics	Bosniak III	Bosniak IV
Patient factors		
▪Age	121 (95.3)	104 (84.5)
●*Cutoff*		
○ *> 55 years old*	6 (5.0)	3 (2.9)
○ *> 65 years old*	35 (28.9)	17 (16.4)
○ *> 75 years old*	80 (66.1)	84 (80.8)
▪Presence of comorbidities	121 (96.0)	105 (85.4)
Tumor factors		
▪Cyst size	72 (56.7)	59 (48.0)
●*Cutoff*		
○ *< 4 cm*	56 (77.8)	54 (91.5)
○ *< 7 cm*	16 (22.2)	5 (8.5)
▪Size of nodular component	N/A	86 (69.9)
●*Upper limit cutoff, median (IQR)*		2 cm (1–3 cm)
▪Number of septa/calcification	32 (25.2)	25 (20.7)
●*Cutoff*		
○ *≤ 2*	7 (22.9)	9 (36.0)
○ *≤ 3*	20 (62.5)	12 (48.0)
○ *≤ 4 or 5*	5 (15.7)	4 (16.0)
▪Thickness of septa/calcification	56 (44.1)	31 (25.2)
●*Upper limit cutoff, median (IQR)*	3 mm (2–5 mm)	5 mm (3–5 mm)
▪Cyst wall nodularity	95 (74.8)	N/A

Table 4 Criteria perceived as being triggers for intervention

Characteristics	Criterion reported as being a trigger for intervention N (%)	
	Bosniak III	Bosniak IV
Progression on imaging from Bosniak III to IV	110 (79.1)	N/A
Growth rate of solid component above threshold (for example: > 0.5 cm/year)	N/A	85 (61.2)
Growth of solid component above threshold (for example: > 3 cm)	N/A	88 (63.3)
Growth rate of cysts above threshold (for example: > 0.5 cm/year)	48 (34.5)	28 (20.1)
Doubling time of calculated volume ≤ 12 months	39 (28.1)	39 (28.1)
Progression in the number of septa or calcifications	29 (20.9)	28 (20.1)
Progression in the thickness of septa or calcifications	60 (43.2)	43 (30.9)
Worsening or change in the wall or septa enhancement	70 (50.4)	N/A
Progression or development of cyst wall nodularity	94 (67.6)	N/A
None of the above	2 (1.4)	3 (2.2)
I do not offer active surveillance	1 (0.7)	25 (18.0)

partial nephrectomy approach to patients with a complex cyst as the surgical management of choice. No significant differences in terms of surgical management were observed between academic and non-academic urologists (Additional file 2). When compared to the management of small non-cystic renal masses, the majority of surveyed urologists managed Bosniak III and IV cysts in a similar fashion to how they manage small non-cystic renal masses. However, 20.7% of respondents were more inclined to offer an open surgical approach, while 14.6% were more inclined to perform a radical nephrectomy as opposed to a partial nephrectomy. Again, there were no statistically significant differences observed in the management of academic and community urologists (Additional file 3).

Discussion

Indirect evidence from the small non-cystic renal mass literature has supported the role of active surveillance as a management option for complex renal cysts [5, 8, 10, 11, 16, 21–24]. Two recent retrospective studies have also reported the outcomes of patients with a complex renal cyst who opted to be managed by active surveillance [17, 18]. The average cyst sizes in the two studies were 4.1 cm and 3.5 cm for Bosniak III cysts, and 3.1 cm and 3.8 cm for Bosniak IV lesions, respectively. Both studies have suggested that this approach could be safely used in this population, with only one death due to kidney cancer observed after 5 years of follow-up in these studies. Moreover, only two patients with a Bosniak IV cyst developed a metastasis out of 243 patients with a Bosniak III or IV cyst (0.8%) – both of whom had refused surgery despite evidence of local progression. Criteria for lesion progression included increase in cyst size, increase in vascularity, and increase in size of the solid component. Importantly, during the 5-year observation period, 65% of patients avoided surgery given the absence of lesion progression, and among patients who progressed, 16.5% were found to have a benign tumor on final pathology. While these results are encouraging, given the low quality of existing evidence, current guidelines on the management of complex renal cysts continue to recommend surgery as the mainstay treatment and suggest that the use of active surveillance should be reserved for select patients [6, 16].

This study sought out to assess the adoption of active surveillance in Canada and to examine barriers to more widespread use. We found that approximately one third of Canadian urologists stated that they offered active surveillance as a treatment option in greater than 50% of patients who are diagnosed with a Bosniak III cyst, while only 10% of urologists offered surveillance in the majority of Bosniak IV cases. Importantly, over 60% of urologists did not consider or rarely considered active surveillance as a treatment option for a Bosniak IV cyst. Furthermore, the adoption of active surveillance for both Bosniak III and IV cysts was significantly greater among academic urologists compared to non-academic urologists. Likely reflecting the confidence of urologists for active surveillance, a greater proportion of urologists felt that, when offered to a patient, the chance of surveillance being chosen as management strategy was greater among patients diagnosed with a Bosniak III cyst than those with a Bosniak IV cyst.

When respondents were questioned on potential barriers preventing a more widespread use of active surveillance, the most common perceived concerns were [1] the lack of data supporting this strategy in this population, [2] the oncologic safety and benefits of active surveillance and [3] the lack of guidance on how to perform active surveillance and which specific triggers should be used to recommend discontinuation of active surveillance. We asked respondents what patient and tumor characteristics increased their likelihood of recommending active surveillance. As expected, a number of factors seemed to influence the urologist's decision, highlighting the fact that treatment decision for Bosniak III and IV cysts is a challenging one. We identified that a personal or familial history of kidney cancer, as well as the patient's treatment preference, influenced the likelihood that a physician would offer active surveillance. Multiple tumor characteristics also seemed to influence the likelihood of offering surveillance, with the most reported features being cyst size, size of nodular component, and presence of cyst wall nodularity. Importantly, the respondents also identified criteria perceived as triggers to offer discontinuation of active surveillance. For Bosniak III, the most common triggers were progression of cyst on imaging from Bosniak III to IV or development of cyst wall nodularity, and worsening or change in the wall or septa enhancement. For Bosniak IV cysts, the most common criteria identified were growth rate of solid component and overall growth of solid component. Interestingly, for both Bosniak III and IV cysts, the growth of the cystic component was not considered by most urologists as being worrisome enough to warrant treatment.

Although this study offers insight into the current management of complex renal cysts in Canada, it is not devoid of limitations. First, the results are based on Canadian urologists' perceptions, and the identified criteria for initiation and discontinuation of active surveillance have never been properly studied. Therefore, the reported use of active surveillance may not necessarily be generalized to all clinicians' real-life practice. The reported patterns of active surveillance may provide a starting point for future studies, but criteria need to be validated before being applied in clinical practice. Second, there might be a selection bias in our cohort, as urologists interested in active surveillance of complex cysts may have responded to the survey more readily.

On the other hand, the study carries several strengths. First, the survey was pilot tested and validated by 20 experts in the field of urology. Second, the response rate to this survey was 24%, which is similar, and even higher than in other Canadian urology surveys [25, 26]. Third, this study was designed, conducted and reported according to appropriate recommendations for survey research [19, 20]. Most of the questions were structured in a closed format (binary, ordinal, nominal) in order to lower the bias of the responses.

Conclusions

This study supports that, despite the lack of high-quality evidence, many Canadian urologists offer active surveillance as an option to patients with complex renal cysts, especially if they have a Bosniak III cyst. However, the lack of sufficient data or guidelines on safety seems to prevent widespread adoption of active surveillance. Prospective studies should be conducted to provide evidence on the oncologic safety, benefits, harms, cost, eligibility criteria, and guidelines for the discontinuation of active surveillance in the management of Bosniak III and IV cysts.

Supplementary information

Additional file 1. Survey questions.

Additional file 2. Surgical management of choice for a patient with a Bosniak III or IV cyst ($N = 131$).

Additional file 3. Surgical management of complex cysts compared to the surgical management of solid small renal masses ($N = 130$).

Abbreviation

IQR: Interquartile range

Acknowledgements

The authors would like to thank l'Unité de recherche clinique et épidémiologique of the Centre de Recherche CHUS for their support in the design of the study and the revision of the manuscript.

Authors' contributions

AF, AT, LL, PDV, and POR conceived the study and the survey. AT and POR collected and analysed the data. FC and POR wrote the manuscript. AF, AT, BB, RHB, AK, WK, LL, ST, and PDV reviewed and contributed to the manuscript. All authors read and approved the final manuscript.

Author details

[1]Division of Urology, Department of Surgery, Centre Hospitalier Universitaire de Sherbrooke, 3001, 12e avenue N, Sherbrooke, Quebec J1H 5N4, Canada. [2]Division of Urology, Department of Surgery, Princess Margaret Cancer Centre, University Health Network and the University of Toronto, Toronto, Canada. [3]Unité de recherche clinique et épidémiologique, Centre de Recherche, Centre Hospitalier Universitaire de Sherbrooke, Sherbrooke, Canada. [4]Division of Urology, Department of Surgery, Southern Alberta Institute of Urology, Calgary, Canada. [5]Division of Urology, Department of Surgery, Ottawa Hospital, Ottawa Hospital Research Institute and University of Ottawa, Ottawa, Canada. [6]Division of Urology, Department of Surgery, Juravinski Hospital, St. Joseph Healthcare, McMaster University, Hamilton, Canada. [7]Division of Urology, Department of Surgery, McGill University Health Centre, McGill University, Montreal, Canada. [8]Division of Urology, Department of Surgery, Woodstock Hospital, Woodstock, Canada.

References

1. Marumo K, Horiguchi Y, Nakagawa K, Oya M, Ohigashi T, Asakura H, et al. Incidence and growth pattern of simple cysts of the kidney in patients with asymptomatic microscopic hematuria. Int J Urol. 2003;10:63–7.
2. Bosniak M. The current radiological approach to renal cysts. Radiology. 1986; 158:1–10.
3. Bosniak M. Diagnosis and Management of Patients with complicated cystic lesions of the kidney. AJR. 1997;169:819–21.
4. Israel GM, Bosniak MA. An update on the Bosniak renal cyst classification system. Urology. 2005;66:484–9.
5. Bhatt JR, Jewett M, Richard PO, Kawaguchi S, Timilshina N, Evans A, et al. Multilocular cystic renal cell carcinoma: pathological T staging makes no difference to favorable outcomes and should be reclassified. J Urol. 2016; 196:1350–5.
6. Richard PO, Violette PD, Jewett MAS, Pouliot F, Leveridge MJ, So A, et al. CUA guideline on the management of cystic renal lesions. Can Urol Assoc J. 2017;11:E66–73.
7. Schoots IG, Zaccai K, Hunink MG, Verhagen P. Bosniak classification for complex renal cysts reevaluated: a systematic review. J Urol. 2017;198:12–21.
8. Donin NM, Mohan S, Pham H, Chandarana H, Doshi A, Deng F-M, et al. Clinicopathologic outcomes of cystic renal cell carcinoma. Clin Genitourin Cancer. 2015;13:67–70.
9. Gong K, Zhang N, He Z, Zhou L, Lin G, Na Y. Multilocular cystic renal cell carcinoma: an experience of clinical management for 31 cases. J Cancer Res Clin Oncol. 2008;134:433–7.

10. Nassir A, Jollimore J, Gupta R, Bell D, Norman R. Multilocular cystic renal cell carcinoma: a series of 12 cases and review of the literature. Urology. 2002; 60:421–7.
11. Winters BR, Gore JL, Holt SK, Harper JD, Lin DW, Wright JL. Cystic renal cell carcinoma carries an excellent prognosis regardless of tumor size. Urol Oncol. 2015;33:e9–13.
12. Bielsa O, Lloreta J, Gelabert-Mas A. Cystic renal cell carcinoma: pathological features, survival and implications for treatment. Br J Urol. 1998;82:16–20.
13. Corica FA, Iczkowski KA, Cheng L, Zincke H, Blute ML, Wendel A, et al. Cystic renal cell carcinoma is cured by resection: a study of 24 cases with long-term followup. J Urol. 1999;161:408–11.
14. Koga S, Nishikido M, Hayashi T, Matsuya F, Saito Y, Kanetake H. Outcome of surgery in cystic renal cell carcinoma. Urology. 2000;56:67–70.
15. Murad T, Komaiko W, Oyasu R, Bauer K. Multilocular cystic renal cell carcinoma. Am J Clin Pathol. 1991;95:633–7.
16. Ljungberg B, Albiges L, Abu-Ghanem Y, Bensalah K, Dabestani S, Fernandez-Pello S, et al. European Association of Urology Guidelines on Renal Cell Carcinoma: The 2019 Update. Eur Urol. 2019;75(5):799–810.
17. Chandrasekar T, Ahmad A, Fadaak K, Jhaveri K, Bhatt J, Jewett M, et al. Natural history of complex renal cysts: clinical evidence supporting active surveillance. J Urol. 2018;199:633–40.
18. Pruthi D, Liu Q, Kirkpatrick I, Gelfond J, Drachenberg D. Long-term surveillance of complex cystic renal masses and heterogeneity of Bosniak 3 lesions. J Urol. 2018;200:1192–9.
19. Burns KE, Duffett M, Kho ME, Meade MO, Adhikari NK, Sinuff T, et al. A guide for the design and conduct of self-administered surveys of clinicians. CMAJ. 2008;179(3):245–52.
20. Eysenbach G. Improving the quality of web surveys: the checklist for reporting results of internet E-surveys (CHERRIES). J Med Internet Res. 2004; 6(3):e34.
21. Bhindi B, Thompson R, Lohse C, Mason R, Frank I, Costello B, et al. The probability of aggressive versus indolent histology based on renal tumor size: implications for surveillance and treatment. Eur Urol. 2018;74:489–97.
22. Finelli A, Ismaila N, Bro B, Durack J, Eggener S, Evans A, et al. Management of small renal masses: American Society of Clinical Oncology clinical practice guideline. J Clin Oncol. 2017;35:668–80.
23. Jewett MA, Mattar K, Basiuk J, Morash CG, Pautler SE, Siemens DR, et al. Active surveillance of small renal masses: progression patterns of early stage kidney cancer. Eur Urol. 2011;60:39–44.
24. Pierorazio PM, Johnson MH, Ball MW, Gorin MA, Trock BJ, Chang P, et al. Five-year analysis of a multi-institutional prospective clinical trial of delayed intervention and surveillance for small renal masses: the DISSRM registry. Eur Urol. 2015;68:408–15.
25. Richard PO, Martin L, Lavallee LT, Violette PD, Komisarenko M, Evans AJ, et al. Identifying the use and barriers to the adoption of renal tumour biopsy in the management of small renal masses. Can Urol Assoc J. 2018; 12(8):260–6.
26. Millar AC, Elterman DS, Goldenberg L, Van Asseldonk B, Curtis A, Jarvi K. A survey of Canadian urologists' opinions and prescribing patterns of testosterone replacement therapy in men on active surveillance for low-risk prostate cancer. Can Urol Assoc J. 2016;10(5–6):181–4.

11

Relationship of endoscopic lesions of the renal papilla with type of renal stone and 24 h urine analysis

X. A. Sabaté Arroyo[1*], F. Grases Freixedas[2], J. L. Bauzà Quetglas[1], J. Guimerà Garcia[1] and E. Pieras Ayala[1]

Abstract

Background: Our purpose was to study the relationship of the 3 different types of endoscopic calcifications of the renal papilla (Randall's plaque, intratubular calcification, papillary crater) with the type of stone and urine analysis.

Methods: This prospective study examined 41 patients (age range: 18 to 80 years) who received retrograde intrarenal surgery (RIRS) for renal lithiasis (mean stone size: 15.3 ± 7.2 mm). The renal papilla injuries were endoscopically classified as Randall's plaque, intratubular calcification, or papillary crater. Calculi were classified as uric acid, calcium oxalate monohydrate (COM; papillary and cavity), calcium oxalate dihydrate (COD), or calcium phosphate (CP). A 24 h urine analysis of calcium, oxalate, citrate, phosphate, and pH was performed in all patients. The relationship of each type of papillary injury with type of stone and urine chemistry was determined. Fisher's exact test and Student's t-test were used to determine the significance of relationships, and a p value below 0.05 was considered significant.

Results: The most common injury was tubular calcification (78%), followed by Randall's plaque (58%), and papillary crater (39%). There was no significant relationship of Randall's plaque with type of stone. However, endoscopic intratubular calcification ($p = 0.025$) and papillary crater ($p = 0.041$) were more common in patients with COD and CP stones. There were also significant relationships of papillary crater with hypercalciuria ($p = 0.036$) and hyperoxaluria ($p = 0.024$), and of Randall's plaque with hypocitraturia ($p = 0.005$).

Conclusions: There are certain specific relationships between the different types of papillary calcifications that were endoscopically detected with stone chemistry and urine analysis. COD and CP stones were associated with endoscopic tubular calcifications and papillary craters. Hypercalciuria was associated with tubular calcification, and hypocitraturia was associated with Randall's plaque.

Keywords: Randall's plaque, Tubular calcification, Papillary crater, Hypercalciuria, Hypocitraturia

Background

In 1937 Alexander Randall first established a relationship between a non-inflammatory subepithelial calcification and the onset of kidney stone formation [1]. Although many subsequent studies have examined the mechanisms and causes of Randall's plaques, the conclusions of many of these studies still require verification [2].

Papillary calculi can initiate in the papillary tissue or inside the Bellini ducts, and there are therefore two different types of stone formation. First, calculi may initiate in papillary tissue following oxidative stress, exposure to cytotoxic substances, or other factors that injure collagen-rich areas near the loop of Henle and the cubic

* Correspondence: sabate.arnau@gmail.com
[1]Hospital Universitari Son Espases, Ctra. Valldemossa, 79, Palma de Mallorca, Spain
Full list of author information is available at the end of the article

epithelium, which covers the papilla. Because the interstitial fluid has a pH of 7.4, and is therefore always supersaturated with calcium phosphate, cellular detritus or oxidized cellular collagen can act as a heterogeneous nucleant, leading to the deposit of hydroxyapatite (HAP). If this deposit grows enough to break through the epithelium that covers the papilla, it can contact the urine. Because the urine is always supersaturated with calcium oxalate, a calcium oxalate monohydrate (COM) calculus will form when there is a deficiency of crystallization inhibitors and/or an alteration of the immune system. Stones can also form when there is intratubular injury of the Bellini ducts and urine supersaturation, in which there are large amounts of calcium oxalate dihydrate (COD) and/or HAP crystals. In this case, obstruction of the collecting tubules and deposits that form in the most distal part of the tubule, upon contacting the urine, generate the renal calculi [3–5].

Obviously, not all kidney stones develop by processes that involve the renal papillae. Thus, the presence of morpho-anatomical factors, such as cavities that have low urodynamic efficacy and anatomical malformations, can lead to urine stasis, the accumulation of stagnant urine, and stone formation, as also occurs in the urinary bladder. The renal papillae have no role in the formation of these stones [5–7].

Because of advances in urological technologies and endoscopy, and the increasing comfort and dexterity of the surgeons in performing endoscopic procedures, retrograde intrarenal surgery (RIRS) has become a common method for treatment of renal stones. These techniques of renal exploration allow better treatment of renal stones and more thorough examination of the renal papillae [8, 9]. Although endoscopic renal surgery can detect a wide range of injuries to the renal papilla surface, the relationships of these different injuries with the etiopathogenic mechanisms of renal stone formation are unclear [10].

The purpose of this paper is to study the relationship between injuries detected endoscopically of the renal papilla detected by endoscopy with the type of renal calculus and 24 h urine analysis.

Methods

Forty-one consecutive patients with renal lithiasis and indications for RIRS were recruited prospectively from our institution. All patients provided informed consent for participation in the study, and the study was approved by the ethics committee of our hospital (No. 3105/15P, Comité de Ética de la Investigación de las Islas Baleares- CEI-IB). All research was performed in accordance with relevant guidelines/regulations.

We measured stone size using computed tomography prior to surgery. Systematic endoscopic examination of the renal papilla was performed using a flexible digital ureteroscope (Olympus URF-V and Karl Storz Flex Xc). The procedure started with examination of the upper calyx, ended in the lower calyx, and photographs were taken in the area of the renal papillae. The 3 types of injury in the papilla were defined as previously described [11]:

- Randall's plaque (Fig. 1): White deposits of intrarenal HAP calcifications, near the epithelium of the papilla, with irregular shape.
- Intratubular calcification or Randall's plug (Fig. 2): Yellow punctate deposit on the surface of the renal papilla or at the end of a dilated terminal collection tubule.
- Papillary crater (Fig. 3): Slit-shaped injury or crater in the surface of a renal papilla.

After laser lithotripsy, some stone fragments were extracted to determine calculus type. In particular, electron microscopy and infrared spectroscopy were used to classify stones into 1 of 4 groups: calcium oxalate monohydrate (COM; papillary and cavity), calcium oxalate dihydrate (COD), uric acid, and calcium phosphate (HAP and mixed stones) [12, 13]. Struvite and brushite stones were not considered because their mechanisms of formation are completely different.

At 30 to 60 days after surgery, 24 h urinary chemistry was analyzed in each patient. The results were used to

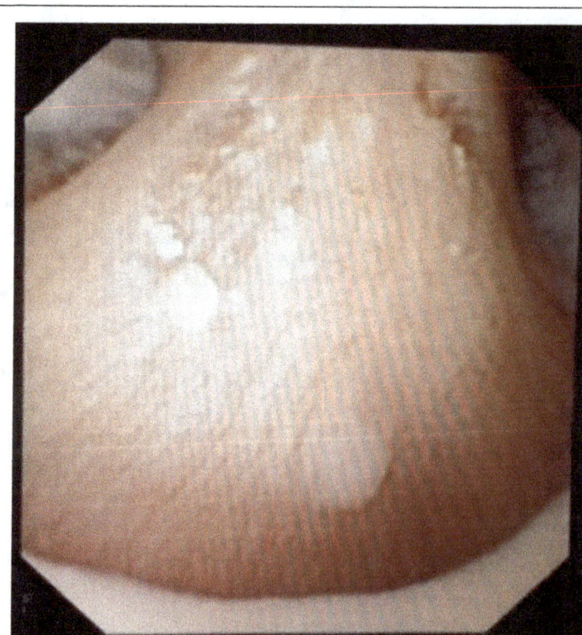

Fig. 1 Example of Randall's plaque

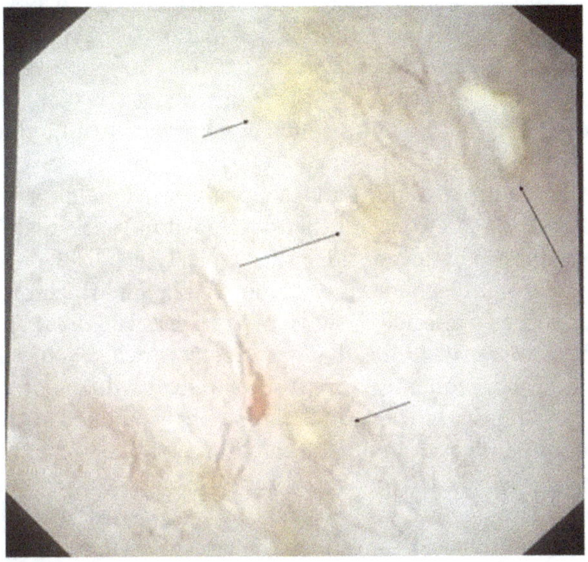

Fig. 2 Example of Intratubular calcifications

classify patients as having hypercalciuria (> 220 mg/24 h or > 17 mg/dL), hyperoxaluria (> 40 mg/24 h or > 3 mg/dL), hypocitraturia (< 350 mg/24 h or < 23 mg/dL), or hyperphosphaturia (> 1100 mg/24 h or > 100 mg/dL), as previously described [12–14].

The relationships of each endoscopic papillary injury with type of stone, urinary biochemical parameters, and urinary pH were determined. Each value is reported as mean ± standard deviation. Fisher's exact test was used for the analysis of qualitative variables, and the Student's *t*-test for the comparison of means. A *p* value below 0.05 was considered significant.

Results

The average patient age was 48 years (±13), and 54% of the patients were male. A total of 58% of the patients had Randall's plaque, 78% had intratubular calcification, and 39% had a papillary crater. Thus, 54% of the patients had 2 or more different types of renal injury, and 46% only had one kind of renal injury.

The stone mean size (i.e., largest diameter) was 15.4 mm (±7.4). Urinary biochemistry indicated the mean pH was 6.0 (±0.79), mean 24 h urine volume was 1863 mL (±901), mean calcium level was 218 mg/24 h (±127), mean phosphate level was 835 mg/24 h (±312), mean oxalate level was 27 mg/24 h (±12), and mean citrate level was 398 mg/24 h (±300).

There was no significant relationship of Randall's plaque with the type of stone ($p = 0{,}39$) (Table 1). However, there were significant relationships of endoscopic intratubular calcification ($p = 0.025$) and papillary crater ($p = 0.041$) with type of stone, in that COD and calcium phosphate stones were more common in both groups (Tables 2 and 3).

There were also significant relationships between papillary crater and hypercalciuria ($p = 0.036$) and hyperoxaluria ($p = 0.024$), and between Randall's plaque and hypocitraturia ($p = 0.005$). None of the other relationships were statistically significant.

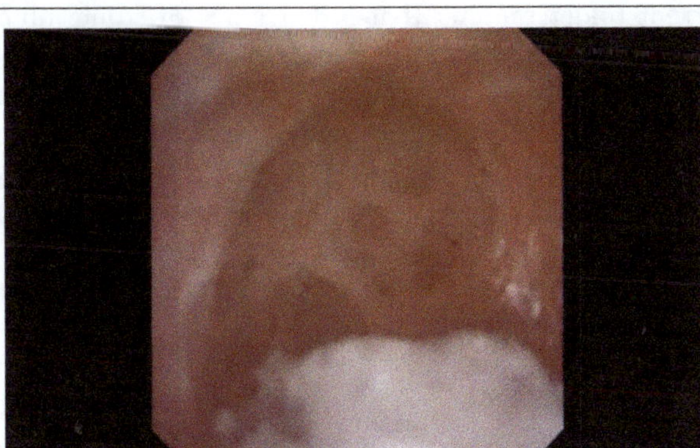

Fig. 3 Example of Papillary cráter

Discussion

Our results suggest that the type of papillary injury identified by endoscopy is associated with the type of stone and with certain disorders in urinary analysis. This suggests that different mechanisms are responsible for these different endoscopic papillary injuries.

Coe et al. [15] hypothesized that the direct contact of a plug blocking Bellini's duct in an environment with hypercalciuric urine favors the formation of HAP and calcium oxalate stones, although this relationship has not

Table 1 Randall's Plaque

	RANDALL'S PLAQUE		
	YES	NO	Significance
Patients (*N* = 41)	**24 (59%)**	**17 (40%)**	
COM	**5 (71%)**	**2 (28%)**	**0,390**
COD	**7 (77%)**	**2 (22%)**	
Uric Acid	**3 (50%)**	**3 (50%)**	
Calcium Phosphate	**9 (47%)**	**10 (52%)**	
pH	**6,0 ± 0,81**	**6,19 ± 0,78**	**0,48**
Diuresis (mL)	**1965 ± 966**	**1580 ± 487**	**0,56**
Calcium (mg/24 h)	**202,09 ± 119,78**	**247,0 ± 140,53**	**0,37**
Oxalate (mg/24 h)	**28,35 ± 13,54**	**26,77 ± 9,32**	**0,72**
Citratoe (mg/24 h)	**391,77 ± 326,12**	**409,69 ± 260,37**	**0,86**
Calcium (mg/dL)	**11,21 ± 7,11**	**15,76 ± 10,13**	**0,09**
Phosphate (mg/dL)	**52,60 ± 30,31**	**59,21 ± 32,59**	**0,62**
Citrate (mg/dL)	**21,35 ± 19,90**	**28,37 ± 14,82**	**0,005***
Oxalate (mg/dL)	**1,83 ± 1,19**	**1,79 ± 0,91**	**0,98**
Uric acid (mg/dL)	**30,07 ± 16,91**	**39,31 ± 21,69**	**0,16**

Table 2 Tubular calcification

	TUBULAR CALCIFICATION		
	YES	NO	Significance
Patients (*N* = 41)	32 (78%)	9 (21%)	
COM	3 (42%)	4 (57%)	0,02*
COD	9 (100%)	0	
Uric Acid	4 (66%)	2 (33%)	
Calcium Phosphate	16 (84%)	3 (15%)	
pH	6,1 ± 0,75	5,6 ± 0,89	0,12
Diuresis (mL)	1990 ± 963	1619 ± 742	0,67
Calcium (mg/24 h)	234,21 ± 123,98	162,63 ± 132,29	0,16
Oxalate (mg/24 h)	28,52 ± 11,6	25,19 ± 14,05	0,49
Citrate (mg/24 h)	416,29 ± 283,35	335,08 ± 367,86	0,50
Calcium (mg/dL)	14,15 ± 9,51	9,68 ± 3,67	0,036*
Phosphate (mg/dL)	55,23 ± 31,29	56,01 ± 32,08	0,49
Citrate (mg/dL)	23,60 ± 16,41	26,86 ± 23,87	0,42
Oxalate (mg/dL)	1,74 ± 1,07	2,06 ± 1,07	0,67
Uric acid (mg/dL)	34,27 ± 19,91	33,06 ± 18,55	0,90

been demonstrated previously. Our results are consistent with this hypothesis. In particular, we observed that intratubular calcification and papillary crater each had significant associations with the type of lithiasis, in that they were more prevalent in patients with COD and CP stones. Moreover, we found that Randall's Plaque was mainly associated with COM calculi.

We also found that intratubular calcification was significantly associated with urinary calcium concentration.

Table 3 Papillary crater

	PAPILLARY CRATER		
	YES	NO	Significance
Patients (*N* = 41)	16 (39%)	25 (61%)	
COM	1 (14%)	6 (85%)	0,04*
COD	7 (77%)	2 (22%)	
Uric Acid	2 (33%)	4 (66%)	
Calcium Phosphate	6 (31%)	13 (68%)	
pH	6,22 ± 0,82)	5,97 ± 0,77	0,33
Diuresis (mL)	2328 ± 1092	1560 ± 603	0,45
Calcium (mg/24 h)	265,87 ± 128,55	184,33 ± 118,27	0,05*
Oxalate (mg/24 h)	28,79 ± 12,84	27,05 ± 11,75	0,67
Citrate (mg/24 h)	501,80 ± 363,51	324,27 ± 226,96	0,08
Calcium (mg/dL)	13,12 ± 10,31	13,17 ± 7,82	0,52
Phosphate (mg/dL)	51,31 ± 40,24	57,86 ± 24,64	0,58
Citrate (mg/dL)	25,96 ± 20,77	23,36 ± 16,59	0,41
Oxalate (mg/dL)	1,33 ± 0,69	2,11 ± 1,19	0,024*
Uric Acid (mg/dL)	30,21 ± 23,74	36,27 ± 16,35	0,58

This result confirms that Bellini's duct must be exposed to supersaturated urine for the formation of HAP stones ($pH > 6$) and to hypercalciuria for the formation of an intratubular obstruction. When this deposit reaches the end of Bellini's duct and contacts the urine, it can induce the development of COD or COD+HAP calculi.

On the other hand, Randall's plaque was mainly associated with COM calculi that developed in renal cavities. It is important to consider that typical calculi of papillary COM are generated on Randall's plaque, which originates from internal lesions of intrapapillar tissue [6]. These are small stones that are usually expelled spontaneously. Consequently, this type of calculus does not require surgery. However, all the stones examined in the present study required RIRS for elimination because they were larger, developed on the most distal part of Bellini's ducts, and had fast growth due to the existence of hypercalciuria and sometimes high urinary pH. Therefore, we expected that none of the included patients had typical COM papillary calculi. We did observe the presence of Randall's plaques, which in principle are related to the formation of COM stones. However, recent studies showed that not all of Randall's plaques generate papillary COM calculi [6].

In fact, Randall's plaque seems to occur without symptoms in most individuals, and stone formation only occurs when there are large numbers of these plaques [6]. It is thus possible that the small number of Randall's plaque lesions and their total area in these patients were insufficient to lead to the development of papillary COM stones. We did not evaluate the percentage of surface affected by Randall's plaque. However, other studies reported that the surface affected by Randall's plaque was 7.4% in those who developed papillary calculi, but only 0.5% in those who did not develop calculi [16–22].

We found that Randall's plaque was significantly associated with hypocitraturia ($p = 0.005$) and that urinary calcium concentration was significantly lower than those detected in the presence of intratubular calcification and / or renal crater. These data are consistent with the current understanding that a deficiency of stone inhibitors and normocalciuria can lead to the development of COM calculi [6]. Thus, citrate inhibits the crystallization of oxalate and calcium phosphate, preventing the formation of the lithiasic core and posterior growth. Interestingly, regardless of the type of injury, the presence of uric acid stones is more likely when the urinary pH is below 5.5, and the presence of HAP stones is more likely when the urinary pH is above 6.0 [23–29].

There were some limitations in our study. First, we only described the experience of 41 patients at a single center. Second, the identification of papillary injury was somewhat subjective, even though we used previously described criteria to define the different types of injuries.

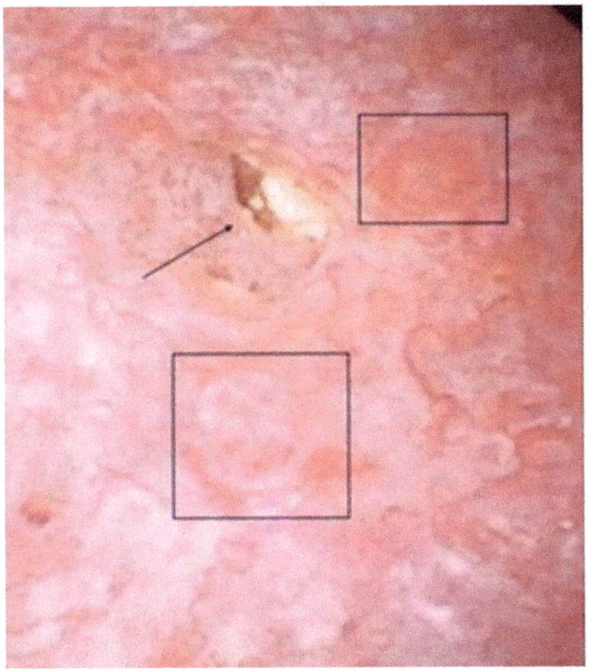

Fig. 4 Intratubular calcification and Papillary crater in same papilla

Third, we did not consider the severity of papillary injuries, and only considered the presence or absence of a lesion. Another possible limitation is that there may have been some overlap in the different types of lesions if they were at different stages of disease progression. For example, we found an association of intratubular calcification with papillary crater. This can occur if lithiasis begins in an intratubular calcification, but detachment of the calculus from the renal papilla leads to the formation of a papillary crater (Fig. 4). The last limitation of the study is that the urine analysis was done at the 30–60 day after surgery and this could make changes in the urine chemistry.

Our study identified several significant relationships of endoscopic papillary injuries with the type of stone and urine chemistry. The characterization of a papillary endoscopic injury may help a urologist to better understand the underlying mechanism of stone formation in individual patients. Further studies with larger numbers of patients are needed to confirm this hypothesis.

Conclusions

We identified certain specific relationships between different endoscopic types of papillary calcifications with stone and urine chemistry. In particular, COD and CP stones are associated with endoscopic tubular calcifications and papillary craters; hypercalciuria is associated with endoscopic tubular calcification; and COM calculi, hypocitraturia, and normocalciuria are associated with Randall's plaque.

Abbreviations

UA: Uric Acid; COM: Calcium oxalate monohydrate; COD: Calcium oxalate dihydrate; CP: Calcium phosphate

Acknowledgements

IUNICS lab. Universitat de les Illes Balears.

Authors' contributions

SA, XA: Project development, Data Collection, Data analysis, Manuscript writing. GF, F.: Project development, Manuscript Writing. BQ, JL.: Data Collection. GG, J: Data Collection. PA, E: Project development, Data Collection, Data analysis, Manuscript writing. All Authors read and approved the manuscript.

Author details

[1]Hospital Universitari Son Espases, Ctra. Valldemossa, 79, Palma de Mallorca, Spain. [2]Universitat de les Illes Balears. IUNICS, Ctra. de Valldemossa, Km. 7.5, Palma de Mallorca, Spain.

References

1. Randall A. The origin and growth of renal calculi. Ann Surg. 1937;105(6):1009–27.
2. Evan AP. Physiopathology and etiology of stone formation in the kidney and the urinary tract. Pediatr Nephrol. 2010;25(5):831–41.
3. Evan AP, Worcester EM, Coe FL, Williams J, Lingeman JE. Mechanisms of human kidney stone formation. Urolithiasis. 2015;43(S1):19–32.
4. Coe FL, Evan AP, Worcester EM, Lingeman JE. Three pathways for human kidney stone formation. Urol Res. 2010 Jun 22;38(3):147–60.
5. Bird VY, Khan SR. How do stones form? Is unification of theories on stone formation possible? Arch Esp Urol. 2017;70(1):12–27.
6. Grases F, Costa-Bauza A, Ramis M, Montesinos V, Conte A. Simple classification of renal calculi closely related to their micromorphology and etiology. Clin Chim Acta. 2002;322:29–36.
7. Gambaro G, Trinchieri A. Recent advances in managing and understanding nephrolithiasis/nephrocalcinosis. F1000Research. 2016;5:695.
8. Reis Santos JM. Ureteroscopy from the recent past to the near future. Urolithiasis. 2018;46:31–7.
9. Rassweiler J, Fiedler M, Charalampogiannis N, et al. Robot assisted flexible ureteroscopy: an update. Urolithiasis. 2018;46:69–77.
10. Almeras C, Daudon M, Ploussard G, Gautier JR, Traxer O, Meria P. Endoscopic description of renal papillary abnormalities in stone disease by flexible ureteroscopy: a proposed classification of severity and type. World J Urol. 2016 Nov;34(11):1575–82.
11. Borofsky MS, Paonessa JE, Evan AP, Williams JC, Coe FL, Worcester EM, et al. A proposed grading system to standardize the description of renal papillary appearance at the time of endoscopy in patients with nephrolithiasis. J Endourol. 2016;30(1):122–7.
12. Norman RW, Bath SS, Robertson WG, Peacock M. When should patients with symptomatic urinary stone disease be evaluated metabolically? J Urol. 1984;132(6):1137–9.
13. Levy FL, Adams-Huet B, Pak CY. Ambulatory evaluation of nephrolithiasis: an update of a 1980 protocol. Am J Med. 1995 Jan;98(1):50–9.
14. Tiselius HG. An improved method for the routine biochemical evaluation of patients with recurrent calcium oxalate stone disease. Clin Chim Acta. 1982;122(3):409–18.
15. Coe FL, Worcester EM, Evan AP. Idiopathic hypercalciuria and formation of calcium renal stones. Nat Rev Nephrol. 2016;12(9):519–33.
16. Aggarwal KP, Narula S, Kakkar M, Tandon C. Nephrolithiasis: Molecular Mechanism of Renal Stone Formation and the Critical Role Played by Modulators. Biomed Res Int. 2013;2013:1–21.
17. Chung H. The role of Randall plaques on kidney stone formation. Transl Androl Urol. 2014;3(3):251–4.
18. Haggitt RC, Pitcock JA. Renal medullary calcifications: a light and electron microscopic study. J Urol. 1971 Sep;106(3):342–7.

19. Williams JC, Matlaga BR, Kim SC, Jackson ME, Sommer AJ, McAteer JA, et al. Calcium oxalate calculi found attached to the renal papilla: preliminary evidence for early mechanisms in stone formation. J Endourol. 2006;20(11): 885–90.
20. Evan A, Lingeman J, Coe FL, Worcester E. Randall's plaque: pathogenesis and role in calcium oxalate nephrolithiasis. Kidney Int. 2006;69(8):1313–8.
21. Daudon M, Bazin D, Letavernier E. Randall's plaque as the origin of calcium oxalate kidney stones. Urolithiasis. 2015;43(S1):5–11.
22. Kuo RL, Lingeman JE, Evan AP, Paterson RF, Parks JH, Bledsoe SB, et al. Urine calcium and volume predict coverage of renal papilla by Randall's plaque. Kidney Int. 2003;64(6):2150–4.
23. Low RK, Stoller ML. Endoscopic mapping of renal papillae for Randall's plaques in patients with urinary stone disease. J Urol. 1997;158(6):2062–4.
24. Wang X, Krambeck AE, Williams JC, Tang X, Rule AD, Zhao F, et al. Distinguishing characteristics of idiopathic calcium oxalate kidney stone formers with low amounts of Randall's plaque. Clin J Am Soc Nephrol. 2014 Oct 7;9(10):1757–63.
25. Strohmaier WL, et al. Papillary calcifications: a new prognostic factor in idiopathic calcium oxalate urolithiasis. Urolithiasis. 2013;41:475–9.
26. Daudon M, Dessombz A, Frochot V, Letavernier E, Haymann J-P, Jungers P, et al. Comprehensive morpho-constitutional analysis of urinary stones improves etiological diagnosis and therapeutic strategy of nephrolithiasis. Int J Surg. 2016;36(Part D):624–32.
27. Hesse A, Kruse R, Geilenkeuser W-J, Schmidt M. Quality control in urinary stone analysis: results of 44 ring trials (1980–2001). Clin Chem Lab Med. 2005;43(3):298–303.
28. Evan AP, Lingeman JE, Coe FL, Parks JH, Bledsoe SB, Shao Y, et al. Randall's plaque of patients with nephrolithiasis begins in basement membranes of thin loops of Henle. J Clin Invest. 2003;111(5):607–16.
29. Evan AP, Lingeman JE, Worcester EM, Sommer AJ, Phillips CL, Williams JC, et al. Contrasting histopathology and crystal deposits in kidneys of idiopathic stone formers who produce hydroxy apatite, brushite, or calcium oxalate stones. Anat Rec (Hoboken). 2014;297(4):731–48.

12

Axitinib as a third or further line of treatment in renal cancer: A single institution experience

G. Tsironis[1†], M. Liontos[1†], A. Kyriazoglou[1*], K. Koutsoukos[1], A. Tsiara[1], M. Kaparelou[1], R. Zakopoulou[1], A. Cohen[1], E. Skafida[1], S. Fontara[2], F. Zagouri[1], A. Bamias[1] and M. A. Dimopoulos[1]

Abstract

Background: Kidney cancer is a lethal neoplasm that affects several thousands of people every year. Renal cell carcinoma (RCC) is the most common histologic type. Recent developments in the therapeutic approach include antiangiogenic targeted approaches and Immunotherapy. Thus, the therapeutic algorithm of RCC patients and the survival outcomes have changed dramatically.

Methods: Herein we present a retrospective study of the patients treated in our Department with an antiangiogenic agent -Axitinib, a tyrosine kinase inhibitor- as a third or further line treatment. Statistical analysis was performed with SPSS, including the available clinicopathological data of the patients included.

Results: Axitinib was found to be active in patients who received this treatment beyond second line. The toxicity profile of this regimen did not reveal any unknown adverse events.

Conclusions: Our real world data reflect that axitinib is a safe and effective option, even beyond the second line.

Keywords: Axitinib;beyond second line, mRCC, Long responders, TKIs

Background

Kidney cancer represents the ninth most common cancer with an estimation of 63.990 new cases and 14.400 deaths in US for 2017 [1]. Renal cancer is most often diagnosed in males than in females and the median age at diagnosis is 64 years [1]. Five year survival estimates about 74% for all stages ranging from 12% for patients with distant metastasis to 93% for patients with localized disease [2]. Renal cell carcinoma is the most common histological type of kidney cancer, accounting for about 85–90% of cases, whereas clear cell carcinoma (80%), papillary (10–15%) and chromophobe (4–5%) are its three most common subtypes [3, 4].

* Correspondence: tassoskyr@gmail.com
†G. Tsironis and M. Liontos contributed equally to this work.
[1]Oncology Unit, Department of Clinical Therapeutics, Alexandra Hospital, Athens, Greece
Full list of author information is available at the end of the article

Antiangiogenetic agents [5–9] along with mTOR inhibitors [10, 11] or their combination [12] and immune checkpoint inhibitors [13], led to the regulatory approval of 10 different agents for metastatic RCC patients the last 12 years resulting in a significant increase of overall survival of RCC patients [14, 15]. Available treatments have not only increased survival of patients, but also improved their quality of life and performance status allowing more lines of therapy [16]. The latter also correlates with improved survival [16]. The plethora of available treatment options is depicted to the European Association of Urology guidelines (EAU) which include Immunotherapy, antiangiogenic agents and mTOR inhibitors [17].

Little data exist though to guide therapy decisions beyond 2nd line and are limited to the results of GOLD trial, a subanalysis of RECORD-1 trial and subgroups of patients in the cabozatinib and nivolumab studies [9, 13, 18, 19]. This field is further complicated by the recent approval of immunotherapy/VEGF-TKIs combination as frontline treatment. As a result, it is very common in everyday clinical practice "first and second line" agents that have not been given before to be used beyond second line.

Axitinib is a selective inhibitor of VEGF receptors 1,2 and 3 that has been approved in patients with mRCC progressing after sunitinib or cytokines as a result of AXIS trial [20]. This second generation TKI was found superior to sorafenib in terms of PFS regardless of prior treatment (6.7 months vs 4.7 months, HR: 0.665; 95% CI 0.544–0.812; one-sided $p < 0.0001$), in partial responses (19.4 vs. 9.4%, $p < 0.001$) whereas in OS did not reach significance (mOS 20.1 months, 95% CI 16.7–23.4 vs 19.2 months 17.5–22.3, HR: 0.969, 95% CI 0.800–1.174; one-sided $p = 0.3744$) [21]. Although its approval is in second line, axitinib has been found to be the most common treatment option, in real-world treatment patterns in the USA, in patients with mRCC progressing after TKI and mTOR [22].

Under this perspective, we hypothesized that axitinib might be an active and safe option for patients with mRCC who receive this treatment later on their treatment sequence. We conducted a retrospective study of patients with mRCC treated in our department that received axitinib beyond second line aiming to study the efficacy and safety of this agent in this subgroup of patients.

Methods

This is a single-institutional, retrospective study, which was carried out in Hematology-Oncology Unit of Clinical Therapeutics Department of University of Athens in Alexandra General Hospital. Medical records of patients who were treated with axitinib beyond second line, between August 2013 and January 2017 were retrospectively reviewed. All subjects had given written informed consent. Only patients aged above 18 years old that had received at least two treatment lines for metastatic, histologically confirmed RCC, before the initiation of axitinib were recorded. Data was collected through a single institution database consisted of demographic, clinicopahtological and treatment-related and survival data.

Statistical analysis

Descriptive statistics were used to assess clinicopathological parameters of the patients. OS was calculated from the initiation of axitinib treatment until death or last follow-up. The effect of the expression of the various clinicopathological parameters on clinical outcome was assessed by plotting survival curves according to the Kaplan–Meier method and comparing groups using the log-rank test. Patients with PFS on axitinib treatment > 12 months were considered as having long term benefit from the treatment and were also analyzed separately to identify possible factors related to this response. The associations of each of the above-indicated factors and clinicopathological parameters with OS were assessed through hazard ratios estimated from univariate Cox proportional hazards models. Factors for which the hazard ratios were statistically significant at the level of significance 0.1 were then included simultaneously in a multivariate Cox proportional hazards model using the backward-stepwise method with removal criterion $p >$ 0.10. All results with a two-sided p level ≤ 0.05 were considered statistically significant, whereas a p value between 0.05 and 0.10 was considered of borderline significance. Statistical analyses were performed using SPSS software package, version 21 (Computing Resource Centre, Santa Monica, California, USA) and GraphPad Prism software (GraphPad Software Inc., La Jolla, California, USA).

Results

Clinicopathological characteristics and previous treatments

22 patients initiated Axitinib in our institution as third or further line of treatment for their renal cancer from December 2013 to January 2017 and were recorded in our study. Clinicopathological characteristics of the patients as well as data regarding their previous treatments are presented in Table 1. All patients had undergone radical nephrectomy and the histological diagnosis was predominant Clear Cell Renal cell carcinoma (ccRCC) in 17 (77%) patients, while 5 (23%) patients had non-ccRCC tumors At the beginning of 1st line treatment 20 patients (91%) were evaluable for categorizing into Heng prognostic groups, resulting in 6 (30%), 13 (65%), and 1 (5%), good, intermediate and poor prognostic scores respectively. The majority of patients (12 patients, 54,5%) received axitinib as third line treatment, while 4 patients (18,2%) received drug as fourth line treatment and 6 patients (27,3%) beyond fourth line of treatment. At the beginning of axitinib treatment, 19 patients (85,3%) had already received VEGF-TKIs and mTOR inhibitors as previous lines of therapy, 1 patients (4,5%) VEGF-TKIs only and 2 patients (9,1%) VEGF-TKIs and immune checkpoint inhibitors. Also, 11 patients (50%) had received only one prior VEGF-TKI, while the remaining 11 patients two or more different drugs of this class of agents (Table 2). The duration of treatment with axitinib was 6.15 months (range 3.26–8.2 months). Patients were followed after the initiation of axitinib for a median period of 13.5 months (range 2.6–39.18 months). The majority of patients that started axitinib treatment had significant burden of disease. More specifically, 18 patients (81,8%) had multiple sites of metastases, while 9 patients (40,9%) had liver disease and 5 patients (22,7%) had bone disease. As a result, at the beginning of axitinib

Table 1 Clinicopathological and treatment-related characteristics of the patients

Characterstics	Median	Range
Age	55,4	30,2-73,5
	N	%
Sex		
Male	11	50
Female	11	50
Histology		
ccRCC	17	77,3
non-ccRCC	5	22,7
Nephrectomy		
Yes	22	100
No	0	0
Fuhrman grade		
< 3	6	27,3
≥ 3	13	59,1
NA	3	13,6
Heng prognostic group at 1st line		
Good	6	27,3
Intermediate	13	59,1
Poor	1	4,5
NA	2	9,1
Heng prognostic group at axitinib line		
Good	0	0
Intermediate	9	40,9
Poor	11	50
NA	2	9,1
Axitinb line of treatment		
3	12	54,5
4	4	18,2
> 4	6	27,3
Previous treatments		
TKI only	1	4,5
TKI/IO	2	9,1
TKI/mTOR inhibitor	19	85,3
No of previous TKIs received		
< 2	11	50
≥ 2	11	50
No of metastatic sites at axitinib treatment		
solitary	4	18,2
multiple	18	81,8
Sites of metastases at axitinib treatment		
lymph nodes	12	54,5
lung	19	85,3
liver	9	40,9
bone	5	22,7
local relapse	8	36,4

treatment, 9 patients were classified as intermediate risk (40,9%) and 11 patients (50%) as poor prognosis according to Heng criteria.

Efficacy results

At the time of data cut off only 1 patient (4,5%) remained on treatment with axitinib. The majority of patients (13/68%) had clinical benefit from axitinib therapy resulting in 6 (27%) partial responses and 9 (41%) stabilizations of disease by RECIST 1.1 criteria, while 7 patients (32%) had disease progression as best response to the treatment. Median PFS was 6.27 months (95% CI 3.62–8.91 months) (Fig. 1a) and median OS after initiation of axitinib treatment was not reached (Fig. 1b). No clinicopathological factor (sex, histology, sites of metastases, Heng criteria) or treatment related factors [line of axitinib treatment (3rd line or beyond 3rd line), number of previous TKIs (1 or ≥ 2), type of previous treatment (TKI only, TKI/mTORi, TKI/IO) and dose reduction] had predictive significance in the univariate analysis (Table 3).

Four patients (18.2%) gained long-term benefit from axitinib treatment exceeding 12 months. mPFS in this group of patients was 14.3 months (95% CI 8.7–19.9), while in the remaining patients mPFS was 4.3 months (95% CI 2.5–6.1) (Fig. 2). Two of these patients achieved Partial Response with axitinib treatment, while the other two had Stable Disease. Again, no specific correlation was found between long-term responders and previously described clinicopathological and treatment-related parameters. However, the small number of patients is a limitation of this statistical analysis.

Safety

Regarding safety, all but one patients (95.8%) experienced adverse events during axitinib treatment (Table 4). The majority of them were grade 1–2 (69%) while ≥ grade 3 toxicities were recorded in 31% of patients. Dose reduction and drug discontinuation had to be performed for 5 (22%) and 3 patients (13%) respectively. The five more common toxicities independently of grade were fatigue (11 patients/50%), hypertension (5 patients/ 23%), hypothyroidism (5 patients/ 23%), hand foot syndrome (HFS) (4 patients/ 18%) and hoarseness (4 patients/ 18%) whereas the two more common grade ≥ 3 toxicities

Table 2 Treatments before Axitinib

	1st line (*n* = 22)		2nd line (*n* = 22)		3rd line (*n* = 10)		4th line (*n* = 6)		5th line (*n* = 3)	
Agent(s)	n	%	n	%	n	%	n	%	n	%
Sunitinib	14	63.6	0	0	1	10	0	0	0	0
Pazopanib	3	13.6	3	13.6	1	10	4	66.6	1	33.3
Sunitinib- Everolimus (Sequential)	4	18.2	4	18.2	0	0	0	0	0	0
Bevacizumab	1	4.5	0	0	1	10	0	0	0	0
Temsirolimus- Bevacizumab (Concurrent)	0	0	2	9	0	0	0	0	0	0
Nivolumab	0	0	1	4.5	1	10	0	0	0	0
Sorafenib	0	0	1	4.5	3	30	0	0	0	0
Dovitinib	0	0	0	0	1	10	0	0	0	0
Everolimus	0	0	11	50	2	20	2	33.3	0	0
Temsirolimus	0	0	0	0	0	0	0	0	2	66.6
Total	22	100	22	100	10	100	6	100	3	100

were HFS (4 patients/ 18%) and hypertension (3 patients/ 14%).

Discussion

Renal cell carcinoma is a common malignancy with many treatment options developed during the last decade. Targeting VEGF and PD-L1 signaling have enriched the armamentarium of the therapeutic options and have prolonged both OS and PFS [5, 6, 8, 9, 13]. However, the existence of several TKIs and the addition of Immunotherapy (IO) resulted to a more complex therapeutic algorithm in the treatment of metastatic RCC [13]. Further it should be noted that TKIs are still studied. Clinical trial NCT02330783 studies the combination of sorafenib and bevacizumab in third line treatment of mRCC. Clinical trial NCT02627963 compares tivozanib and sorafenib in third or fourth line of treatment of patients with mRCC.

Under this perspective data regarding the efficacy of TKIs in the later lines of therapy are important. This is also the case for axitinib that lacks randomized data for efficacy beyond second line and very few published data exist regarding its administration beyond second line. Our study aimed at providing efficacy and safety data for axitinib in this setting. These data provide evidence that axitinib is an active agent even in latter lines of therapy in mRCC as objective responses and mPFS is favorably compared to those achieved in second line in the AXIS trial. Our data are also in agreement with other case series presented in the literature. A large retrospective study with real world data from the United States, regarding axitinib administration resulted that axitinib was

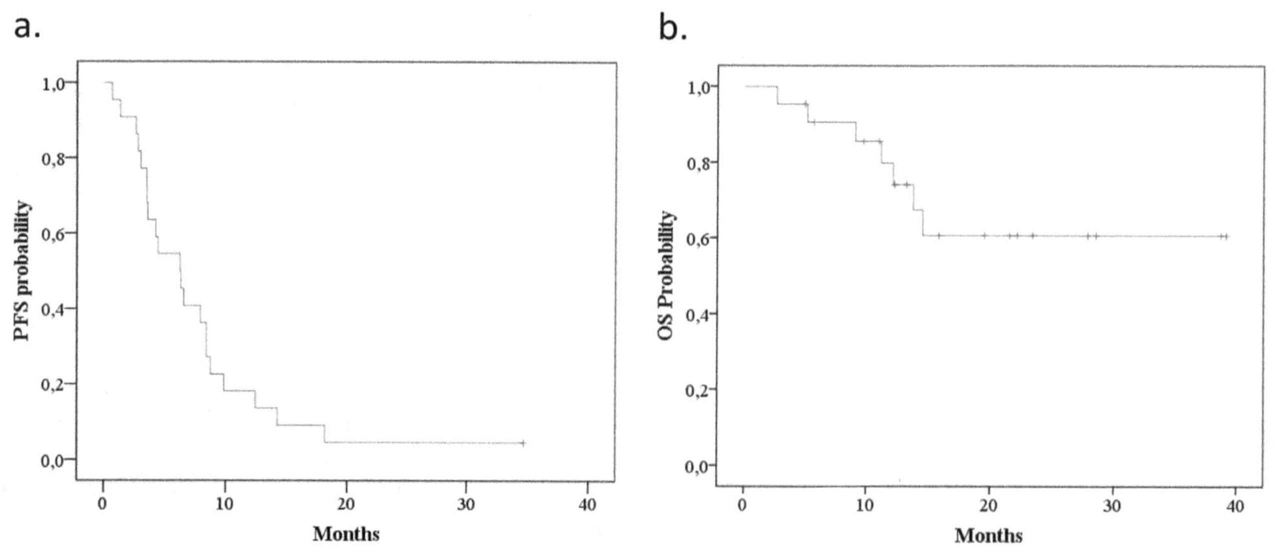

Fig. 1 Progression Free Survival (**a**) and Overall Survival (**b**) after axitinib initiation

Table 3 Univariate analysis of Progression Free Survival

Variables	*N*	mPFS	95% CI	*P* value
Sex				
Male	10	4267	0,000 - 11,085	0,936
Female	11	6267	3318 - 9216	
Histology				
Clear Cell	16	4267	2568 - 5965	0,227
Non Clear-Cell	5	8433	7360 - 9507	
Heng Group				
Good	5	3.5	2498 - 4502	0,027
Intermediate	13	6.567	1478 - 11,655	
Poor	1	18.167	. .	
Sites Of Metastasis (Baseline)				0,738
1	8	4467	1695 - 7239	
2	6	3533	0,000 7214	
3	5	3,6	2383 - 4817	
Sites Of Metastasis (Axitinib)				
1	4	3033	0,000- 8064	0,963
2	2	3,5	. .	
3	12	4267	2796 - 5738	
4	3	6333	6227–6440	
Previous TKIs				
< 2	11	4467	1158 - 7775	0,704
≥ 2	11	6267	3064 - 9469	
Axitinib line of treatment				
3	12	4467	0,000 - 9615	0,443
> 3	9	6267	0,423 - 12,110	
Dose Reduction				
Yes	5	8133	7360 - 9507	0,216
No	16	3,6	2163 - 5037	
Type of previous treatment				
TKI only	1	9866		0,183
TKI/IO	2	2,8		
TKI/mTORi	19	6333	1524-3347	

most commonly prescribed as a third line treatment [23], while another cohort of patients that received axitinib as either a 2nd line or 3rd line treatment, showed similar activity and tolerability with clinical trials [24]. The efficacy of axitinib beyond second line in our study prompt us to further investigate possible clinicopathological or treatment-related factors that could influence this result. However, no predictive factor was indicated by the analysis, possibly due to the small number of patients. We should also take into consideration that the population of patients that receive treatment beyond second line is usually already selected for improved survival.

The role of axitinib beyond second line was studied retrospectively in a study of Mclean et al. using linked datasets from 22 specialty pharmacies that dispense axitinib with databases of longitudinal medical and pharmacy claims [23]. In this study axitinib was prescribed as third-line therapy in 326 patients and as fourth-line or later therapy in 190 patients resulting in a median duration of treatment of 122 (7–644) and 111 days (10–642). In another retrospective study of third line targeted treatment among 1012 patients with mRCC treated at 25 centers from all over the world axitinib was given in 90 patients resulting in 5.9 months PFS (4.6–8.0), 19.2 months OS (13.5–22.7) and 66% RR [25].

Finally in another retrospective analysis of the data of patients participated in NCT00835978 and NCT00920816 studies revealed a subgroup of long- term responders whereas the duration of treatment with axitinib -as a second line treatment- have been found to be associated with increased frequency of early tumor shrinkage, greater magnitude of tumor shrinkage, and a favorable OS [26].

An important finding of our study was though that four out of the 22 patients had clinical benefit from the axitinib treatment for more than a year. Again previous therapeutic options or other clinicopathological data included to our study, failed to prove any predictive value. This kind of analysis, even though it is retrospective and includes a limited number of patients, is a unique attempt to discover predictive factors; in order to choose the responsive subgroup of patients with mRCC to axitinb treatment, beyond second line. A retrospective analysis of two clinical trials with patients with mRCC who received axitinib as a first line treatment, revealed a population of 37.8% who were long responders [26]. This response was related ECOG performance status 0, no liver or bone metastases, favorable hematology characteristics and baseline tumor burden below the overall median [26].

The molecular pathway that drives this response to axitinib is unknown. Long-term responses have also been described to other TKIs. Long term response to sunitinib has been studied retrospectively from several authors concluding that the absence of adverse disease characteristics (poor PS, poor MSKCC risk, absence of bone or liver metastases) may predict long responders [27–29]. Analogous results have been presented for Pazopanib [30, 31] and Sorafenib [32], but in no case they could provide clinical guidance for the optimal use of these agents in latter lines of therapy.

No new safety signals were recognized in our cohort of patients. Toxicity profile, dose reductions and treatment discontinuation of our patients was similar to the registrational trial of axitinib as a second line treatment [20]. The most frequent adverse events occurring in more than 30% of patients in Axis study; associated with

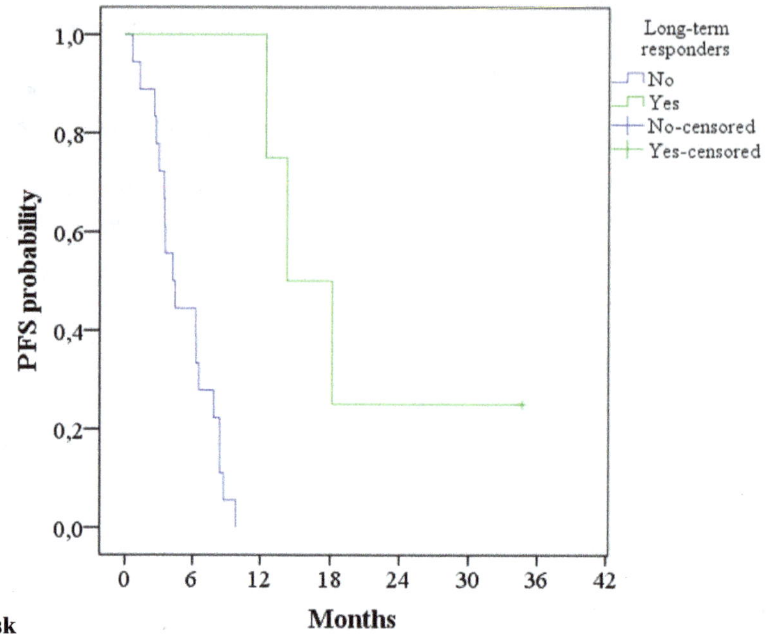

Numbers at risk

Short-term responders	18	7	0	0	0	0	0	0
Long-term responders	4	4	4	1	1	1	0	0

Fig. 2 Progression Free Survival in Long-Term responders and the remaining patients in our cohort

axitinib were diarrhea, hypertension, fatigue, decreased appetite, nausea, and dysphonia, while grade 3 or higher toxicity included hypertension, diarrhea and fatigue [20]. The five most common toxicities independently of grade in our analysis were fatigue, hypertension, hypothyroidism, hand foot syndrome and hoarseness, with grade 3 or higher toxicities including hypertension and hand foot syndrome. It is evident that axitinib administration beyond second line, even in heavily pretreated patients; is not accompanied by a more severe pattern of adverse effects.

Table 4 Adverse Events recorded in patients during axitinib treatment

Adverse Event	Any Grade ***N***(%)	Grade >=3 ***N***(%)
Hypertension	5 (22,72)	3 (13,63)
Arthralgia	2 (9,09)	1 (4,54)
Fatigue	11 (50)	1 (4,54)
Hypothyreoidism	5 (22,72)	0 (0)
Increased Liver Function Tests	3 (13,63)	1 (4,54)
Diarrhea	3 (13,63)	0 (0)
Hand Foot Syndrom	4 (18,18)	4 (18,18)
Anorexia	1 (4,54)	1 (4,54)
Mucositis	2 (9,09)	1 (4,54)
Muscle paitn	1 (4,54)	1 (4,54)
Hoarseness	4 (18,18)	1 (4,54)
Proteinurua	2 (9,09)	0 (0)
Anemia	2 (9,09)	0 (0)

We must highlight the caveats of our study, which is a retrospective non randomized study with a small number of patients included. Several confounding factors such as selection bias, heterogeneous treatments prior to axitinib and a relatively short period of follow up are crucial limitations that should be reported. Further, this analysis is based only to clinicopathological data without any translational studies and assessment of quality of life to accompany and support the clinical outcome.

In conclusion, axitinib is an effective treatment option for patients with mRCC beyond second line. Axitinib is well tolerated from patients, even heavily pretreated. Further studies including larger numbers of patients, combined with translational research analyses; are needed to discover the subgroup of patients who are responsive to this treatment beyond second line.

Conclusions

Antiangiogenic targeted therapy still remains an important element of RCC treatment. Axitinib is a tyrosine kinase inhibitor with proven efficacy in RCC as a 2nd line treatment. Our retrospective study highlights Axitinib's efficacy and safety in third and further line treatment in RCC.

Abbreviations

mRCC: Metastatic renal cell carcinoma; mTOR: *Mammalian target of rapamycin*; VEGF: Vascular endothelial growth factor; TKI: Tyrosine kinase inhibitor; EAU: European association of urology; OS: Overall survival; PFS: Progression free survival; PS: Performance status; ECOG: Eastern Cooperative Oncology Group; MSKCC: Memorial Sloan kettering cancer center

Acknowledgements

Not applicable.

Authors' contributions

GK was the primary writer of the article and with ML and AK codirected the study including data analysis and interpretation. GT with ML performed statistical analysis. FZ, KK, AK, MK, AT, RZ contributed to conception and design and acquisition of data. CA, ES, SF made substantial contributions to conception and design, acquisition of data, analysis and interpretation of data. AB with MAD contributed to conception and design and were involved in drafting the manuscript and revising it critically for important intellectual content. All authors have read and approved the final manuscript.

Author details

[1]Oncology Unit, Department of Clinical Therapeutics, Alexandra Hospital, Athens, Greece. [2]1st Department of Radiology, Aretaieio University hospital, Athens, Greece.

References

1. Zagouri F, Peroukidis S, Tzannis K, Kouloulias V, Bamias A, Hellenic Genito-Urinary Cancer G. Current clinical practice guidelines on chemotherapy and radiotherapy for the treatment of non-metastatic muscle-invasive urothelial cancer: a systematic review and critical evaluation by the Hellenic Genito-urinary Cancer group (HGUCG). Crit Rev Oncol Hematol. 2015;93(1):36–49.
2. Bamias A, Escudier B, Sternberg CN, Zagouri F, Dellis A, Djavan B, Tzannis K, Kontovinis L, Stravodimos K, Papatsoris A, et al. Current clinical practice guidelines for the treatment of renal cell carcinoma: a systematic review and critical evaluation. Oncologist. 2017;22(6):667–79.
3. Cohen HT, McGovern FJ. Renal-cell carcinoma. N Engl J Med. 2005;353(23): 2477–90.
4. Shingarev R, Jaimes EA. Renal cell carcinoma: new insights and challenges for a clinician scientist. Am J Physiol Renal Physiol. 2017;313(2):F145–54.
5. Motzer RJ, Hutson TE, Tomczak P, Michaelson MD, Bukowski RM, Rixe O, Oudard S, Negrier S, Szczylik C, Kim ST, et al. Sunitinib versus interferon alfa in metastatic renal-cell carcinoma. N Engl J Med. 2007;356(2):115–24.
6. Sternberg CN, Davis ID, Mardiak J, Szczylik C, Lee E, Wagstaff J, Barrios CH, Salman P, Gladkov OA, Kavina A, et al. Pazopanib in locally advanced or metastatic renal cell carcinoma: results of a randomized phase III trial. J Clin Oncol. 2010;28(6):1061–8.
7. Escudier B, Eisen T, Stadler WM, Szczylik C, Oudard S, Siebels M, Negrier S, Chevreau C, Solska E, Desai AA, et al. Sorafenib in advanced clear-cell renal-cell carcinoma. N Engl J Med. 2007;356(2):125–34.
8. Escudier B, Pluzanska A, Koralewski P, Ravaud A, Bracarda S, Szczylik C, Chevreau C, Filipek M, Melichar B, Bajetta E, et al. Bevacizumab plus interferon alfa-2a for treatment of metastatic renal cell carcinoma: a randomised, double-blind phase III trial. Lancet. 2007;370(9605):2103–11.
9. Choueiri TK, Escudier B, Powles T, Mainwaring PN, Rini BI, Donskov F, Hammers H, Hutson TE, Lee JL, Peltola K, et al. Cabozantinib versus Everolimus in advanced renal-cell carcinoma. N Engl J Med. 2015;373(19): 1814–23.
10. Motzer RJ, Escudier B, Oudard S, Hutson TE, Porta C, Bracarda S, Grunwald V, Thompson JA, Figlin RA, Hollaender N, et al. Efficacy of everolimus in advanced renal cell carcinoma: a double-blind, randomised, placebo-controlled phase III trial. Lancet. 2008;372(9637):449–56.
11. Hudes G, Carducci M, Tomczak P, Dutcher J, Figlin R, Kapoor A, Staroslawska E, Sosman J, McDermott D, Bodrogi I, et al. Temsirolimus, interferon alfa, or both for advanced renal-cell carcinoma. N Engl J Med. 2007;356(22):2271–81.
12. Motzer RJ, Hutson TE, Glen H, Michaelson MD, Molina A, Eisen T, Jassem J, Zolnierek J, Maroto JP, Mellado B, et al. Lenvatinib, everolimus, and the combination in patients with metastatic renal cell carcinoma: a randomised, phase 2, open-label, multicentre trial. Lancet Oncol. 2015;16(15):1473–82.
13. Motzer RJ, Escudier B, McDermott DF, George S, Hammers HJ, Srinivas S, Tykodi SS, Sosman JA, Procopio G, Plimack ER, et al. Nivolumab versus Everolimus in advanced renal-cell carcinoma. N Engl J Med. 2015;373(19): 1803–13.
14. Fogli S, Porta C, Del Re M, Crucitta S, Gianfilippo G, Danesi R, Rini BI, Schmidinger M. Optimizing treatment of renal cell carcinoma with VEGFR-TKIs: a comparison of clinical pharmacology and drug-drug interactions of anti-angiogenic drugs. Cancer Treat Rev. 2020;84:101966.
15. Gulati S, Vaishampayan U. Current state of systemic therapies for advanced renal cell carcinoma. Curr Oncol Rep. 2020;22(3):26.
16. Angulo JC, Shapiro O. The Changing Therapeutic Landscape of Metastatic Renal Cancer. Cancers (Basel). 2019;11(9):1227.
17. Ljungberg B, Bensalah K, Canfield S, Dabestani S, Hofmann F, Hora M, Kuczyk MA, Lam T, Marconi L, Merseburger AS, et al. EAU guidelines on renal cell carcinoma: 2014 update. Eur Urol. 2015;67(5):913–24.
18. Motzer RJ, Porta C, Vogelzang NJ, Sternberg CN, Szczylik C, Zolnierek J, Kollmannsberger C, Rha SY, Bjarnason GA, Melichar B, et al. Dovitinib versus sorafenib for third-line targeted treatment of patients with metastatic renal cell carcinoma: an open-label, randomised phase 3 trial. Lancet Oncol. 2014; 15(3):286–96.
19. Calvo E, Escudier B, Motzer RJ, Oudard S, Hutson TE, Porta C, Bracarda S, Grunwald V, Thompson JA, Ravaud A, et al. Everolimus in metastatic renal cell carcinoma: subgroup analysis of patients with 1 or 2 previous vascular endothelial growth factor receptor-tyrosine kinase inhibitor therapies enrolled in the phase III RECORD-1 study. Eur J Cancer. 2012;48(3):333–9.
20. Rini BI, Escudier B, Tomczak P, Kaprin A, Szczylik C, Hutson TE, Michaelson MD, Gorbunova VA, Gore ME, Rusakov IG, et al. Comparative effectiveness of axitinib versus sorafenib in advanced renal cell carcinoma (AXIS): a randomised phase 3 trial. Lancet. 2011;378(9807):1931–9.
21. Motzer RJ, Escudier B, Tomczak P, Hutson TE, Michaelson MD, Negrier S, Oudard S, Gore ME, Tarazi J, Hariharan S, et al. Axitinib versus sorafenib as second-line treatment for advanced renal cell carcinoma: overall survival analysis and updated results from a randomised phase 3 trial. Lancet Oncol. 2013;14(6):552–62.
22. Pal SK, Signorovitch JE, Li N, Zichlin ML, Liu Z, Ghate SR, Perez JR, Vogelzang NJ. Patterns of care among patients receiving sequential targeted therapies for advanced renal cell carcinoma: a retrospective chart review in the USA. Int J Urol. 2017;24(4):272–8.
23. MacLean E, Cisar L, Mehle K, Eremina D, Quigley JM. Real-World Axitinib Use in the United States: A Retrospective Study Using Linked Datasets. J Manag Care Spec Pharm. 2016;22(6):723–732u.
24. Hutson TE, Jiao X, Wilson T, Cisar L, MacLean EA. Axitinib in metastatic renal cell carcinoma: patient characteristics and treatment patterns in US community oncology centers. Future Oncol. 2017;13(15):1323–32.
25. Kyriakopoulos CE, Chittoria N, Choueiri TK, Kroeger N, Lee JL, Srinivas S, Knox JJ, Bjarnason GA, Ernst SD, Wood LA, et al. Outcome of patients with metastatic sarcomatoid renal cell carcinoma: results from the international metastatic renal cell carcinoma database consortium. Clin Genitourin Cancer. 2015;13(2):e79–85.
26. Rini BI, Gruenwald V, Jonasch E, Fishman MN, Tomita Y, Michaelson MD, Tarazi J, Cisar L, Hariharan S, Bair AH, et al. Long-term duration of first-line Axitinib treatment in advanced renal cell carcinoma. Target Oncol. 2017; 12(3):333–40.
27. Molina AM, Jia X, Feldman DR, Hsieh JJ, Ginsberg MS, Velasco S, Patil S, Motzer RJ. Long-term response to sunitinib therapy for metastatic renal cell carcinoma. Clin Genitourin Cancer. 2013;11(3):297–302.
28. Smaletz O, Chacon M, de Oliveira KL, de Carvalho Rocha DR, Cardoso FC. Long-term benefit of sunitinib in patients with metastatic renal cell carcinoma in Latin America: retrospective analysis of patient clinical characteristics. Onco Targets Ther. 2016;9:7309–14.
29. Tannir NM, Figlin RA, Gore ME, Michaelson MD, Motzer RJ, Porta C, Rini BI, Hoang C, Lin X, Escudier B. Long-term response to Sunitinib treatment in metastatic renal cell carcinoma: a pooled analysis of clinical trials. Clin Genitourin Cancer. 2017;S1558-7673(17)30171–4.
30. Park J, Jiao X, Ghate S, Wilson T, Ahmad QI, Vogelzang NJ. Predictors of long-term response with Pazopanib in patients with advanced renal-cell carcinoma. Clin Genitourin Cancer. 2018;16(4):293–7.

31. Sbrana A, Biasco E, Paolieri F, Palesandro E, Caserta C, Iacovelli R, Detti B, Santini D, Mosca A, Morelli F, et al. Long-term response to first-line Pazopanib therapy in mRCC patients: a multicenter Italian experience. Anticancer Res. 2018;38(8):4913–8.
32. Zhang HL, Qin XJ, Wang HK, Gu WJ, Ma CG, Shi GH, Zhou LP, Ye DW. Clinicopathological and prognostic factors for long-term survival in Chinese patients with metastatic renal cell carcinoma treated with sorafenib: a single-center retrospective study. Oncotarget. 2015;6(34):36870–83.

13

LithoVue™ for renal stone therapy – A perfect fit for high volume academic centers: A retrospective evaluation of 108 cases

Maximilian Pallauf[1], Sabina Sevcenco[2], Christopher Steiner[1], Martin Drerup[1], Michael Mitterberger[1], Daniela Colleselli[1], Lukas Lusuardi[1] and Thomas Kunit[1*]

Abstract

Background: Over the last few years the number of flexible ureterorenoscopies, used for renal stone treatment, has risen steadily. This was associated with an increase in costs for maintenance and repair of the fragile ureterorenoscopes used. To overcome this problem single-use devices have been introduced to the market. The aim of this study was to assess surgical outcome and workability for LithoVue™, a single-use flexible ureterorenoscope.

Methods: We retrospectively analyzed all flexible ureterorenoscopies performed at our department between January and October 2017. We included a total of 108 interventions for renal stone therapy, all performed using the single-use device LithoVue™. We assessed patients' characteristics including stone size, count and location. We evaluated the surgical outcome, analyzing stone-free rates, reintervention rates, complication rates, as well as surgery time. Learning curve for single-use ureterorenoscopes was evaluated by comparing the surgical outcome between residents and consultants.

Results: The average time needed per intervention was 52,31 min ± 28,11. In 77 out of 108 (71,30%) patients we were able to remove all stones by a single intervention. In 8 patients (7,41%) intra- or postoperative complications occurred, none of which was graded higher than Clavien-Dindo III B. We did not find any statistical differences comparing the surgical outcome between residents and consultants. No technical difficulties occurred during surgery.

Conclusion: Single-use flexible ureterorenoscopes provide decent working properties resulting in good surgical outcome. Furthermore, they are proven to be easy to handle even for unexperienced surgeons, making them a feasible choice for high volume academic centers.

Keywords: Nephrolithiasis, Flexible ureterorenoscopy, Single-use flexible ureterorenoscope, LithoVue™

* Correspondence: t.kunit@salk.at
[1]Landeskrankenhaus Salzburg - Universitätsklinikum der Paracelsus Medizinischen Privatuniversität, Universitätsklinik für Urologie und Andrologie, Müllner Hauptstraße 48, 5020 Salzburg, Austria
Full list of author information is available at the end of the article

Background

Over the last decade flexible ureterorenoscopy became more and more popular for upper urinary tract stone treatment, leading to numerous innovations in the field of flexible ureterorenoscopy. Several different types of flexible ureterorenoscopes are available, using fiber optics or digital imaging for image transmission. Whereas digital ureterorenoscopes have shown to have better image quality [1], fiber optic ones have better end-tip deflection providing better access to sharp angled calices [2]. As numbers of flexible ureterorenoscopies are constantly rising [3], costs for flexible ureterorenoscopy have become of great importance for health care providers. High costs per surgery can be explained by the purchase price of the flexible ureterorenoscope as well as high maintenance costs, including sterilization and repair. Since durability of reusable flexible ureterorenoscopes is low, needing substantial repair every 6 [4]-31 [5] interventions, single-use flexible ureterorenoscopes have been introduced.

There are several different single-use flexible ureterorenoscopes available. The most tested one is LithoVue™, a digital flexible ureterorenoscope manufactured by Boston Scientific®, showing similar working properties as well tested reusable ones [6–8]. Whereas maneuverability as well as image quality of LithoVue™ have been proven not to be inferior to those of reusable ones, [9] it is still debatable whether single-use flexible ureterorenoscopes are more cost-effective than their reusable counterparts. Several previous studies compared the costs for both instruments, showing that single-use flexible ureterorenoscopes are only cost-effective for institutions where less than 99–118 interventions are being performed per year [10, 11]. Nevertheless, the authors do not take into consideration that repair rates for reusable ureterorenoscopes might differ depending on the type of institution where they are being used. For example, it seems plausible that hospitals that fulfill a training assignment and teach young doctors might experience a higher rate of instrument breakage than centers where only experienced surgeons perform flexible ureterorenoscopy.

In our department we experienced a high number of instrument breakage using reusable ureterorenoscopes. Whether this was due to inappropriate handling intraoperatively or postoperatively was not clear. However, considering that approximately one third of all flexible ureterorenoscopies had been carried out by a resident, introduction of a single-use device appeared to be a reasonable choice. Following one year of experience in using LithoVue™ we finally wanted to evaluate its impact on renal stone treatment and verify whether it had any effects on residents' surgical skills. Therefore we retrospectively assessed surgical outcome and complications in all flexible ureterorenoscopies performed between January and October 2017.

Methods

We retrospectively reviewed all flexible ureterorenoscopies performed at our department between January and October 2017. Data was collected from patient medical records. Personal data was encrypted. Since this is a retrospective study, no patient consent could be obtained in advance. Permission to collect the data was given by the department. We only included flexible ureterorenoscopies performed for renal and ureteral stone therapy using the single-use device LithoVue™. We excluded all diagnostic flexible ureterorenoscopies or flexible ureterorenoscopies performed for upper tract urothelial carcinoma (UTUC) therapy. Age, gender, comorbidities, health status or long-term medication were not part of the exclusion criteria. Since we do not treat children in our department, all patients were of age. A total of 108 flexible ureterorenoscopies were found to be eligible for our study.

We examined whether the surgery was performed by a resident or a consultant and recorded surgery time of every intervention. Furthermore, we assessed stone size, count and location in all patients using preoperative computerized tomography (CT) scans and surgery reports. Patients were considered to be free of renal stones when no residuum was found either by endoscopic inspection of the pelvicalyceal system or in the retrograde pyelogram at the end of the intervention. In addition, we recorded whether ureteral stones were present and whether they had been removed. Furthermore, we recorded whether a laser was needed for fragmentation of large stones. Also, we noted if any intraoperative complication occurred. The information mentioned above, except for preoperative stone size, location and count, was taken from the surgery report. By additionally studying the patients' hospital record, we revealed whether a patient needed any further surgeries for renal stone therapy or if any postoperative complication occurred. The decision whether a patient needed a second intervention was made on a case to case basis. As this is a retrospective study there was no form where physicians declared their reason for planning reintervention. Therefore, we cannot provide more precise information on this. If a complication occurred, regardless of whether this was noticed intra- or postoperatively, it was classified according to the Clavien-Dindo (CD) classification.

Furthermore, we investigated whether any statistically significant differences can be found comparing surgery time, complication rates, stone-free rates and rates of reintervention between residents and consultants. To prevent any statistical bias caused by differences in stone size and count we compared stone characteristics between residents and consultants as well.

For comparing surgery times and differences in stone size and count we used Mann-Whitney-U Test or students T-Test depending on whether the samples were normally distributed. Study samples were tested for normal distribution using Shapiro-Wilks test. To evaluate the effect size of the tests, we calculated Cohen's d. For comparing complication rates, stone-free rates and rates of reintervention we used Fisher's exact test. Odd's ratio was calculated to evaluate the tests' effect size.

Differences were considered to be statistically significant at $p < 0.05$. All statistical analyzes were performed using XLSTAT by Addinsoft.

Results

Patient characteristics, surgery specific characteristics and stone characteristics

Patient characteristics, surgery specific characteristics and stone characteristics are listed in Table 1.

Results of surgery

Results of surgery are listed in Table 2.

Complications

In 8 out of 108 patients (7,41%) an intra- or postoperative complication occurred, none of which was graded higher than CD III B. Four times leakage of contrast media from the efferent urinary tract into the retroperitoneal space was observed intraoperatively, leading to a prolonged course of urethral stenting (CD I; Residents 2, Consultants 2). One patient suffered of pyelonephritis due to a subcapsular hematoma. The patient had to be treated with antibiotics intravenously (CD II; Residents 1, Consultants 0). No surgical intervention was necessary. In one patient (female) the ureteral stent was dislocated and needed to be relocated under local anesthesia (CD III A; Residents 0, Consultants 1). Two patients needed an intervention under general anesthesia due to postoperative complications (CD III B; Residents 0, Consultants 2). One patient (male) developed high fever after the ureteral stent was removed. A new ureteral stent had to be inserted, therefore needing general anesthesia. One patient developed ureteral stenosis following flexible ureterorenoscopy needing temporary ureteral stenting and laparoscopic surgery of the ureter.

In 68 out of 108 patients (62,96%) a laser was needed to fragment renal stones. The use of a laser did not increase the risk for intraoperative complications (7,35% vs.7,5%; $p = 1$).

Resident versus consultant

Surgery time

108 interventions have been included in our study. 77 interventions were performed by a consultant, 31 by a resident. The average time needed to perform a flexible ureterorenoscopy was 52,31 min ± 28,11. The average surgery time for a consultant was 52,34 min ± 28,11 and 52,23 min ± 28,56 for a resident, showing no statistically significant difference ($p = 0{,}865$; Cohen's d = 0,004) Fig. 1. In 27 out of 108 surgeries an additional rigid ureterorenoscopy was performed in order to remove an ureteral calculus. The average surgery time was 55,78 min ± 31, 27. The average surgery time for patients without an ureteral calculus was 51,15 min ± 26,85. No statistically significant difference in surgery time was found for those patients comparing surgery time between residents, 52, 95 min ± 30,97, and consultants, 50,47 min ± 25,50 ($p = 0{,}795$; Cohen's d = 0,088) Fig. 2. Furthermore, we investigated whether it took residents longer than consultants to perform a flexible ureterorenoscopy depending on the location of the renal calculus. No difference in surgery time between residents and consultants was found when stones were located only at one site of the pelvicalyceal system (renal pelvis, upper calyx, middle calyx, lower calyx) ($p = 0{,}241$; Cohen's d 0,007) Fig. 3. The average time needed to remove stones by flexible ureterorenoscopy solely at a single site of the pelvicalyceal system was calculated to be 42,29 min ± 12,3 for residents, 42, 17 min ± 21,83 for consultants, and 42,21 min ± 18,99 for consultants and residents together. Hence 56,5% of all removed stones were located in the lower calyx, we calculated the time needed to remove solely stones in the lower calyx. The average time needed was 42,33 min ± 21,54. It took residents 40,77 min ± 12,67 and consultants 42,35 min ± 26,02 to remove solely one stone from the lower calyx, showing no statistically significant difference ($p = 0{,}532$; Cohen's d = 0,126) Fig. 4.

Stone-free rate, rate of reintervention, complications

To assess surgical outcome, we measured stone-free rates, rates of reintervention and complication rates. Following flexible ureterorenoscopy 77 out of 108 patients (71,3%) were considered radiologically or endoscopically free of renal stones. When comparing stone-free rates between residents (77,41%) and consultants (68,83%) we did not find any statistically significant difference ($p = 0{,}482$). We found an odds ratio of 1,55, favoring stone-free rates for residents.

18 out of 108 patients (17,6%) needed at least one more surgical intervention to be considered free of renal stones. As for stone-free rates, no statistical difference was discovered when comparing rates of reintervention between residents (12,9%) and consultants (18,18%) ($p = 0{,}582$). However, we found an odds ratio of 0,67 favoring a lower likelihood of reintervention for residents.

More severe complications (>CD II) were found in the consultants' group. Hence this group made up for 71,3% of the cases this does not surprise. However, when comparing complication rates between residents (9,68%) and consultants (6,49%), we did not find a statistically significant difference ($p = 0{,}687$). We found an odds ratio of 0,

Table 1 Patient characteristics, surgery specific characteristics and stone characteristics. The first part of the table gives information about general characteristics of the patients such as gender and age. The information on gender distribution is given in absolute numbers and percentages in relation to the total number of patients. The average age of the patients is given in years and is represented by the mean value together with the standard deviation. The second part of the table summarizes surgery specific characteristics for example in how many patients an ureteral stent was placed pre- and postoperatively, whether an access sheath was needed, whether an additional rigid ureterorenoscopy was performed in the same surgery and whether a laser was needed for stone fragmentation. The information is given in absolute numbers and percentages in relation to the total number of patients. The third part of the table provides detailed information on the characteristics of the patients' renal stones. The total number of renal stones found in all patients is given as well as the average number of stones found per patient and group. The latter is represented by the mean value together with the standard deviation. Furthermore, it provides an overview on the local distribution of the stones in the pelvicalyceal system (ureter, renal pelvis, upper calyx, middle calyx, lower calyx). For each location the number of stones found as well as their percentage in relation to the total number of stones are given. Additionally, the table provides information on the average size of the renal stones found and is given for each group and each location in the pelvicalyceal system. Average stone size is given in millimeters and is represented by its mean value together with the standard deviation.

Patient characteristics	Number of patients (n) and percentage (%) or mean ± standard deviation (SD)
Number of patients	108 (100%)
Male	59 (54,63%)
Female	49 (45,37%)
Age (years)	54,55 ± 15,55
Surgery specific characteristics	Number of patients (n) and percentage (%)
Ureteral stent was placed preoperatively	96 (88,89%)
Ureteral stent was placed postoperatively	103 (95,37%)
Ureteral access sheath was used intraoperatively	107 (99,07%)
An additional rigid ureterorenoscopy was performed to remove an ureteral stone	27 (25,00%)
Laser fragmentation was needed	68 (62,96%)
Stone characteristics[1]	
Stone count	Number of stones (n) or mean number of stones ± standard deviation (SD)
Number of stones found in all patients	223
Mean number of stones per patient-All	2,35 ± 1,92
Mean number of stones per patient-Consultants group	2,47 ± 2
Mean number of stones per patient-Residents group	2,04 ± 1,7
Stone size	Mean size of the stones in mm ± standard deviation (SD)
Mean size of the stones-All	6,21 ± 2,46
Mean size of the stones-Consultants group	6,21 ± 2,39
Mean size of the stones-Residents group	6,21 ± 2,5
Stone location	Number of stones (n) and percentage or mean size of stones in mm ± standard deviation (SD)
Number of ureteral stones[2] in all patients	1 (0,45%)
Mean size of the stones found in the ureter	3 ± 0
Number of stones in the renal pelvis in all patients	23 (10,31%)
Mean size of the stones found in the renal pelvis	8,20 ± 3,67
Number of stones in the upper calyx in all patients	14 (6,28%)
Mean size of the stones found in the upper calyx	5,41 ± 3,81
Number of stones in the middle calyx in all patients	62 (27,80%)
Mean size of the stones found in the middle calyx	5,83 ± 2,84
Number of stones in the lower calyx in all patients	126 (56,50%)
Mean size of the stones found in the lower calyx	5,86 ± 2,44
[1]we were able to assess reliable stone characteristics in 95 out of 108 patients only	
[2]ureteral stones that were removed using a single-use flexible ureterorenoscope	

Table 2 Results of surgery. The first part of this table provides detailed information on the time needed to perform a flexible ureterorenoscopy. The mean surgery time for each group (all, consultants and residents) is given in minutes together with the standard deviation. The second part of this table summarizes the surgical outcome. For each event (stone-free rate, rate of reintervention and complications) and each group (all, consultants and residents) the number of patients as well as their percentage in relation to the total number of patients are given. Furthermore, complications are classified according to the Clavien-Dindo Classification. For each grade the total number of patients is given.

Surgery time	
Surgery time - All	Mean surgery time in min. ± standard deviation (SD)
Mean surgery time all patients	52,31 (±28,11)
Mean surgery time without removing an ureteral stone	51,15 (±28,11)
Mean surgery time removing 1 stone in the pelvicalyceal system	42,21 (±19,17)
Mean surgery time removing 2 stones in the pelvicalyceal system	65,96 (±33,07)
Mean surgery time removing 1 stone in the lower calyx	42,33 (±21,54)
Surgery time - Consultants group	Mean surgery time in min. ± standard deviation (SD)
Mean surgery time all patients	52,34 (±28,11)
Mean surgery time without removing an ureteral stone	50,47 (±25,50)
Mean surgery time removing 1 stone in the pelvicalyceal system	42,17 (±21,83)
Mean surgery time removing 1 stone in the lower calyx	42,35 (±26,02)
Surgery time – Residents group	Mean surgery time in min. ± standard deviation (SD)
Mean surgery time all patients	52,23 (±28,56)
Mean surgery time without removing an ureteral stone	52,95 (±30,97)
Mean surgery time removing 1 stone in the pelvicalyceal system	42,29 (±12,33)
Mean surgery time removing 1 stone in the lower calyx	40,77 (±12,67)
Surgical outcome	
Stone-free rate	Number (n) and percentage (%) of patients
Patients postoperatively free of renal stones in both the Residents group and the Consultants group (n=108)	77 (71,30%)
Patients postoperatively free of renal stones in the Consultants group (n=77)	53 (68,83%)
Patients postoperatively free of renal stones in the Residents group (n=31)	31 (77,41%)
Rate of reintervention	Number (n) and percentage (%) of patients
Patients receiving a second intervention for renal stones in both the Residents group and the Consultants group (n=108)	18 (17,60%)
Patients receiving a second intervention for renal stones in the Consultants group (n=77)	14 (18,18%)
Patients receiving a second intervention for renal stones in the Residents group (n=31)	4 (12,9%)
Complications	Number (n) and percentage (%) of patients
Patients having intra- postoperative complications in both the Residents group and the Consultants group (n=108)	8 (7,41%)
Patients having intra- postoperative complications in the Consultants group (n=77)	5 (6,49%)
Patients having intra- postoperative complications in the Residents group (n=31)	3 (9,68%)
Complications classified according to the Clavien-Dindo Classification	Number (n) of patients
Clavien-Dindo I	4
Clavien-Dindo II	1
Clavien-Dindo III A	1
Clavien-Dindo III B	2
Clavien-Dindo IV	0
Clavien-Dindo V	0

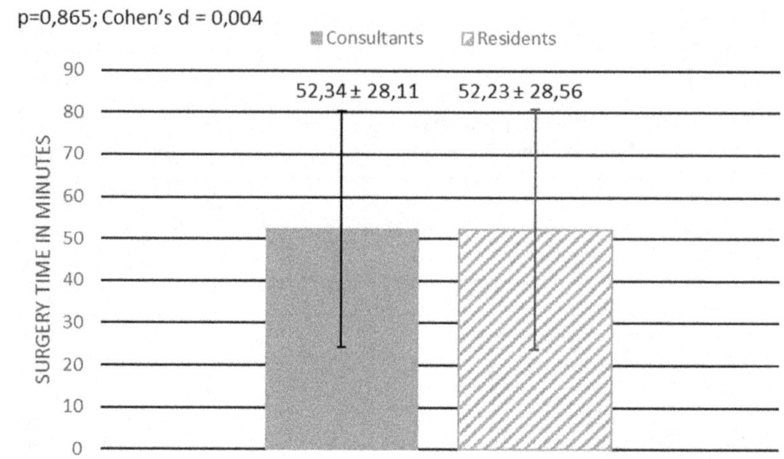

Fig. 1 Surgery time – all patients. This figure shows a bar chart comparing surgery time between consultants and residents. Surgery time is given in minutes. The dark grey box indicates mean surgery time for consultants, the grey and white stripped box indicates mean surgery time for residents. The vertical black line indicates the standard deviation for each group. Additionally, the mean surgery time including the standard deviation is shown for both groups. The result of the statistical comparison between both groups is shown in the left upper corner (*p*-value, Cohen's d)

65 favoring a lower risk for complications for consultants. An overview of the results is given in Table 3.

Technical difficulties

No technical difficulties occurred.

Discussion

In recent years flexible ureterorenoscopy has constantly gained in importance for renal stone therapy [3]. One probable reason therefor are the many improvements made for flexible ureterorenoscopes. As a matter of fact, rising numbers of flexible ureterorenoscopies promote the need for cost-effective devices. However, reusable digital or fiber optic flexible ureterorenoscopes demand high maintenance costs. This is partly due to the costs for sterilization but mainly due to the need for regular repairs. Several studies analyzed the average amount of interventions which can be performed before substantial repair is needed. Depending on the ureterorenoscope in use, repairs were necessary every 6 [4] to 31 [5] interventions. However, the large variance of the study results can not only be attributed to differences in the

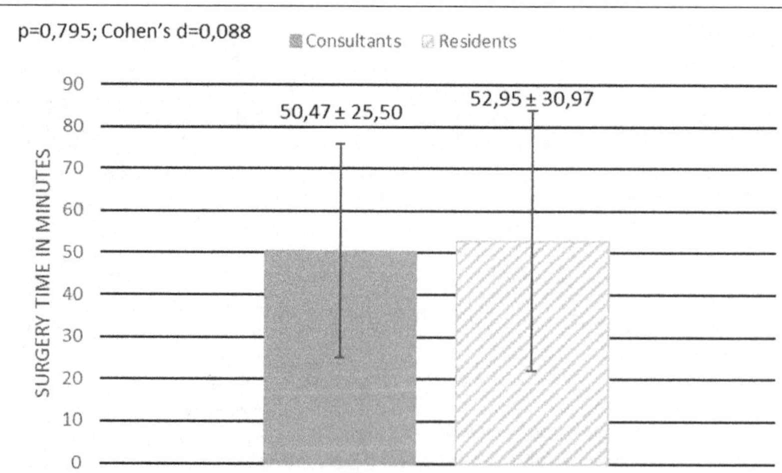

Fig. 2 Surgery time – all patients without an ureteral stone. This figure shows a bar chart comparing surgery time between consultants and residents in patients where solely stones in the pelvicalyceal system have been removed. Surgery time is given in minutes. The dark grey box indicates mean surgery time for consultants, the grey and white stripped box indicates mean surgery time for residents. The vertical black line indicates the standard deviation for each group. Additionally, the mean surgery time including the standard deviation is shown for both groups. The result of the statistical comparison between both groups is shown in the left upper corner (*p*-value, Cohen's d)

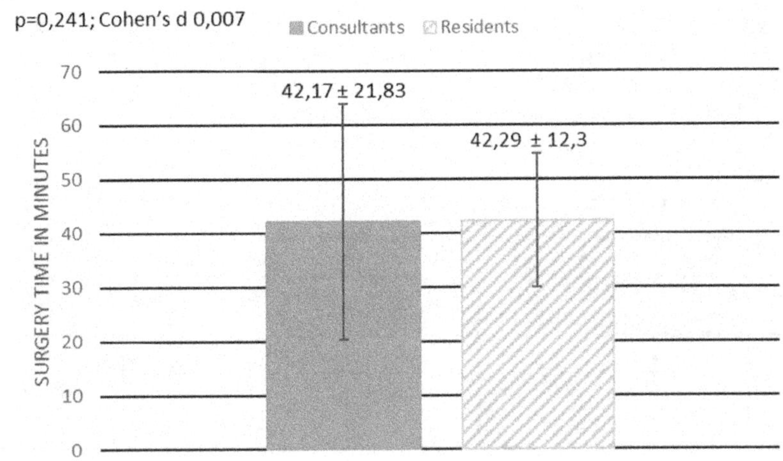

Fig. 3 Surgery time – all patients with only one kidney stone removed. This figure shows a bar chart comparing surgery time between consultants and residents in patients where only one kidney stone has been removed. Surgery time is given in minutes. The dark grey box indicates mean surgery time for consultants, the grey and white stripped box indicates mean surgery time for residents. The vertical black line indicates the standard deviation for each group. Additionally, the mean surgery time including the standard deviation is shown for both groups. The result of the statistical comparison between both groups is shown in the left upper corner (*p*-value, Cohen's d)

manufacturing quality of the devices. This can also be partly explained by the inaccuracy of the selected measurand. Because it is not the number of interventions, but rather the absolute operating time that influences the ureterorenoscopes' durability. As the latter accumulates, the risk of equipment damage increases as well [12]. Still, there are also several other risk factors promoting ureterorenoscope damage. The most important ones are found to be a steep infundibulopelvic angle (IPA) [13] and the use of an ureteral access sheath (UAS) [14]. Steep IPA varies among patients and is often difficult to assess preoperatively. The use of an UAS increases irrigation flow while additionally reduces intrapelvic pressure and therefore is used routinely [15]. This illustrates that scope breakage is difficult to prevent, as risk factors can hardly be avoided in clinical practice. This applies above all to tertiary and reference centers as well as clinics that fulfil a training assignment. Especially for the latter, as prolonged surgery time, that might be due to teaching purposes, bears the risk of promoting ureterorenoscope damage [12]. To make matters worse, refurbishment of the devices seems to further increase their vulnerability and intensify this problem. Carey et al. showed, that once an reusable flexible

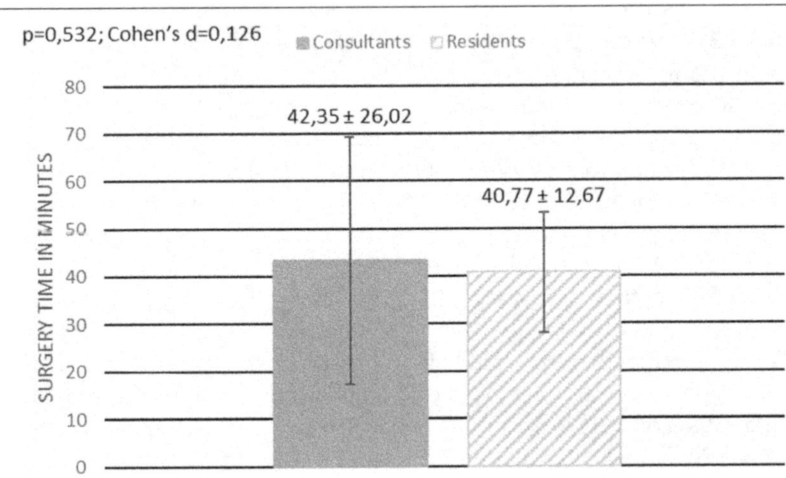

Fig. 4 Surgery time – all patients with only one stone in the lower calyx. This figure shows a bar chart comparing surgery time between consultants and residents in patients when solely one stone in the lower calyx has been removed. Surgery time is given in minutes. The dark grey box indicates mean surgery time for consultants, the grey and white stripped box indicates mean surgery time for residents. The vertical black line indicates the standard deviation for each group. Additionally, the mean surgery time including the standard deviation is shown for both groups. The result of the statistical comparison between both groups is shown in the left upper corner (*p*-value, Cohen's d)

Table 3 Surgical outcome – comparison between consultants and residents. This table provides detailed information on the statistical evaluation of the surgical outcome between consultants and residents. Surgical outcome was evaluated by comparing the stone-free rate, the rate of reintervention and the rate of complications between residents and consultants. For each event (stone-free rate, rate of reintervention, rate of complication) and each group (consultants and residents) the number of patients (n) meeting the criteria as well as their percentage in relation to the total number of patients for each group, are given. Differences between both groups (residents and consultants) on each event (stone-free rate, rate of reintervention, rate of complication) were calculated using Fisher's exact test. The odd's ratio was calculated to evaluate the tests' effect size. For each event the *p*-value and the odds ratio for both groups (residents and consultants) are given.

	Residents Group (n=31)		Consultants Group (n=77)		Residents versus Consultants		
Surgical outcome	*Number of patients (n)*	*Percentage of patients (%)*	*Numberof patients (n)*	*Percentage of patients (%)*	*p-value*	*Odds Ratio Residents*	*Odds Ratio Consultants*
Stone-free rate	24	77,41	53	68,83	0,482	1,55	0,64
Rate of reintervention	4	12,9	14	18,18	0,582	0,67	1,5
Complication rate	3	9,68	5	6,49	0,687	1,54	0,65

ureterorenoscope undergoes substantial repair, an additional repair was needed much more often [16]. This again underlines the need for a robust and cost-effective alternative to reusable flexible ureterorenoscopes.

To address this problem, single-use flexible ureterorenoscopes have been introduced in 2009 [17]. Since the time they first became available, investigators analyzed their working properties in vitro [1, 7, 18] and in vivo [9], attesting single-use flexible ureterorenoscopes similar maneuverability and image quality as reusable ones. Furthermore, a recently published systematic review demonstrated that surgical outcome and complication rates do not differ between single-use and reusable flexible ureterorenoscopes [19].

Our study confirms the high functionality of disposable devices in stone therapy as its results are comparable to those found in the literature. In a large meta-analysis Davis et al. showed that rate of stone clearance and rate of complication for single-use flexible ureterorenoscopes are 87% ± 15 and 9,3% ± 9 respectively [19]. In all those studies, included in the meta-analysis, an average of 66 min ± 29 was needed to remove a single stone measuring 1,13 cm ± 0,26 cm [19]. In our study, stone clearance was reached in 71,3%, leading to only 17,6% of patients needing an additional treatment. Complications only occurred in 7,41% of interventions, none of which was graded higher than CD III B. A mean surgery time of 52,31 min ± 28,11 was needed to treat in average 2, 35 ± 1,92 stones per patient, each calculated to be 6,21 mm ± 2,46 in diameter. When all patients were excluded who additionally received a rigid ureterorenoscopy, the mean surgery time was calculated to be as low as 51,15 min ± 26,85. Therefore we conclude, that introduction of single-use flexible ureterorenoscopes did not deteriorate surgical outcome at our department.

Since 28,7% of all interventions were performed by a resident, we tried to figure out whether the use of single-use flexible ureterorenoscopes worsens surgical outcome or prolongs surgery when used by an unexperienced surgeon. Therefore, we compared complication rates, stone-free rates and rates of reintervention between residents and consultants, showing no statistically significant difference. Furthermore, no statistical difference was found comparing surgery time between residents and consultants. This leads to the assumption, that single-use flexible ureterorenoscopes are easy to handle, also for less experienced surgeons. This is highlighted by the fact, that stone size and stone count did not differ between residents and consultants. Easy maneuverability might be partly due to the low weight of disposable ureterorenoscopes. As they are not meant to last for several interventions, less robust, but in fact, much lighter products can be used, thereby reducing physical effort [20].

However, the informative value of this study is limited due to its retrospective approach. In order to compare the user-friendliness between single-use and reusable flexible ureterorenoscopes a prospective randomized trial will be needed.

Even more controversial than the debate about the functionality of disposable devices is the debate about their cost efficiency. The question remains whether disposable devices are just an overpriced and unnecessary tool, or whether they can really help to reduce the increasing costs in stone therapy. Therefore, several investigators analyzed the costs for reusable ureterorenoscopes (purchase, sterilization, repair) and compared them with those (purchase) for single-use ones. As expected, their projected costs per intervention for reusable scopes differed significantly, ranging between 436$ (393,13€ - 01/2020) [11] and 848,1$ (769,22€ - 01/2020) [10], excluding costs of acquisition. This gap can be explained by the different number of repairs as well as costs for maintenance, storage and sterilization of the devices. This highlights the multiple difficulties, when trying to compare costs per intervention. However, the frequency and the extent of the repairs account for the largest amount and can therefore be used as a benchmark for cost comparison. In other words, if the repair rates are the same than this will be true for the operating costs as well.

As for our department, we experienced high rates of ureterorenoscope breakage prior to the introduction of single-use devices. In 2016 when we were still using solely reusable flexible ureterorenoscopes, substantial repair was needed every 9,2 interventions. This is similar to the rates that have been used in the previously mentioned studies to calculate operating costs for reusable devices 7,5 [11] – 12,5 [10]. By taking over their operating costs we can calculate the costs that would have incurred if we had performed the 108 interventions using a reusable instead of a disposable ureterorenoscope. The calculation is as follows: Due to the high number of cases we are covering every year, six reusable flexible ureterorenoscopes are in use in our department. The acquisition costs per device were 18544,99$ (16720€ - 01/2020) amounting to a total of 111269,93$ (100320€ - 01/2020). If the lower of the two reference values $436 (393,13€ - 01/2020) [11] is used to calculate the devices operating costs, this results in additional expenses of 47088$ (42457,98€ - 01/2020) for 108 interventions. Thus, the theoretical costs for 108 interventions using a reusable flexible ureterorenoscope sum up to 158357,93$ (142775,51€ - 01/2020) which is 1466,28$ (13220€ - 01/2020) per procedure. This amount roughly corresponds to the usual sales price for LithoVue™, which is 1500$ (1360,49€ - 01/2020) [21]. Therefore we can conclude that the use of LithoVue™ is also a cost-effective choice for our department. However, the final proof is still pending.

Conclusion

We were able to show that the introduction of single-use flexible ureterorenoscopes at our department neither did deteriorate surgical outcome for renal stone therapy nor did it raise costs per intervention. Furthermore, single-use devices are proven to be easy to handle even for unexperienced surgeons, making them a feasible choice for high volume academic centers.

Abbreviations

CD: Clavien-Dindo; CT: Computerized tomography; IPA: Infundibulopelvic Angle; n: Number; SD: Standard Deviation; UAS: Ureteral Access Sheath; UTUC: Upper Tract Urothelial Carcinoma

Acknowledgements

Not applicable.

Authors' contributions

MP: Project development; Data collection and management; Data analysis; Manuscript writing. SS: Manuscript editing. CS: Data collection and management; Data analysis. MD: Manuscript editing. MM: Manuscript editing. DC: Manuscript editing. LL: Manuscript editing. TK: Project development; Manuscript editing. All Authors read and approved the manuscript.

Author details

[1]Landeskrankenhaus Salzburg - Universitätsklinikum der Paracelsus Medizinischen Privatuniversität, Universitätsklinik für Urologie und Andrologie, Müllner Hauptstraße 48, 5020 Salzburg, Austria. [2]Abteilung für Urologie und Andrologie, Sozialmedizinisches Zentrum Ost – Donauspital, Langobardenstraße 122, 1220 Wien, Austria.

References

1. Talso M, Proietti S, Emiliani E, Gallioli A, Dragos L, Orosa A, et al. Comparison of Flexible Ureterorenoscope Quality of Vision. An In Vitro Study. J Endourol. 2018;32(6):523–8.
2. Dragos LB, Somani BK, Sener ET, Buttice S, Proietti S, Ploumidis A, et al. Which flexible Ureteroscopes (digital vs. Fiber-optic) can easily reach the difficult lower pole calices and have better end-tip deflection: in vitro study on K-box. A PETRA evaluation. J Endourol. 2017;31(7):630–7.
3. Heers H, Turney BW. Trends in urological stone disease: a 5-year update of hospital episode statistics. BJU Int. 2016;118(5):785–9.
4. Cenk Gurbuz GA, Arikan O, Efilioglu O, Yıldırım A, Danacıoglu O, Caskurlu T. The cost analyisis of flexible ureteroscopic lithotripsy in 302 cases. Urolithiasis. 2014;42:155–8.
5. Eugene Kramolowsky M, MSHA, Zachary McDowell, MD, Blake Moore, MD, Brigette Booth, MHA, and Nada Wood, PhD. Cost Analysis of Flexible Ureteroscope Repairs: Evaluation of 655 Procedures in a Community-Based Practice. J Endourol Volume 30, Number 3. 2016:254–256.
6. Dale J, Kaplan AG, Radvak D, Shin R, Ackerman A, Chen T, Scales CD Jr, Ferrandino MN, Simmons WN, Preminger GM, Lipkin ME. Evaluation of a novel single-use flexible Ureteroscope. J Endourol. 2017. https://doi.org/10.1089/end.2016.0237.
7. Proietti S, Dragos L, Molina W, Doizi S, Giusti G, Traxer O. Comparison of new single-use digital flexible Ureteroscope versus nondisposable Fiber optic and digital Ureteroscope in a cadaveric model. J Endourol. 2016;30(6):655–9.
8. Doizi S, Kamphuis G, Giusti G, Andreassen KH, Knoll T, Osther PJ, et al. First clinical evaluation of a new single-use flexible ureteroscope (LithoVue™): a European prospective multicentric feasibility study. World J Urol. 2017;35(5):809–18.
9. Usawachintachit M, Isaacson DS, Taguchi K, Tzou DT, Hsi RS, Sherer BA, et al. A prospective case-control study comparing LithoVue, a single-use, flexible disposable Ureteroscope, with flexible. Reusable Fiber Optic Ureteroscopes J Endourol. 2017;31(5):468–75.
10. Martin CJ, McAdams SB, Abdul-Muhsin H, Lim VM, Nunez-Nateras R, Tyson MD, et al. The economic implications of a reusable flexible digital Ureteroscope: a cost-benefit analysis. J Urol. 2017;197(3 Pt 1):730–5
11. Mager R, Kurosch M, Höfner T, Frees S, Haferkamp A, Neisius A. Clinical outcomes and costs of reusable and single-use flexible ureterorenoscopes: a prospective cohort study. Urolithiasis. 2018;46(6):587–93.
12. Lasselin J, Viart L, Lasselin-Boyard P, Raynal G, Saint F. Flexible ureteroscope damages. Evaluation of university hospital service equipment. Prog Urol. 2015;25(5):265–73.
13. Ozimek T, Cordes J, Wiessmeyer JR, Schneider MH, Hupe MC, Gilbert N, et al. Steep Infundibulopelvic angle (IPA) as a new risk factor for flexible Ureteroscope damage and complicated postoperative course. J Endourol. 2018.
14. Taguchi K, Harper JD, Stoller ML, Duty BD, Sorensen MD, Sur RL, et al. Identifying factors associated with need for flexible ureteroscope repair: a Western Endourology STone (WEST) research consortium prospective cohort study. Urolithiasis. 2018;46(6):559–66. https://doi.org/10.1007/s00240-017-1013-y. Epub 2017 Dec 9.
15. De Coninck V, Keller EX, Rodríguez-Monsalve M, Audouin M, Doizi S, Traxer O. Systematic review on ureteral access sheaths: facts and myths. BJU Int. 2018;122(6):959–69.
16. Carey RI, Martin CJ, Knego JR. Prospective evaluation of refurbished flexible ureteroscope durability seen in a large public tertiary care center with multiple surgeons. Urology. 2014;84(1):42–5.
17. Boylu U, Oommen M, Thomas R, Lee BR. In vitro comparison of a disposable flexible ureteroscope and conventional flexible ureteroscopes. J Urol. 2009;182(5):2347–51.
18. Marchini GS, Batagello CA, Monga M, Torricelli FCM, Vicentini FC, Danilovic A, et al. In vitro evaluation of single-use digital flexible Ureteroscopes: a practical comparison for a patient-centered approach. J Endourol. 2018;32(3):184–91.

19. Davis NF, Quinlan MR, Browne C, Bhatt NR, Manecksha RP, D'Arcy FT, et al. Single-use flexible ureteropyeloscopy: a systematic review. World J Urol. 2018;36(4):529–36.
20. Cho SY, Lee JY, Shin DG, Seo IY, Yoo S, Park HK. Evaluation of performance parameters of the disposable flexible Ureterorenoscope (LITHOVUE) in patients with renal stones: a prospective, observational, single-arm. Multicenter Study Sci Rep. 2018;8(1):9795.
21. Taguchi K, Usawachintachit M, Tzou DT, Sherer BA, Metzler I, Isaacson D, et al. Micro-costing analysis demonstrates comparable costs for LithoVue compared to reusable flexible Fiberoptic Ureteroscopes. J Endourol. 2018; 32(4):267–73.

14

Atypical focal xanthogranulomatous pyelonephritis without clinical symptoms presenting as infiltrative renal cancer

Xiaobo Ding[1], Gang Wang[2], Tiejun Wang[3], Xiaobo Ma[4] and Yanbo Wang[5*]

Abstract

Background: Xanthogranulomatous pyelonephritis (XGP) is an uncommon form of chronic pyelonephritis. Most patients of XGP are diffuse in radiology and the clinical features are typical.

Case presentation: We present a case of 24-year-old female with the absence of symptoms and normal laboratory examinations. Contrast computed tomography and intravenous pyelography demonstrate infiltrative renal mass and renal cell carcinoma is presumed. Laparoscopic right radical nephrectomy is performed, but the final pathological result shows XGP.

Conclusions: As far as we know, this is the first case report of XGP without any symptoms/signs and with normal laboratory examinations. The diagnosis of atypical XGP is challenging and preoperative renal mass biopsy should be considered in special cases.

Keywords: Xanthogranulomatous pyelonephritis, Infiltrative renal cancer, Renal cancer, Kidney, Case report

Background

Xanthogranulomatous pyelonephritis (XGP) is one kind of chronic pyelonephritis and assumed as a complication of urinary tract obstruction or bacterial infection [1]. Typical characteristics of XGP are destruction of normal renal parenchyma and replacement of xanthoma cells [1, 2]. XGP has been reported from neonate to 84 years old patient and middle aged women are more common [1, 3]. Presence of clinical symptoms and typical radiologic features exist in most of XGP patients [4, 5]. Typical clinical symptoms of XGP patients are fever of unknown origin, abdomen/flank pain, weight loss, anemia or palpable renal mass, which are presented in most of the reported cases. Korkes F and colleagues retrospectively reviewed 41 cases of XGP, all patients were symptomatic [6]. Laboratory tests changes, C-reactive protein or leukocytosis, are shown in 88% of all patients [7]. The present report describes a rare case who presented without any symptoms and with normal laboratory findings, whose radiologic features show renal cancer.

Case presentation

A 24-year-old unmarried woman was incidentally admitted to our hospital during routine ultrasound examination, which showing a homogeneous solid-cystic mass with internal echoes and without well-defined margins in the right kidney. The patient was healthy and refused history of hematuria, frequency, fever, abdominal/flank pain and weight loss. Physical examination and routine laboratory tests were both

* Correspondence: wangyanb@jlu.edu.cn
[5]Department of Urology, First Hospital of Jilin University, Changchun, Jilin 130021, P.R. China
Full list of author information is available at the end of the article

normal. Contrast-enhanced computed tomography (CT) scan of the abdomen revealed a heterogeneous enhancing right renal mass with internal hypodense lesion with a diameter of 6.0 cm × 4.9 cm (Fig. 1a, b and c). Renal cancer was clinical considered but urothelial carcinoma was also possible. Intravenous pyelogram (IVP) demonstrated absence of dilatation or filling defects in the calyces (Fig. 1d). Infiltrative renal cell carcinoma was presumed and retroperitoneal laparoscopic right radical nephrectomy was performed. Pathologic examination reported macroscopically 5.5 cm × 5 cm × 3 cm sized yellow-white lesion and microscopically a granulomatous inflammation with a large number of lipid-laden xanthomatous cells, multinucleated giant cells lymphoplasmacytic as well as some neutrophile cells, supporting a diagnosis of XGP (Fig. 2). Immunohistochemical examination was not necessary based on the typical pathological characteristics of hematoxylin-eosin staining. The patient recovered uneventfully after surgery. Ultrasound was performed every year and the patient went well at follow-up 3 year later.

Discussion and conclusions

XGP is an uncommon chronic inflammation of renal parenchyma, firstly described in 1916 [8]. XGP occurs approximately 1% of pyelonephritis in adults and 16% of pediatric nephrectomy specimens [9, 10]. Recently, Stoica I and colleagues retrospectively reviewed XGP cases from 1963 to 2016. Sixty-three patients (95.5%) underwent nephrectomy and 3 patients (4.5%) underwent partial nephrectomy [4]. XGP is frequently unilateral and bilateral cases of XGP are extremely rare. Shah K and colleagues reported one bilateral XGP child case managed non-surgically [11]. Hyla-Klekot L and colleagues reported one bilateral XGP patient managed by intensive therapy and partial nephrectomy [12].

The exact etiology of XGP is unclear and most of common associated factors are long term urinary tract obstruction or infection. Renal calculi, frequently staghorn stones, may be seen in up to 100% of the published cases [6]. Altered immune response and intrinsic disturbance of leukocyte function are other possible factors [1, 5, 10].

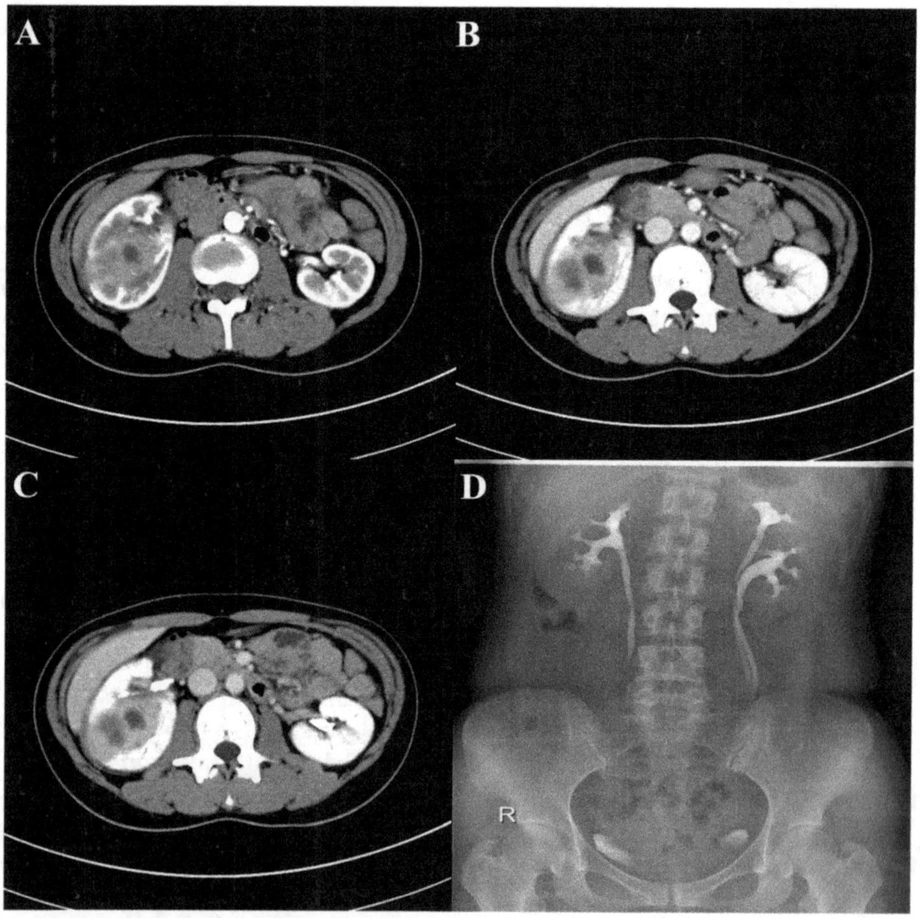

Fig. 1 Contrast-enhanced CT scan showing a 6.0 cm × 4.9 cm heterogeneous enhancing mass with hypodense areas within it in the middle of right kidney (**a**, **b** and **c**). Intravenous pyelogram showing absence of dilatation or filling defects in the right renal calyces or pelvis (**d**)

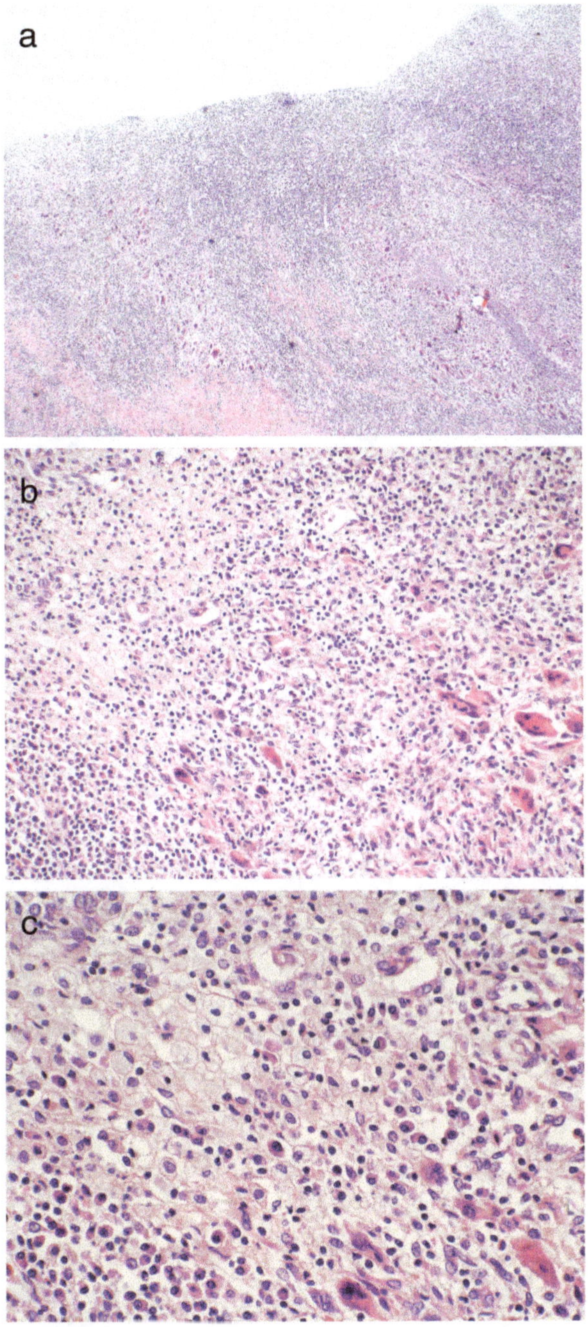

Fig. 2 Microscopically, the majority of urothelium of the renal pelvis and calyceal is necrotic and scaled (**a**). At low power, the kidney shows a granulomatous inflammation with a large number of chronic inflammatory cell infiltration and focal abscess formation (hematoxylin-eosin, original magnification × 4) (**b**). At high power, the inflammatory infiltration is composed of a large number of lipid-laden xanthomatous cells, multinucleated giant cells, lymphoplasmacytic as well as some neutrophile cells (hematoxylin-eosin, original magnification × 40) (**c**)

CT scan is priority for preoperative evaluation of XGP. Based on CT findings, XGP can be divided into diffuse type (92%) or focal type (8%) [13, 14]. Typical CT features of diffuse XGP patients are destruction of renal parenchyma and replacement by multiple, low-attenuation lesions with strong enhancement, described as "bear paw sign". Depending on the extension of inflammation, XGP can be classified as three stages: nephric XGP (stage I), perinephric XGP (stage II) and paranephric XGP (stage III). In focal XGP patients, CT frequently reveal a well-defined localized intra renal lesion with hypo-attenuation [15].

The management of XGP is different for diffuse versus focal. Nephrectomy is the standard treatment approach for diffuse XGP patients, while medical therapy with antibiotics or nephron sparring surgery is priority for focal XGP patients. In the study of Korkes F et al., all 41 cases of XGP underwent nephrectomy [6]. In the study of Çaliskan S et al., one patient underwent partial nephrectomy and 12 patients were performed nephrectomy in all 13 cases of XGP [5].

In the study of Korkes F et al, 41 cases of XGP were retrospectively reviewed and all patients were symptomatic [6]. In the study of Chlif et al., 12 pseudotumoural XGP cases were reviewed [13]. An obstructive renal stone was shown in nine patients and one patient presented with loin pain. Blood investigations showed higher C-reactive protein in one patient and gram-negative organisms in four patients. In our study, the present case did not have any abnormal clinical symptoms and/or signs. Routine laboratory tests were normal. CT and IVP revealed renal cancer rather than XGP. Atypical clinical and radiologic characteristics make the preoperatively correct diagnosis difficult. In order to avoid misdiagnosis and mistreatment, preoperative renal mass biopsy is priority, although the inevitable false negative results were objectively existed [16]. Fitouri Z reported a XGP case which was confirmed by percutaneous renal lesion biopsy. The patient was successfully treated with 8 weeks' antibiotic therapy [17]. Ho CI et al. also reported a XGP patient diagnosed by renal mass biopsy, who recovered by antibiotic therapy for 2 months [18]. Renal tumor biopsy can be used for treatment decision making, especially when a mass is suspected to be infectious, hematologic or metastatic [19, 20]. However, the indications of preoperative needle biopsy are still unclear and vary among centers.

In summary, we reported a case of focal XGP without typical clinical and radiological characteristics, which can mimic infiltrative renal cancer. In special cases, preoperative renal mass biopsy could be performed to avoid misdiagnosis and mistreatment.

Abbreviations

CT: Computed tomography; IVP: Intravenous pyelogram; XGP: Xanthogranulomatous pyelonephritis

Acknowledgements

Not Applicable.

Authors' contributions

XBD, GW, TJW reviewed the literature and drafted the manuscript; XBM performed the histopathological analysis; YBW revised the manuscript. All authors read and approved the final manuscript.

Author details

[1]Department of Radiology, First Hospital of Jilin University, Changchun, Jilin 130021, P.R. China. [2]Second Operating Room, First Hospital of Jilin University, Changchun, Jilin 130021, P.R. China. [3]Department of Orthopedic Traumatology, First Hospital of Jilin University, Changchun, Jilin 130021, P.R. China. [4]Department of Pathology, First Hospital of Jilin University, Changchun, Jilin 130021, P.R. China. [5]Department of Urology, First Hospital of Jilin University, Changchun, Jilin 130021, P.R. China.

References

1. Li L, Parwani AV. Xanthogranulomatous pyelonephritis. Arch Pathol Lab Med. 2011;135(5):671–4.
2. Sangüesa Nebot C, Picó Aliaga S, Serrano Durbá A, Roca MJ. Xantogranulomatous pyeloneprhritis in children. Insights Imaging. 2018;9(5): 643–51.
3. Ayad A, Ettouhami B, Thami B, Bentahila A. Abdominal mass revealing xanthogranulomatous pyelonephritis in an infant. Pan Afr Med J. 2017;27:17.
4. Stoica I, O'Kelly F, McDermott MB, Quinn FMJ. Xanthogranulomatous pyelonephritis in a paediatric cohort (1963–2016): Outcomes from a large single-center series. J Pediatr Urol. 2018;14(2):169.e1–7.
5. Çaliskan S, Özsoy E, Kaba S, Koca O, Öztürk MI. Xanthogranulomatous pyelonephritis. Arch Iran Med. 2016;19(10):712–4.
6. Schlagenhaufer F. Uber eigentumliche staphylomykosen der nieren und des pararenalen bindewebes. Frankf Z Pathol. 1916;19:139–48.
7. Bingöl-Koloğlu M, Ciftçi AO, Senocak ME, Tanyel FC, Karnak I, Büyükpamukçu N. Xanthogranulomatous pyelonephritis in children: diagnostic and therapeutic aspects. Eur J Pediatr Surg. 2002;12(1):42–8.
8. Schlagenhaufer F. Uber epigentumliche Staphylmykosen der Nieven und der pararenalen Bindegewebes. Frankfurt Z Pathol. 1916:139–48..
9. Siddappa S, Ramprasad K, Muddegowda MK. Xanthogranulomatous pyelonephritis: a retrospective review of 16 cases. Korean J Urol. 2011;52(6): 421–4.
10. Rao AG, Eberts PT. Xanthogranulomatous pyelonephritis: an uncommon pediatric renal mass. Pediatr Radiol. 2011;41(5):671–2.
11. Shah K, Parikh M, Pal B, Modi P. Bilateral focal xanthogranulomatous pyelonephritis in a child presenting as complex cystic renal mass: a report on non-surgical treatment. Eur J Pediatr Surg. 2011;21(3):207–8.
12. Hyla-Klekot L, Paradysz A, Kucharska G, Lipka K, Zajecki W. Successfully treated bilateral xanthogranulomatous pyelonephritis in a child. Pediatr Nephrol. 2008;23(10):1895–6.
13. Chlif M, Chakroun M, Ben Rhouma S, Ben Chehida MA, Sellami A, Gargouri MM, Nouira Y. Xanthogranulomatous pyelonephritis presenting as a pseudotumour. Can Urol Assoc J. 2016;10(1–2):E36–40.
14. Shah K, Parikh M, Gharia P, Modi PR. Xanthogranulomatous pyelonephritis-mimicking renal mass in 5-month-old child. Urology. 2012;79(6):1360–2.
15. Hendrickson RJ, Lutfiyya WL, Karrer FM, Furness PD 3rd, Mengshol S, Bensard DD. Xanthogranulomatous pyelonephritis. J Pediatr Surg. 2006; 41(2):e15–7.
16. Posielski NM, Bui A, Wells SA, Best SL, Gettle LM, Ziemlewicz TJ, Lubner MG, Hinshaw JL, Lee FT Jr, Allen GO, Nakada SY, Abel EJ. Risk factors for complications and nondiagnostic results following 1,155 consecutive percutaneous Core renal mass biopsies. J Urol. 2019;201(6):1080–7.
17. Fitouri Z, Nouira Y, Nouira K, Sallami S, Hmidi M, El Fekih N, Horchani A. Focal xanthogranulomatous pyelonephritis: success of conservative treatment. A case report. Tunis Med. 2008;86(10):912–5.
18. Ho CI, Wen YK, Chen ML. Xanthogranulomatous pyelonephritis successfully treated with antibiotics only. J Chin Med Assoc. 2008;71(12):643–5.
19. Herrera-Caceres JO, Finelli A, Jewett MAS. Renal tumor biopsy: indicators, technique, safety, accuracy results, and impact on treatment decision management. World J Urol. 2019;37(3):437–43.
20. Campbell S, Uzzo RG, Allaf ME, Bass EB, Cadeddu JA, Chang A, Clark PE, Davis BJ, Derweesh IH, Giambarresi L, Gervais DA, Hu SL, Lane BR, Leibovich BC, Pierorazio PM. Renal mass and localized renal Cancer: AUA guideline. J Urol. 2017;198(3):520–9.

15

Systemic inflammatory response syndrome in patients with acute obstructive upper tract urinary stone: A risk factor for urgent renal drainage and revisit to the emergency department

Spencer Larkin[1], Jeremy Johnson[1], Trisha Venkatesh[2], Joel Vetter[3] and Ramakrishna Venkatesh[3*]

Abstract

Background: In patients seen in the emergency department (ED) with acute stone obstruction many risk factors that indicate need for urgent renal drainage are known. However, in patients discharged from ED without renal drainage factors that can minimize revisit to the emergency department are not fully identified. We evaluated SIRS (systemic inflammatory response syndrome) as a risk factor for urgent renal drainage and revisit to the ED in patients with acute stone colic during their ED visit.

Methods: Retrospective review was performed of patients presenting to a tertiary academic emergency department (ED) from an obstructing ureteral or UPJ stone with hydronephrosis confirmed on an abdominal and pelvic CT scan. Data evaluated over a 3-year period included stone size, presence of UTI, presence or absence of SIRS and other clinical variables as risk factors for urgent renal drainage and ED revisits.

Results: 1983 patients with urolithiasis were seen at the ED and 649 patients had obstructive urolithiasis on CT scan. SIRS was diagnosed in 15% (99/649) patients. 54/99 (55%) patients with SIRS underwent urgent renal drainage compared to 99/550 (17%) in non-SIRS patients. In a multivariate analysis SIRS was a predictor of urgent intervention compared to non-SIRS patients (odds ratio 4.6, $p < 0.05$). SIRS was also associated with increased risk for revisits to the ED (6.9% with SIRS vs. 2.4% with no SIRS, odds ratio 2.9, $p = 0.05$).

Conclusions: Presence of SIRS in obstructive urolithiasis patients was an independent risk factor of acute urologic intervention and revisits to the ED. A timely consultation with a urologist following discharge from ED for obstructive stone patients with SIRS who had no acute renal drainage may prevent revisit to the ED. Evaluation for SIRS in addition to other clinical risk factors should be considered while making management decision in patients with acute stone obstruction.

Keywords: SIRS, Urolithiasis, Renal obstruction, Emergency department, Ureteral colic

* Correspondence: venkateshr1@wustl.edu
[3]Division of Urology Surgery, Washington University School of Medicine, 4960, Children's place, Campus Box 8242, St. Louis, MO 63110, USA
Full list of author information is available at the end of the article

Background

Obstructive urolithiasis is a common problem resulting in nearly 1.2 million ED visits per year in the United States [1]. A study using a nationwide emergency department sample, the largest all-payer ED database in the United States, reported an average of 19% hospital admission rate for patients presenting with ureteral colic [1]. With high prevalence rates, hospital admissions and enormous inpatient costs, identifying risk factors that affect patient revisit to the ED can help making improvements towards an efficient and safe management of ureteral stone colic patients presenting to the emergency department.

A previous study identified some of the risk factors associated with the need for acute urological intervention in patients presenting with ureteral colic [2]. These included stone size of ≥5 mm, proximal ureteral stone, presence of nitrites or leucocyte esterase on chem-strip urinalysis, age over 50 years, tachycardia at triage and abnormal serum WBC count. The above factors were independently associated with urologic intervention within 90 days in renal colic patients presenting to the ED. Another study reported on the association of pregnancy, diabetes and presence of urinary infection with higher hospital admission rates from the ED and greater cost [1]. In our cohort we studied risk factors at the initial evaluation in the emergency room including SIRS for an urgent need for renal drainage and patient disposition in patients presenting with an obstructive ureteral or UPJ stone. For patients who revisit the ED, pain is the most common variable in addition to symptoms of uti.

Systemic inflammatory response syndrome (SIRS) has been used by many clinicians as a predictor of early sign of severe sepsis in the ICU and the ED settings [3, 4]. The newer sepsis prediction assessment qSOFA (quick Sequential Organ Failure Assessment) has been well studied in an ICU setting but not so much in an ED setting. In a comparative study on predicting mortality from sepsis in an ED setting, qSOFA has shown to be less sensitive compared to SIRS, although it has better specificity [5]. The significance of the presence of SIRS in patients presenting to the ED with obstructing stone has not be previously reported. This includes questions such as 'in the presence or absence of SIRS how safe is it to discharge patients from ED with obstructing stones'. Studying SIRS during the early evaluation process in the ED may help with better management of obstructive stone patients including predicting the need for urgent urologic intervention, minimizing ED revisits and plan proper patient disposition. In the above cohort we hypothesized that presence of SIRS impacts the need for urgent renal drainage and revisit to the ED in patients presenting with an obstructing urinary stone.

Methods

After obtaining the University of Kentucky IRB approval, we performed a retrospective chart review of patients at our tertiary care academic emergency department. We identified patients using ICD-9 codes 592.0 (calculus of kidney), 592.1 (calculus of ureter) and 592.9 (urinary calculus, unspecified) and a database query was performed for 3 years (2013–2016) of adult patients presenting to the ED and included all patients that had ureteral stone or UPJ stone and hydronephrosis on CT scan. We excluded all patients who did not have a CT scan available, patients who did not have all the SIRS criteria recorded and all pediatric patients (< 18 years old). Data collected included age, gender, vital signs, WBC count, stone size, presence of urinary infection, disposition (home, inpatient admission, operating room visit for ureteral stenting), readmission to the ED and subsequent surgical intervention. The concept of SIRS was developed in 1992 and the goal was to identify risk factors for the development of severe sepsis by using common, easy-to-use clinical parameters [1]. There are four components of SIRS (temperature < 36°or > 38 °C, heart rate > 90 bpm, respiratory rate > 20 per minute, WBC# < 4000 or > 12, 000 cells/mm^3) and patients with SIRS meet at least two of these criteria. SIRS in the presence of a source of infection is sepsis. Severe sepsis is sepsis with one or more organ dysfunction. Septic shock is hypotension despite adequate fluid resuscitation along with perfusion abnormalities. We evaluated patients for the presence of UTI on urine dipstix test and urine culture, patients with sepsis (SIRS with infection), and septic shock. We also compared the outcomes in patients with and without SIRS, including positive and negative for urinary infection on dipstix test and culture. Of note, we followed as best we could, the checklist for best practice of reporting observational studies as per STROBE (The Strengthening the Reporting of Observational Studies in Epidemiology) statement [6].

Univariate and multivariate analyses was performed. A p-value of < 0.05 was considered statistically significant. For univariate analysis, Fisher's exact test was used for qualitative data and Wilcoxon sum-rank test for quantitative data. Multivariate logistic regression models were used to calculate the odds of patients needing an operative procedure and ED revisits with case wise deletion used for missing data. All analysis was performed using R version 3.2.2.

Results

A total of 5002 patients with urolithiasis were identified who visited ED that had urolithiasis among other diagnosis codes. Of these, 1983 patients were included because of their primary diagnosis was either ICD-9 code 592.0, 592.1 or 592.9. Chart reviews were performed on these 1983 patients and 649 patients were identified as having a ureteral stone or UPJ stone with hydronephrosis on CT scan and the required SIRS criteria data available. Majority of patients (77%) from ED were discharged and 23% underwent urgent renal drainage.

SIRS was present in 15% (99/649) of patients seen at the ED with obstructive urolithiasis. Only 45% of patients with SIRS were discharged from ED compared to 83% of non-SIRS patients. Over half of SIRS patients (54/99, 55%) underwent emergent surgical renal drainage compared to 17% (94/550) of non-SIRS patients. Of patients discharged home, 13% of SIRS patients and 8% of non-SIRS patients returned to ED. Clinically significant factors that predicted patients going to OR for ureteral stenting were larger stone size (7 mm vs. 4 mm, $p < 0.001$), presence of SIRS (36% vs. 9%, $p < 0.001$), presence of UTI (14% vs 0.3%, $p < 0.001$). Table 1 represents on uni and multivariate analysis the odds ratio of independent predictors requiring urgent renal drainage. Not surprisingly, sepsis had the highest odds ratio of 28, followed by urine dipstick positive for infection (odds ration of 5.5), presence of SIRS (odds ratio 4.6), and stone size (odd ratio 1.4). Among the SIRS criteria, WBC count, elevated temperature and HR had increased odds ratio of going to the operating room. Of note, all our patients in the above cohort underwent ureteral stenting for stone obstruction due to local hospital practice pattern and none had percutaneous nephrostomy. Patients with SIRS compared to non-SIRS patients are more likely to be admitted to hospital, undergo surgical intervention, had UTI (odds ratio 6.4). In our cohort presence of SIRS was indicative of UTI compared to those without SIRS. SIRS patients were also more likely to go into severe sepsis or septic shock, but the number of patients was small to make valid conclusions.

Table 2 represents patients with and without SIRS with odds ratios of different variables. Patients with SIRS had higher odds of hospital admission, surgical intervention, presence of UTI and revisit to the ED. Of note, patients with SIRS with negative urine dipstix for infection had lesser incidence of surgical intervention (23%) compared to those who had SIRS with positive dipstix (73%). Of note, 7% of patients with SIRS who were discharged from the ED had revisits to the ED compared to 2% of patients with no SIRS that were discharged from the ED ($p = 0.05$).

In a subgroup of SIRS and non-SIRS patients we compared patients with urine dipstix positive and negative for infection (Tables 3 and 4). Urine dipstix data was available in 72/99 SIRS patients (39 had negative and 33 had positive dipstix for infection) and 411/550 non-SIRS patients (356 had negative and 55 had positive dipstix for infection). Notably, 72% of SIRS patients with negative urine dipstix were discharged home compared to 21% of positive urine dipstix patients ($p < 0.001$). In comparison 88% of non-SIRS patients with negative urine dipstix was discharged home compared to 47% with positive urine dipstix. We evaluated urine dipstix, as this is a readily available test for decision-making in the ED about patient disposition, as urine culture typically is available 48–72 h later. In the non-SIRS patients with positive urine dipstix 52% underwent ureteral stenting compared to 10% with negative urine dipsitx. In our study more number of SIRS patients with dipstix negative for infection had ureteral stenting compared to non-SIRS patients ($p < 0.05$) also suggesting SIRS was an independent predictor of patients going to the OR with or without UTI. This was also confirmed by multivariate analysis. Table 5 represents patients who revisited ER and those who did not. It shows presence of SIRS was an independent risk factor (odds ratio 2.9) for revisit to the ED.

Discussion

In our tertiary hospital ED there was a 15% incidence of SIRS in the above population. Obstructing stones

Table 1 Univariate and multivariate analysis of factors for urgent renal drainage

Variable	Univariate Table			Multivariable Model			
	Urgent Drainage (No) Mean (SD) or N (%)	Urgent Drainage (Yes) Mean (SD) or N (%)	*p*-value	Odd's Ratio	95 Lower	95 Higher	*p*-value
n	501	148					
Age	41 (15)	46 (16)	0.003	1.02	1.00	1.03	0.026
Male	322 (64)	60 (40)	< 0.001	0.40	0.26	0.63	< 0.001
SIRS	45 (9)	54 (36)	< 0.001	4.63	2.65	8.09	< 0.001
Sepsis	1 (0.2)	21 (14)	< 0.001	28.47	3.57	226.99	0.002
Stone Size	4 (2.0)	7.3 (6)	< 0.001	1.40	1.28	1.53	< 0.001
Temperature (Celsius)	37 (0.3)	37 (0.6)	< 0.001	2.32	1.31	4.11	0.004
HR	79 (15)	92 (21)	< 0.001	1.03	1.01	1.04	< 0.001
RR	19 (3)	19 (3)	0.074	1.07	0.98	1.16	0.122
WBC#	10 (3)	13 (13)	< 0.001	1.16	1.09	1.23	< 0.001

Table 2 Individual Cohorts and Characteristics of SIRS and Non-SIRS patients where urine dipstix data was available (483 patients)

	Non- SIRS	SIRS	Overall	Odds Ratio for SIRS vs. Non-SIRS	*P*-value
No. patients	411	72	483		
Age (years)	41 (16–91)	44 (22–94)	42 (16–94)	1.01 (0.99–1.03)	0.309
Male (%)	247 (60)	37 (51)	284 (59)	0.70 (0.42–1.16)	0.194
Temp. (Celsius)	37 (36–38)	37 (36–39)	37 (36–39)	2.30 (1.65–3.21)	0.002
Heart Rate (beats/min)	78 (23–142)	104 (59–153)	82 (23–153)	1.09 (1.07–1.12)	< 0.001
Resp. Rate (breaths/min)	18 (10–28)	21 (15–36)	19 (10–36)	1.35 (1.23–1.49)	< 0.001
WBC # (cells/mm^3)	10 (2–159)	14 (6–41)	11 (2–159	1.10 (1.04–1.16)	< 0.001
Stone Size (mm)	5 (1–26)	5 (2–30)	5 (1–30)	1.05 (0.98–1.13)	0.521
D/C'd Home	341 (83)	35 (49)	376 (78)	0.19 (0.11–0.33)	< 0.001
To OR on 1st ED visit	64 (16)	33 (46)	97 (20)	4.59 (2.69–7.83)	< 0.001
Readmitted	10 (2)	5 (7)	15 (3)	2.99 (0.99–9.03)	0.057
Infection source identified	96 (23)	47 (65)	143 (30)	6.17 (3.61–10.55)	< 0.001
Proven infection present	60 (15)	35 (49)	95 (20)	5.53 (3.23–9.47)	< 0.001
UTI present	53 (13)	35 (49)	88 (18)	6.39 (3.71–11.02)	< 0.001
Urine culture positive	30 (7)	19 (27)	49 (10)	4.55 (2.39–8.66)	< 0.001
Urine dipstix positive	55 (14)	33 (46)	88 (18)	5.48 (3.18–9.43)	< 0.001
Severe sepsis	2 (0.5)	5 (7)	7 (1)	15.26 (2.90–80.27)	0.001
Septic shock	1 (0.2)	4 (6)	5 (1)	24.1 (2.7–219.0)	0.002

commonly result in ED visits but the majority of these patients are discharged home. Of the patients that require urgent renal drainage, many are for UTI or uncontrolled pain. There is no debate that patients with sepsis from an obstructing stone require emergent renal drainage. However, in a patient with an obstructing stone in the presence of SIRS, it is unclear what would be the patient outcome or disposition. Reports that biomarkers such as presepsin [7–9] and urine NGAL [10] improve the prognostic sensitivity of SIRS. However, these tests are experimental, costly and not commonly available in the ED in a timely manner.

Nadler et al. highlighted the stone burden on hospital admission rates and cost analysis of patients presenting with obstructing stones to the EDs across the United States [1]. Using a nationwide emergency department data sample they estimated an average of 1.2 million patients per year visiting ED yearly from 2006 to 2009 due to stones with a 19% hospital admissions. They identified infection and diabetes to be highly predictive of the need for admission on multivariate analysis. Theakston and co-authors identified stone size ≥5 mm, nitrites on urine dipstix, age > 50 years, and proximal ureteric stone as risk factors for urologic intervention within 3 months of visit to the ED. [2] Similarly, Papa et al. in addition to stone location and size, pain score upon discharge from ED was associated with urologic intervention within 1

Table 3 SIRS patients with and without urinary infection

	SIRS (dipstix negative)	SIRS (dipstix positive)	*P*-value
No. patients	39	33	
Age (years)	42 (22–73)	46 (23–94)	0.545
Male (%)	28 (72)	9 (27)	< 0.001
Temp. (Celsius)	37 (36–38)	37 (36–39)	0.070
Heart Rate (beats/min)	100 (59–136)	109 (59–153)	0.016
Resp. Rate (breaths/min)	21 (16–32)	20 (15–36)	0.398
WBC # (cells/mm^3)	14 (7–32)	15 (6–41)	0.810
Stone Size (mm)	4 (2–7)	7 (2–30)	0.136
D/C'd Home	28 (72)	7 (21)	< 0.001
To OR on 1st ED visit	9 (23)	24 (73)	< 0.001
Readmitted	3 (8)	2 (6)	1.000

Table 4 Non-SIRS patients with and without urinary infection

	Non-SIRS (dipstix negative)	Non-SIRS (dipstix positive)	*P*-value
No. patients	356	55	
Age (years)	41 (16–86)	44 (19–91)	0.195
Male (%)	229 (64)	18 (33)	< 0.001
Temp. (Celsius)	37 (36–37)	37 (36–38)	0.135
Heart Rate (beats/min)	77 (23–120)	84 (52–142)	0.025
Resp. Rate (breaths/min)	18 (10–28)	19 (16–24)	0.364
WBC # (cells/mm^3)	10 (2.5–159)	10 (2–27.5)	0.738
Stone Size (mm)	4.5 (1–17)	6 (2–26)	< 0.001
D/C'd Home	315 (88.5)	26 (47)	< 0.001
To OR on 1st ED visit	35 (10)	29 (53)	< 0.001
Readmitted	9 (2.5)	1 (2)	1.000

month after initial presentation [11]. In our study apart from SIRS as a risk factor for urgent intervention and ED revisit, we found UTI on dipstix, age, presence of fever, elevated white cell count as other risk factors with OR > 1 (Table 2).

More recently the third international consensus for sepsis and septic shock updated the definitions of sepsis and septic shock [12]. The task force uses the qSOFA (quick Sequential Organ Failure Assessment) criteria RR > 22, altered mentation, systolic ≤ BP100. In the above study, qSOFA was better than SIRS criteria in the intensive care settings but similar to SIRS in an outside the ICU setting in predicting hospital mortality. The task force stresses that SIRS criteria still remain useful for the identification of sepsis. A more recent study, where the authors did a meta-analysis comparing the association of qSOFA and SIRS in predicting patient mortality in an ED setting [5]. Their results showed that both qSOFA score of ≥2 and a SIRS score of ≥2 were strongly associated with mortality in ER patients with infections. They showed qSOFA had higher specificity (88%) but lower sensitivity (42%), compared to SIRS, which had higher sensitivity (81%) and lower specificity (41%). The authors concluded that both are important at this time and that qSOFA cannot replace the use of SIRS in the ED setting until the sensitivity of qSOFA is improved.

Yamamoto et al. revealed that patient age (median 74 years) was an independent risk factor for the development of septic shock from an obstructing stone [13]. This corroborates our findings that advanced age increased the risk for requiring surgery ($p = 0.026$) (Table 2). Friedlander and colleagues reported that for every point increase in WBC count and pulse resulted in a 7 and 3% increase in sepsis, respectively [14]. The development of SIRS after ureteroscopy for stone disease has been reported but the role of SIRS in patients with obstructive urolithiasis presenting to the ED has not been studied [15].

To our knowledge there is no previously reported study evaluating the role of SIRS in obstructing stone patients presenting to the ED. A vast majority (77%) of our patients presenting to ED with an obstructing stone

Table 5 Univariate and multivariate analysis of factors for revisit to the ED

	Revisit to ED = N	Revisit to ED = Y		Multivariable Model			
	Univariate Model						
Variable	Mean (SD) or N (%)	Mean (SD) or N(%)	*p*-value	Odd's Ratio	95 Lower	95 Higher	*p*-value
N	468	15					
Age	42 (16–94)	46 (18–70)	0.187	1.03	1.00	1.04	0.021
Male	277 (59)	7 (46)	0.426	0.50	0.26	0.54	< 0.001
SIRS	67 (14)	5 (33)	0.057	2.90	2.65	8.09	< 0.001
Sepsis	1 (0.1)	7 (1.5)	1.000	2.00	2.20	121.08	0.002
Stone Size	5 (1–30)	5 (3–13)	0.470	1.07	0.98	1.16	0.122
Temp.	37 (36–40)	37 (36–40)	0.830	1.10	1.31	3.11	0.142
Heart Rate	82 (23–153)	90 (58–116)	0.084	1.03	1.01	1.04	< 0.001
Respiratory Rate	19 (10–36)	18 (16–24)	0.370	1.07	0.98	1.16	0.122
WBC	11 (2–159)	11 (7–17)	0.849	1.06	1.08	1.23	0.121

were discharged. However, SIRS patients were less likely (45%) to be discharged home compared to non-SIRS (83%) ($p < 0.01$). This may be because more number of SIRS patients had associated UTI and also other factors such as inadequate pain control might have contributed to this. Also, patients without infection, the presence of SIRS can be a reaction to inflammation, pain or other factors. These non-infective factors may have contributed to SIRS and the need for urgent renal drainage. Patient with SIRS who were discharged from the ED were more likely to revisit the ED (7%) compared to patients with no SIRS (2%, $p = 0.05$). In our cohort, patients with SIRS had higher incidence of UTI (49%)(on urine dipstix and culture) compared to those who did not have SIRS (13%), $p < 0.01$). However, patients with SIRS who were discharged from the ED with negative urine dipstix for infection had higher incidence of ED revisits compared to patients with no SIRS and had negative urine dipstix (Tables 3 and 4). Also, patients with SIRS had a higher likelihood of going into severe sepsis, 7% compared to 0.5% with no SIRS; albeit patients' numbers were small. It is important to note that the judgment whether to drain the kidney or not should not be based solely on positive or negative urine dipstix but to be combined with other clinical factors including the presence of fever or chills, high white cell count etc.

Our hypothesis that SIRS impacts the disposition of patients including surgical intervention with obstructive urolithiasis was confirmed by this observational study. In the multivariate analysis SIRS was an independent factor associated with increased urgent surgical intervention and ED revisit. As our study was retrospective in nature, we could only conclude from our findings that SIRS is an independent risk factor for urgent drainage and revisits to the ED. The number of patients with critical illness (sepsis or septicemia) in our study group was very small and as many of our patients with SIRS had intervention, thereby preventing progression to severe sepsis or septic shock, it is difficult to conclude from the above study that SIRS is a predictor of critical illness in stone patients. Nevertheless, presence of SIRS should be an important factor in decision-making regarding patient disposition.

Limitations of our study include retrospective study design with lack of documentation of pain through a validated pain scale; hence, it is difficult to estimate the impact of pain on the patient disposition. However, all our patients had pain who had intervention and who revisited the ED with or without SIRS. We did not have urine cultures on all patients as many were discharged if the urine dipstix showed no infection. Also, some patients may have followed up at a different hospital following discharge from our ED, nevertheless as our data compared SIRS and non-SIRS patients, we presume the readmission percentage rates at other hospitals may be comparable to our center. Also, we did not have information on the stone type in the majority (> 95%) of our study population, we are not sure whether the stone type can influence which patients had SIRS with or without infection.

Conclusions

SIRS was present in only 15% patients seen in our emergency department with obstructive urolithiasis. Presence of SIRS was indicative of increased need for urgent renal drainage with ureteral stenting and ED revisits. Although patients with SIRS had increased rate of associated UTI, SIRS was an independent risk factor for urgent urologic intervention with or without the presence of urinary infection. Presence of SIRS is one other risk factor to be considered during the early evaluation of patients presenting to the ED with obstructive stone colic while making decisions about treatment. Also, patients discharged who had SIRS but no urologic intervention had increased ED revisits. Revisits to ED may be minimized if a timely urology consultation as quickly as possible is made possible for patients with SIRS who were discharged from ED.

Abbreviations

SIRS: Systemic Inflammatory Response Syndrome; ED: Emergency Department; qSOFA: quick Sequential Organ Failure Assessment); STROBE: The Strengthening the Reporting of Observational Studies in Epidemiology

Acknowledgements

Dr. Daniel Davenport, PhD, Statistician, University of Kentucky, helped with some of the initial statistics for the study.

Authors' contributions

SL contributed for data acquisition, interpretation of data and writing of manuscript. JJ contributed for design of the work, data acquisition, interpretation including analysis and writing manuscript. TV contributed for data acquisition and analysis. JV contributed for statistical analysis for the study. RV contributed for the conception, design of work, interpretation, writing manuscript and revision. Note all the authors have read and approved the above revised manuscript.

Author details

[1]Department of Urology, University of Kentucky, Lexington, KY, USA. [2]Washington University in St. Louis, St. Louis, MO, USA. [3]Division of Urology Surgery, Washington University School of Medicine, 4960, Children's place, Campus Box 8242, St. Louis, MO 63110, USA.

References

1. Eaton S, Cashy J, Pearl J, Stein D, Perry K, Nadler R. Admission rates and costs associated with emergency presentation of urolithiasis: analysis of the Nationwide emergency department sample 2006-2009. J Endourol. 2013; 27(12):1535–8.

2. Yan JW, McLeod SL, Edmonds ML, Sedran RJ, Theakston KD. Risk factors associated with urologic intervention in emergency department patients with suspected renal colic. J Emerg Med. 2015;49(2):130–5.
3. Bone RC, Balk RA, Cerra FB, et al. Definitions for sepsis and organ failure and guidelines for the use of innovative therapies in sepsis. The ACCP/SCCM Consensus Conference Committee. American College of Chest Physicians/ Society of Critical Care Medicine. Chest. 2009;136(5):article e28.
4. Kaukonen KM, Bailey M, Pilcher D, Cooper DJ, Bellomo R. Systemic inflammatory response syndrome criteria in defining severe sepsis. N Engl J Med. 2015;372(17):1629–38.
5. Jiang J, Yang J, Mei J, Jin Y, Youjin L. Head-to-head comparison of qSOFA and SIRS criteria in predicting the mortality of infected patients in the emergency department: a meta-analysis. Scand J Trauma Resusc Emerg Med. 2018;26:56.
6. von Elm E, Altman DG, Egger M, Pocock SJ, Gøtzsche PC, Vandenbroucke JP. The Strengthening the Reporting of Observational Studies in Epidemiology (STROBE) statement: guidelines for reporting observational studies. Lancet. 2007;370(9596):20–6 1453–1457.
7. Hou YS, Wang H, Chen H, Wu LF, Lu LF, He Y. Pathfast presepsin assay for early diagnosis of systemic inflammatory response syndrome in patients with nephrolithiasis. Biomed Res Int. 2015;6(2):25–8.
8. Ulla M, Pizzolato E, Lucchiari M, et al. Diagnostic and prognostic value of presepsin in the management of sepsis in the emergency department: a multicenter prospective study. Critical Care. 2013;17(4):article R168.
9. Shozushima T, Takahashi G, Matsumoto N, Kojika M, Okamura Y, Endo S. Usefulness of presepsin (sCD14-ST) measurements as a marker for the diagnosis and severity of sepsis that satisfied diagnostic criteria of systemic inflammatory response syndrome. J Infect Chemother. 2011;17(6):764–9.
10. Zhu W, Liu M, Wang GC, Che JP, Xu YF, Peng B, Zheng JH. Urinary neutrophil gelatinase-associated lipocalin, a biomarker for systemic inflammatory response syndrome in patients with nephrolithiasis. J Surg Res. 2014;187(1):237–43.
11. Papa L, Stiell IG, Wells GA, et al. Predicting intervention in renal colic patients after emergency department evaluation. CJEM. 2005;7:78–86.
12. Singer M, Deutschman CS, Angus D, et al. The third international consensus definitions for Sepsis and septic shock. JAMA. 2016;315(8):801–10.
13. Yamamoto Y, Fujita K, Nakazawa S, et al. Clinical characteristics and risk factors for septic shock in patients receiving emergency drainage for acute pyelonephritis with upper urinary tract calculi. BMC Urol. 2014;12:4–9.
14. Freidlander J, Jaimes, Garces J, Cuervo J, Ramirez F, Ramirez J, Vargas A, et al. The systemic inflammatory response syndrome (SIRS) to identify infected patients in the emergency room. Intensive Care Med. 2003;29: 1368–71.
15. Southern JB, Higgins AM, Young AJ, Garg T, et al. Risk factors for post-operative fever and SIRS for stone disease. J Endourol. 2019;33([illegible]):[illegible]

Small renal masses in Latin-American population: Characteristics and prognostic factors for survival, recurrence and metastasis – A multi-institutional study from LARCG database

Thiago Camelo Mourão[1*], Diego Abreu[2], Gustavo F. Carvalhal[3], Guillermo Gueglio[4], Walter H. da Costa[1], Vinicius Fernando Calsavara[5], Luis Meza-Montoya[6], Rubén G. Bengió[7], Carlos Scorticati[8], Ricardo Castillejos-Molina[9], Francisco Rodríguez-Covarrubias[9], Ana María Autran-Gómez[10], José Gadu Campos-Salcedo[11], Alejandro Nolazco[12], Carlos Ameri[13], Hamilton Zampolli[14], Raúl Langenhin[15], Diego Muguruza[15], Marcos Tobias Machado[14,16], Pablo Mingote[17], Jorge Clavijo[18], Lucas Nogueira[19], Omar Clark[20], Agustín R. Rovegno[21], Fernando P. Secin[22], Ricardo Decia[2], Gustavo C. Guimarães[23], Sidney Glina[16,24], Oscar Rodríguez-Faba[25], Joan Palou[25] and Stenio C. Zequi[1,26]

Abstract

Background: To evaluate demographic, clinical and pathological characteristics of small renal masses (SRM) (≤ 4 cm) in a Latin-American population provided by LARCG (Latin-American Renal Cancer Group) and analyze predictors of survival, recurrence and metastasis.

Methods: A multi-institutional retrospective cohort study of 1523 patients submitted to surgical treatment for non-metastatic SRM from 1979 to 2016. Comparisons between radical (RN) or partial nephrectomy (PN) and young or elderly patients were performed. Kaplan-Meier curves and log-rank tests estimated 10-year overall survival. Predictors of local recurrence or metastasis were analyzed by a multivariable logistic regression model.

Results: PN and RN were performed in 897 (66%) and 461 (34%) patients. A proportional increase of PN cases from 48.5% (1979–2009) to 75% (after 2009) was evidenced. Stratifying by age, elderly patients (≥ 65 years) had better 10-year OS rates when submitted to PN (83.5%), than RN (54.5%), $p = 0.044$. This disparity was not evidenced in younger patients. On multivariable model, bilaterality, extracapsular extension and ASA (American Society of Anesthesiologists) classification ≥3 were predictors of local recurrence. We did not identify significant predictors for distant metastasis in our series.

(Continued on next page)

* Correspondence: thiagocmourao@gmail.com
[1]A.C. Camargo Cancer Center, Rua Antônio Prudente 211, Liberdade, São Paulo 01509-010, Brazil
Full list of author information is available at the end of the article

(Continued from previous page)
Conclusions: PN is performed in Latin-America in a similar proportion to developed areas and it has been increasing in the last years. Even in elderly individuals, if good functional status, sufficiently fit to surgery, and favorable tumor characteristics, they should be encouraged to perform PN. Intending to an earlier diagnosis of recurrence or distant metastasis, SRM cases with unfavorable characteristics should have a more rigorous follow-up routine.

Keywords: Kidney cancer, Nephron-sparing surgery, Latin America, Renal cell carcinoma, Nephrectomy

Background

Comprehensive approach of renal cell carcinoma (RCC) is a priority in the main cancer centers. Increasing trend in incidence, particularly of incidentally detected small renal masses (SRM), has not been clearly associated to a significant decrease in global mortality. According to the SEER (Surveillance, Epidemiology, and End Results) database, the estimated number of new cases of RCC in the United States in 2019 is 73,820. RCC represents about 4% of all new cancer cases and about 2.5% of all cancer deaths [1–3].

Latin America (LA) represents a large area with about 8.5% of the world population, most of them living in developing countries. GLOBOCAN estimated the RCC incidence and mortality in LA in 4.4/100,000 and 1.5/100,000, respectively [4]. Recently, an elegant study suggested that in 2030, LA countries (Brazil and Ecuador) will experiment the highest burden of increase of new cases in both genders [5]. RCC data in LA are scarce and, over time, miscegenation has impacted this population in a singular ethnicity, which could make unreliable extrapolating biomolecular profiles and guided therapies already stablished in developed world populations [6].

Nephron-sparing surgery (NSS) is the standard of care for SRM, providing equivalent oncological control and a decrease in the non-cancer related mortality [7, 8]. Besides that, even with the improvement of minimally-invasive and robotic techniques, large series continue to evidence a high proportion of radical nephrectomy (RN) in this setting [7, 9–11].

Considering the paucity of information about RCC in LA, the aims of this study were to review the LARCG (Latin-American Renal Cancer Group) database to evaluate demographic, clinical and pathologic features of SRM in this population, correlating the impact in prognosis and survival in comparison to literature.

Methods

Data source

This is a multi-institutional retrospective cohort study involving the registries from 28 institutions in LA and Spain, members of LARCG [6]. Data were collected from patient charts and pathological reports from each institution with a total of 6039 cases of RCC operated from 1979 to 2016 in Argentina, Bolivia, Brazil, Chile, Mexico, Peru, Uruguay, and two Spanish centers. Institutional Review Board of Fundação Antônio Prudente approved this protocol (number 2.478.489, CAAE: 71749917.3.0000.5432/January 30th 2018) and the study did not interfere with the treatment or follow-up of the patients.

Study population and variables definition

We selected patients with renal tumors up to 4 cm on pathological reports and no evidence of distant metastasis at presentation. We found 1523 patients with these characteristics which were stratified by histologic subtype criteria in clear cell, papillary, chromophobe or others (collecting duct carcinoma, TTFE3 gene, unclassified and mixed histologies) and by surgical treatment: partial nephrectomy (PN) or RN. Firstly, we excluded patients with benign histology and those with missing values for histologic subtype. Afterwards, non-surgical management cases were excluded.

Demographic, clinical and pathological variables selected were age, gender, race, body mass index (BMI), smoking status, ECOG (Eastern Cooperative Oncology Group) Performance Status, Karnofsky and ASA (American Society of Anesthesiologists) classifications, symptoms at presentation, tumor size (≤ 3 cm or > 3 – 4 cm), positive surgical margins (PSM), nuclear Fuhrman grade (low or high grade), intratumoral necrosis, sarcomatoid component, extracapsular extension (ECE), multifocality or bilaterality, and admission period (before or after 2009). Patients were considered symptomatic at presentation if they had hematuria, local pain, palpable mass, paraneoplastic syndrome, neurological symptoms, acute onset varicocele and constitutional symptomatology. Nuclear grade was just established for clear cell and papillary RCC [12]. ECE was considered in cases presenting disease in perinephric fat, hilar fat and/or in renal pelvis.

Follow-up was established from the date of surgery to the date of death or to the latest follow-up. Treatment indications and follow-up routine were determined at the discretion of each center. Overall deaths considered deaths due to the renal cancer and deaths from other causes. Local recurrence was defined as recurrence in the renal fossa after RN, and demonstration of recurrent enhancement within the tumor bed or enhancing suspicious lesion in the ipsilateral kidney after PN.

Authors used a multiple imputation method only in variables with a limited proportion of missing data [13]. The data were assumed to be missing completely at random (MCAR) and a method of predictive mean machine (PMM) was adopted [14]. Variables with more than 50% of missing data and non-attributable characteristics (e.g., race, and histological subtype) were not submitted to the imputation method. This method was used for the following variables: perinephric fat invasion (24% of missing data), smoking status (32% of missing data), intratumoral necrosis (41% of missing data), weight (42% of missing data), and ECOG performance status (44% of missing data).

Statistical analysis

Continuous variables were expressed as mean, standard deviation, median and interquartile range. Categorical variables were expressed as absolute relative frequencies. They were compared with a Pearson's chi-squared test or a Fisher's exact test, when appropriate. Student's *t*-test was used to compare continuous variables. Kaplan-Meier curves and log-rank tests were used in 10-year overall survival (OS) estimation, according age, tumor size and surgery performed. Considering that some patients underwent the surgical treatment at a referral center and then return to their communities, survival analysis were performed only for patients with follow-up ≥ 12 months. Univariable and multivariable logistic regression analysis were used to predict independent factors for local recurrence or distant metastasis. Related to these outcomes, it was considered the entire period, including all the patients regardless of the available follow-up time. The analysis was conducted using IBM SPSS®software v.24 (IBM Corp. Armonk, NY, USA) and the packages R-Software v. 3.5 for graphical analysis. The significance level of the tests were fixed at 0.05.

Results

A total of 1008 cases had a defined malignant histologic subtype, being 651 cases (64.6%) of clear cell RCC, 60 (6%) of papillary RCC (types I and II), 238 (23.6%) of chromophobe RCC, and 59 (6%) of other histologies. PN and RN were performed in 897 (66%) patients and 461 (34%), respectively. The proportion of PN cases increased from 48.5% (up to 2009) to almost 75% after that year. Table 1 summarizes the main clinical and pathological characteristics.

Regarding surgical aspects of PN cases, open and minimally-invasive approaches (laparoscopic, retroperitoneoscopic or robot-assisted) were performed in 47.9 and 50.4%, respectively. Median blood loss was 200 mL (5 – 2500 mL), median warm ischemia time was 20 min, and median hospital stay was 4 days (1–37).

The median follow-up time was 24 months (range: 0–289). We reported 72 (4.7%) overall deaths and 30 (2.0%) cancer-specific deaths. Local recurrence occurred in 49 (6.1%) from 804 cases and metastasis during follow-up, in 10 (1.7%) from 588 evaluable cases.

There were no significant differences in 10-year OS rates comparing patients with SRM ≤ 3 cm or > 3 cm. Similarly, OS rates were not different between patients underwent PN or RN. The 5-year and 10-year OS rates for SRM ≤ 3 cm were 95.1 and 80.3%, respectively. For SRM > 3 cm, 5-year and 10-year OS rates were 94.1 and 74.8%, respectively (Fig. 1-a). Patients underwent PN presented the 5-year and 10-year OS of 96.9 and 88.8%, respectively; whereas RN cases achieved 93.2 and 74.2%, respectively (Fig. 1-b).

Stratifying by age, elderly patients (≥ 65 years) had better 10-year OS rates when submitted to PN (83.5%), than RN (54.5%), $p = 0.044$ (Fig. 2-b). This disparity was not evidenced in younger patients (Fig. 2-a). Elderly group presented more comorbidities, ASA ≥ 3, larger SRM, and a higher proportion of RN than younger. A crosstab analysis considering younger and elderly patients is presented in Table 2.

On univariable analysis, extracapsular extension (ECE), ASA classification and bilaterality were associated with recurrence (data not shown). On multivariable model, bilaterality, ECE and ASA classification ≥3 were significant predictors of local recurrence. We did not identify significant predictors for distant metastasis in our series (Table 3).

Discussion

Several reports attempt to provide information regarding predictive clinical, pathological and molecular factors in RCC leading to aggressive histology or unfavorable outcomes. Majority of published literature is provided from developed countries. After the propagation of cross-sectional images, incidence of SRM has increased worldwide, as we verified in LA. Some of them may present adverse clinico-pathological features, potentially compromising the oncological outcomes. NSS demonstrates lower rates of chronic kidney disease or cardiovascular events. However, there are some issues about oncological efficacy of PN in comparison to RN [8, 15, 16].

In literature, benign SRM are found in 13 to 30% of the cases and about 40% correspond to low aggressiveness [17–19]. A recent study from Mexico, involving elderly patients, reported 26% of pT1a [20]. Our series evidenced a similar proportion of pT1a cases (25.2%). However, we were not able to report reliable data about benign SRM, because many centers could have rejected information of benign lesions in their database.

Table 1 Comparison of clinical and pathological data between patients with small renal masses who performed partial or radical nephrectomy

Variable Category	Partial Nephrectomy (*n* = 897)	Radical Nephrectomy (*n* = 461)	*p* Value *
Year of the surgery			
Up to 2009 n (%)	225 (48.5)	239 (51.5)	**< 0.001**
Since 2010 n (%)	637 (74.9)	214 (25.1)	
Age (years)			
Mean (SD)	57.9 (12.7)	61.2 (12.8)	**< 0.001**
Median (Q1 - Q3)	59 (50–67)	63 (53–71)	
BMI (Body Mass Index)			
Mean (SD)	27.6 (4.8)	27.5 (4.9)	0.661
Median (Q1 – Q3)	26.9 (24.2–29.9)	26.7 (24.2–30)	
Blood Transfusion n (%)	107 (12.6)	43 (10.5)	0.317
Serum Creatinine - mg/dL			
Baseline - Mean (SD)	1.02 (0.61)	1.23 (1.23)	**0.011**
Median (Q1 – Q3)	0.96 (0.86–1.1)	1.0 (0.8–1.2)	
Post-operative - Mean (SD)	1.13 (0.51)	1.50 (1.50)	**0.003**
Median (Q1 – Q3)	1.1 (0.9–1.3)	1.3 (1.1–1.5)	
Operation time – min			
Mean (SD)	174.4 (76.6)	197.3 (86.8)	**< 0.001**
Median (Q1 – Q3)	120 (90–180)	180 (120–240)	
ECOG			
0–1 n (%)	862 (96.1)	437 (94.8)	0.329
≥ 2 n (%)	35 (3.9)	24 (5.2)	
Karnofsky			
≤ 80 n (%)	74 (8.2)	46 (10)	0.336
> 80 n (%)	823 (91.8)	415 (90.0)	
ASA classification			
1–2 n (%)	767 (85.5)	359 (77.9)	**0.001**
≥ 3 n (%)	130 (14.5)	102 (22.1)	
Renal tumor			
Exophytic tumor	236 (62.8)	140 (37.2)	**< 0.001**
Totally endophytic tumor	19 (26.0)	54 (74.0)	
≤ 3 cm	538 (74.8)	181 (25.2)	**< 0.001**
3.1 - 4 cm	261 (53.0)	231 (47.0)	
Extracapsular extension n (%)			
Yes	51 (6.9)	87 (20.8)	**< 0.001**
No	686 (93.1)	332 (79.2)	
Surgical Margins n (%)			
Positive	42 (4.7)	7 (1.6)	**0.008**
Negative	844 (95.3)	422 (98.4)	
Nuclear grade			
Low grade n (%)	685 (76.4)	330 (71.6)	0.064
High grade n (%)	212 (23.6)	131 (28.4)	

Table 1 Comparison of clinical and pathological data between patients with small renal masses who performed partial or radical nephrectomy *(Continued)*

Variable Category	Partial Nephrectomy (*n* = 897)	Radical Nephrectomy (*n* = 461)	*p* Value *
Sarcomatoid component n (%)			
Yes	2 (0.6)	3 (1.2)	0.654
No	354 (99.4)	253 (98.8)	
Tumoral necrosis n (%)			
Yes	104 (11.6)	77 (16.7)	**0.011**
No	793 (88.4)	384 (83.3)	
Multifocality n (%)			
Yes	41 (5.0)	33 (7.7)	0.070
No	782 (95.0)	395 (92.3)	
Locoregional recurrence n (%)			
Yes	19 (4.4%)	26 (7.2%)	0.126
No	410 (95.6%)	334 (92.8%)	

* *p*-Value < 0.05 considered statistically significant. Pearson's chi-squared test or Fisher's exact test were used in categorical variables when appropriate. Student's t-test was used in continuous variables

The proportion of PN or RN in the surgical treatment of SRM was clearly heterogeneous comparing this decade with the first period of the study (up to 2009). This can be attributable to the development of minimally invasive techniques, the better expertise of the LA referral centers, and the stage migration with the raise of SRM in the last years [21]. Sun et al. [22] described that PN for SRM increased from 4.7% in 1988 to 40.4% in 2008. A recent British study showed more than 90% of NSS performed in T1 tumors [10]. Cases with lower mean age and less comorbidities had PN performed more frequently. Interestingly, the mean operation time in PN was significantly lower than in RN, maybe due to factors related to the patients or to the participating centers (teaching hospitals or communitarian hospitals).

From 1983 to 2002, overall mortality rose in patients with RCC in the USA. In tumors < 2 cm, this rise was 0.07 to 0.2 deaths per 100,000. In tumors between 2 and 4 cm, this rise was from 0.2 to 1.5 deaths per 100,000 US population [23]. Considering only patients with at least 12-months of follow-up, our 5-year and 10-year OS were 94.7 and 81.3%, respectively. Tumor size in our SRM casuistic did not affect the 10-year OS. Interestingly, Jeon [19] pointed that in studies limited to small tumors, they may not find associations with size and favorable histologic features.

Considering that elderly people have more comorbidities and that RN can proportionate a higher risk of renal dysfunction [20, 24], we found that NSS is associated with a better 10-year OS in this population. Russel [25] analyzed patients ≥80 years of age and described a

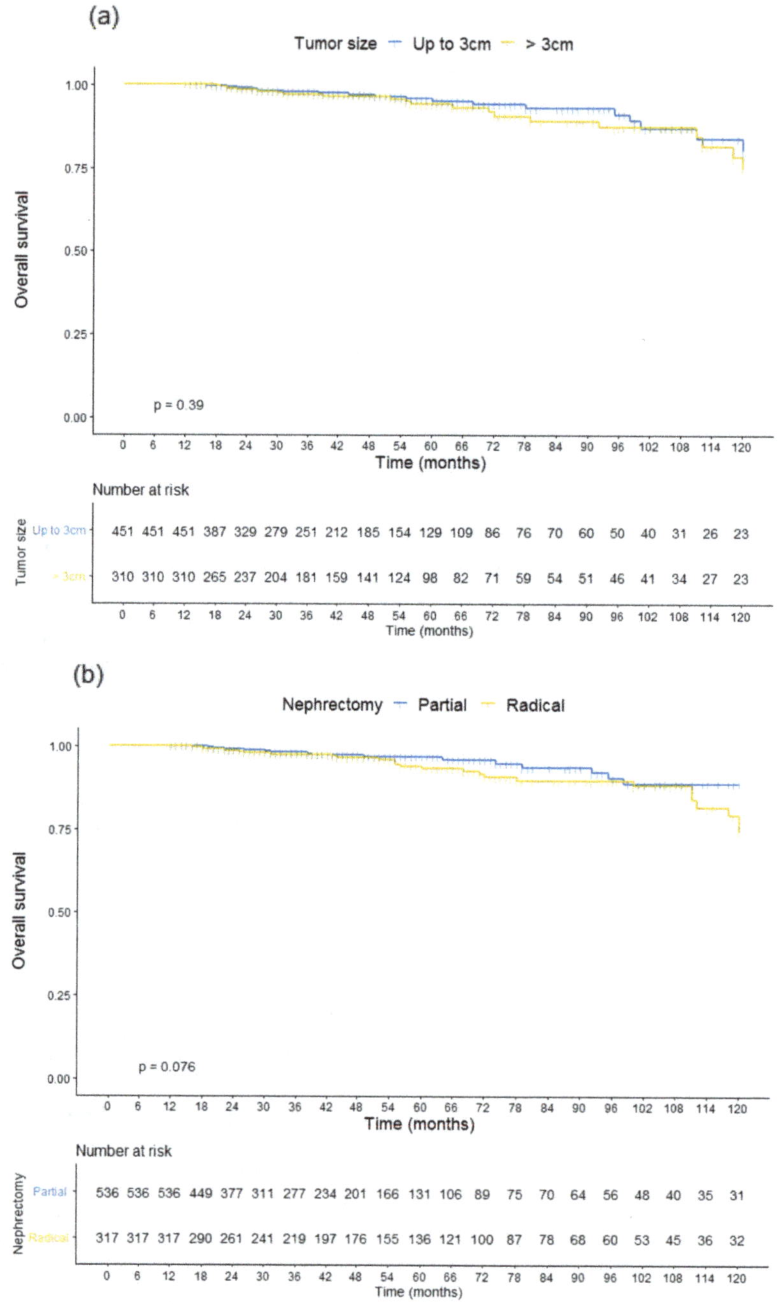

Fig. 1 Kaplan-Meier curve for 10-year overall survival (OS) in evaluable patients according to the tumor size (**a**) and the surgical treatment (**b**)

decreased RCC-specific mortality for tumors larger than 3 cm submitted to surgery. A previous series from Mayo Clinic found also an association of RN for pT1a tumors and a decreased OS, but particularly in younger patients (< 66 years of age) [26]. Similarly, in a recent Cochrane review, PN was associated with a reduced time-to-death of any cause (HR: 1.50, 95%CI: 1.03–2.18) [27]. The effect of age on cancer-specific mortality was tested in a recent study. Elderly patients (≥ 70 years) evidenced larger masses, a higher nuclear grade, and presented worse OS and CSS in comparison with those patients < 70 years [28]. Similarly to our study, elderly patients underwent more frequently to RN than PN. Treatment decisions favoring PN in selected SRM in elderly patients should be discussed, particularly if we consider that reference centers have acquired expertise on minimally invasive techniques.

The benefits of regional or retroperitoneal lymphadenectomy are controversial, particularly in small renal masses, that rarely present positive lymph nodes. The

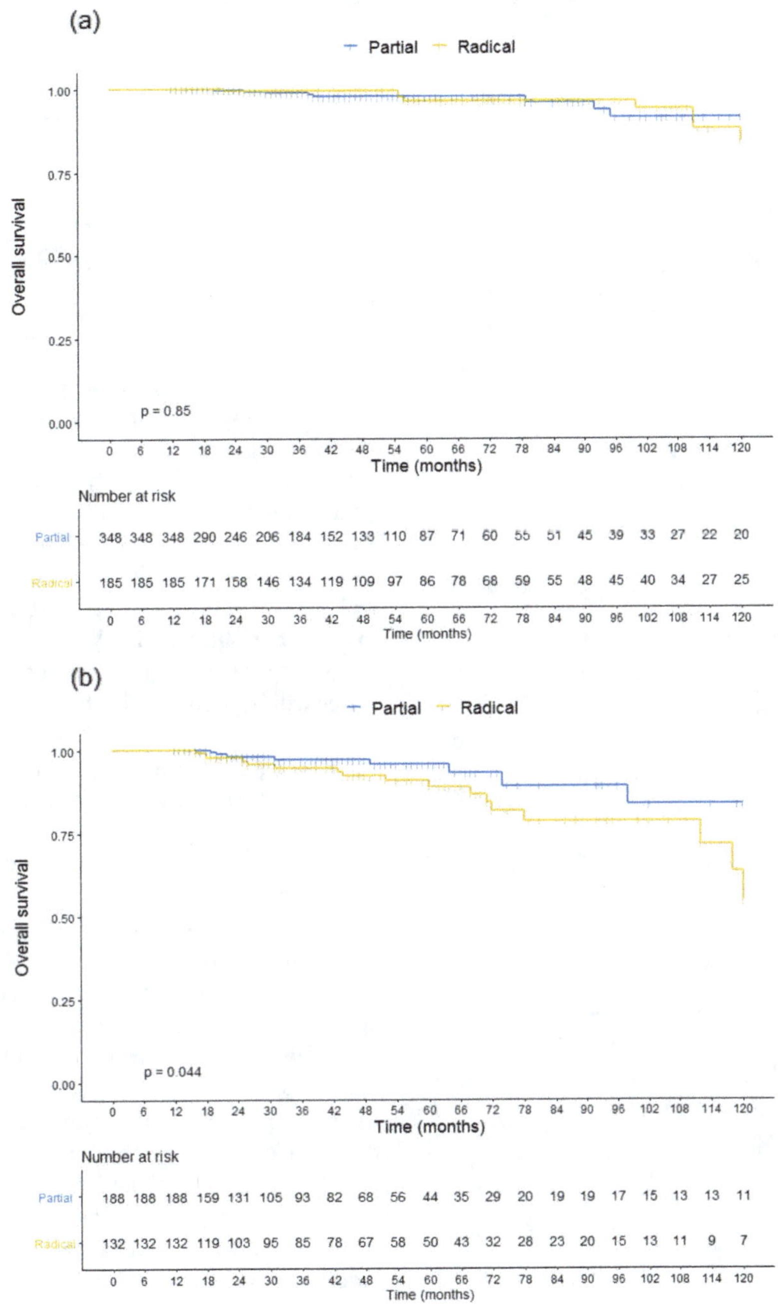

Fig. 2 Kaplan Meier curve for 10-year overall survival (OS) comparing patients submitted to PN or RN according to the group of age. **a** < 65 years **b** ≥ 65 years

extent and number of retroperitoneal lymph nodes removed have no defined templates. Marchioni et al [29] studied pT2-pT3 renal masses treated with RN and evidenced no gain in CSS related to the lymph nodes dissection (LND). In our study, LND was not analyzed because it is not a routine procedure in SRM, even when it is treated with RN.

Ball et al. [30] described that male gender, tumor size ≥3 cm and R.E.N.A.L. nephrometry score ≥ 8 are predictive of unfavorable pathology in cT1a cases. Other recent study with SRM under AS described 2% of distant metastasis during follow-up and associated non-black race, male gender, high nuclear grade, clear cell subtype and tumor size as independent predictors [31]. We were able to find an association of ECE with local recurrence, but not with distant metastasis. ECE is a rare event in SRM, due to this reason, we aggregated perinephric fat invasion, hilar fat invasion, and renal pelvis invasion in

Table 2 Comparison of clinical and surgical data between younger (< 65 years) and elderly patients (≥ 65 years) with small renal masses

	< 65 years (**n** = 949)	≥ 65 years (**n** = 574)	**p** Value *
Gender			
Male n (%)	644 (68.1)	378 (66.3)	0.496
Female n (%)	301 (31.9)	192 (33.7)	
Comorbidities n (%)			
Yes	552 (61.3)	387 (72.6)	**< 0.001**
No	349 (38.7)	146 (27.4)	
Hypertension n (%)	115 (18.0)	128 (37.8)	**< 0.001**
Obesity n (%)			
Yes	229 (24.9)	131 (23.6)	0.634
No	691 (75.1)	423 (76.4)	
Smoking n (%)			
Yes	339 (35.7)	190 (33.1)	0.324
No	610 (64.3)	384 (66.9)	
Symptomatic at presentation n (%)			
Yes	442 (46.6)	260 (45.3)	0.666
No	507 (53.4)	314 (54.7)	
Serum Creatinine - mg/dL			
Baseline - Mean (SD)	1.04 (0.81)	1.17 (0.92)	**0.045**
Median (Q1 – Q3)	0.96 (0.83–1.1)	1.0 (0.83–1.2)	
Post-operative - Mean (SD)	1.20 (0.79)	1.35 (1.22)	0.143
Median (Q1 – Q3)	1.1 (0.9–1.33)	1.2 (1.01–1.41)	
Tumor size			
≤ 3 cm n (%)	487 (62.3)	255 (55.6)	**0.023**
> 3 cm n (%)	295 (37.7)	204 (44.4)	
Surgical treatment			
Partial Nephrectomy n (%)	602 (69.7)	295 (59.7)	**< 0.001**
Radical Nephrectomy n (%)	262 (30.3)	199 (40.3)	
Histologic subtype			
Clear cell n (%)	401 (64.8)	250 (64.3)	0.921
Non-clear cell n (%)	218 (35.2)	139 (35.7)	
Nuclear grade n (%)			
Low grade	224 (23.6)	166 (28.9)	**0.025**
High grade	725 (76.4)	408 (71.1)	
Extracapsular extension n (%)			
Yes	81 (10.9)	60 (14.0)	0.140
No	661 (89.1)	368 (86.0)	
ECOG			
0–1 n (%)	912 (96.1)	543 (94.6)	0.212
≥ 2 n (%)	37 (3.9)	31 (5.4)	
Karnofsky			
≤ 80 n (%)	73 (7.7)	69 (12.0)	**0.006**
> 80 n (%)	876 (92.3)	505 (88.0)	

Table 2 Comparison of clinical and surgical data between younger (< 65 years) and elderly patients (≥ 65 years) with small renal masses *(Continued)*

	< 65 years (**n** = 949)	≥ 65 years (**n** = 574)	**p** Value *
ASA classification			
1–2 n (%)	822 (86.6)	421 (73.3)	**< 0.001**
≥ 3 n (%)	127 (13.4)	153 (26.7)	

* *p*-Value < 0.05 considered statistically significant. Pearson's chi-squared test or Fisher's exact test were used in categorical variables when appropriate. Student's t-test was used in continuous variables

this variable. This feature was seldom evidenced and it demonstrated an ominous factor in the follow-up of these patients.

Furthermore, bilaterality and ASA classification ≥3 associated with local recurrence following surgery. Patients classified with ASA ≥ 3 can present more aggressive tumors [32, 33]. Usually, these patients have routine clinical appointments and, probably, perform more image exams than fit people. We suggest that these patients can have earlier diagnosis of recurrence than others.

Regarding nephrometry, patients with totally endophytic tumors performed RN more than three times than patients with exophytic tumors (76% vs. 24%). Due to the historic long-time design of this series, we have no confident data of nephrometry scores (e.g.: R.E.N.A.L.). We did not find differences between totally endophytic or exophytic tumors in OS neither in our recurrence or distant metastasis analysis (data present in only 449 cases).

There are limitations in our study, including the retrospective design and heterogeneity of each center. Pathologic reports were provided by different pathologists and central pathology review was performed only in Brazilian cases (*N* = 244). Furthermore, the heterogeneity of the different centers and the long period of this series could lead to a selection bias of the elderly patients underwent PN or RN. Proposed protocols regarding surgical approaches have been changed during the last decades. Additionally, we did not include patients treated with non-surgical approaches, such as active surveillance, watchful waiting, or ablative treatments, which are possible options in SRM, particularly in elderly or in patients with multiple comorbidities. Due to the lack of data, we were not able to report the nephrometry score of the cases. Related to the secondary outcomes for local recurrence and distant metastasis, we were unable to define the exact moment of the event. Thus, a logistic regression model was the most appropriate for the analysis of secondary outcomes, instead of a survival analysis. Finally, the short median follow-up time of 24 months could be related to possible influences on survival outcomes. Despite these limitations, this study is one of the

Table 3 Multivariable logistic regression analysis of predictive factors for local recurrence (a) and metastasis during follow-up (b)

(a) Variable	Category	OR	95% CI	*p* Value *
Signs and symptoms at diagnosis	–	1.265	0.593–2.694	0.543
Bilaterality	Bilateral tumors	5.936	2.104–16.746	**0.001**
Extracapsular extension		2.700	1.216–5.995	**0.015**
ASA classification	ASA ≥ 3	3.380	1.643–6.957	**0.001**
(b) Variable	**Category**	**OR**	**95% CI**	***p* Value ***
Gender	Male	4.494	0.545–37.058	0.163
Bilaterality	Bilateral tumors	2.112	0.235–18.954	0.504
Extracapsular extension		3.849	0.881–16.821	0.073
Histologic subtype	Non-clear cell	Ref.	–	–
	Clear Cell	2.464	0.484–12.531	0.277

* *p*-Value < 0.05 considered statistically significant

largest known series of patients with small renal masses in Latin America. Many of the involved institutions are referral centers or teaching institutions. They tend to have skilled uropathologists, more detailed pathology records, and more available data about oncological outcomes. The results are important to recognize particular features of SRM in LA and to counsel patients about appropriate decisions.

Conclusions

RN is still overly done in the SRM setting in LA. However, NSS procedures are performed in a proportion similar to developed areas and has been increasing in the last years. RN might be considered an overtreatment for many of these patients. Even in elderly individuals, if good functional status, sufficiently fit to surgery, and presenting favorable tumor characteristics, they should be encouraged to underwent PN. Posteriorly, a more intense follow-up routine could be discussed in SRM cases with unfavorable characteristics, intend to an earlier diagnosis of recurrence or distant metastasis.

Abbreviations

ASA: American Society of Anesthesiologists; BMI: Body Mass Index; ECE: Extracapsular extension; ECOG: Eastern Cooperative Oncology Group; LA: Latin America; LND: Lymph nodes dissection; NSS: Nephron-sparing surgery; OS: Overall Survival; PN: Partial Nephrectomy; PSM: Positive surgical margins; RCC: Renal Cell Carcinoma; RN: Radical Nephrectomy; SRM: Small Renal Mass

Acknowledgments

We would like to thank, in special, all participants of LARCG who contributed to this database.

Authors' contributions

TCM was involved in data analysis and manuscript writing; GFC, GG, WHC, LM, RB, CS, RC, FR, AMA, JG, AN, CA, HZ, RL, DM, MTM, PM, JC, LN, OC, AR, FPS, RD, GCG, SG, ORF, JP were involved in data collection and project development; VFC was involved in statistical analysis; DA was involved in group and database coordination. SCZ was involved in the idealization of the study, data collection, project development, and manuscript revision. Manuscript was approved by the authors.

Author details

[1]A.C. Camargo Cancer Center, Rua Antônio Prudente 211, Liberdade, São Paulo 01509-010, Brazil. [2]Pasteur Hospital, Montevideo, Uruguay. [3]São Lucas Hospital – PUCRS, Porto Alegre, Brazil. [4]Italian Hospital, Buenos Aires, Argentina. [5]Epidemiology and Statistics Department, International Research Center, A.C.Camargo Cancer Center, São Paulo, Brazil. [6]Instituto Nacional de Enfermedades Neoplásicas, Lima, Peru. [7]Urological Center Profesor Bengió, Cordoba, Argentina. [8]Clinics Hospital José de San Martín, Buenos Aires, Argentina. [9]Instituto Nacional de Ciencias Médicas y Nutrición Salvador Zubirán (INCNSZ), Mexico City, Mexico. [10]Jiménez Díaz Foundation, Madrid, Spain. [11]Military Hospital, Mexico City, Mexico. [12]British Hospital, Buenos Aires, Argentina. [13]German Hospital, Buenos Aires, Argentina. [14]Instituto Arnaldo Vieira de Carvalho, São Paulo, Brazil. [15]Corporación Médica de Paysandú (COMEPA), Paysandu, Uruguay. [16]ABC Medical School, São Paulo, Brazil. [17]Policlinico Neuquén, Neuquen, Argentina. [18]Clinics Hospital, Montevideo, Uruguay. [19]Federal University of Minas Gerais, Belo Horizonte, Brazil. [20]Military Hospital, Montevideo, Uruguay. [21]Centro de Educación Médica e Investigaciones Clínicas (CEMIC), Buenos Aires, Argentina. [22]San Lázaro Foundation and FUNDES, Buenos Aires, Argentina. [23]Surgical Oncology Coordinator at Beneficencia Portuguesa Hospital, São Paulo, Brazil. [24]Ipiranga Hospital, São Paulo, Brazil. [25]Puigvert Foundation, Barcelona, Spain. [26]National Institute for Science and Technology in Oncogenomics and Therapeutic Innovation, AC Camargo Cancer Center, São Paulo, Brazil.

References

1. Siegel RL, Miller KD, Jemal A. Cancer statistics, 2019. CA Cancer J Clin. 2019; 69:7–34 https://doi.org/10.3322/caac.21551.
2. Nguyen MM, Gill IS, Ellison LM. The evolving presentation of renal carcinoma in the United States: trends from the surveillance, epidemiology, and end results program. J Urol. 2006;176:2397–400 https://doi.org/10.1016/j.juro.2006.07.144.
3. Volpe A, Jewett MAS. The natural history of small renal masses. Nat Clin Pract Urol. 2005;2:384–90 https://doi.org/10.1038/ncpuro0254.
4. Bray F, Ferlay J, Soerjomataram I, et al (2018) Global cancer statistics 2018: GLOBOCAN estimates of incidence and mortality worldwide for 36 cancers in 185 countries. CA Cancer J Clin 0:1–31. https://doi.org/10.3322/caac.21492.
5. Wong MCS, Goggins WB, Yip BHK, et al. Incidence and mortality of kidney cancer: temporal patterns and global trends in 39 countries. Sci Rep. 2017;7:1–10 https://doi.org/10.1038/s41598-017-15922-4.
6. Zequi S de C, Clavijo DA, Nolazco A, et al (2017) The creation, development and diffusion of the larcglatin american renal cancer group. Int Braz J Urol 43:3–6. https://doi.org/10.1590/S1677-5538.IBJU.2017.01.02.
7. Zini L, Perrotte P, Capitanio U, et al. Radical versus partial nephrectomy:

effect on overall and noncancer mortality. Cancer. 2009;115:1465–71 https://doi.org/10.1002/cncr.24035.
8. Van Poppel H, Da Pozzo L, Albrecht W, et al. A prospective, randomised EORTC intergroup phase 3 study comparing the oncologic outcome of elective nephron-sparing surgery and radical nephrectomy for low-stage renal cell carcinoma. Eur Urol. 2011;59:543–52 https://doi.org/10.1016/j.eururo.2010.12.013.
9. Sun M, Becker A, Tian Z, et al. Management of localized kidney cancer: calculating cancer-specific mortality and competing risks of death for surgery and nonsurgical management. Eur Urol. 2014;65:235–41 https://doi.org/10.1016/j.eururo.2013.03.034.
10. Hadjipavlou M, Khan F, Fowler S, et al. Partial vs radical nephrectomy for T1 renal tumours: an analysis from the British Association of Urological Surgeons Nephrectomy Audit. BJU Int. 2016; https://doi.org/10.1111/bju.13114.
11. Huang WC, Elkin EB, Levey AS, et al. Partial nephrectomy versus radical nephrectomy in patients with small renal tumors-is there a difference in mortality and cardiovascular outcomes? J Urol. 2009;181:55–62 https://doi.org/10.1016/j.juro.2008.09.017.
12. Delahunt B, Cheville JC, Martignoni G, et al. The International Society of Urological Pathology (ISUP) grading system for renal cell carcinoma and other prognostic parameters. Am J Surg Pathol. 2013;37:1490–504 https://doi.org/10.1097/PAS.0b013e318299f0fb.
13. Rubin DB. Multiple imputation for nonresponse in surveys. 1st ed. New York: Wiley; 1987.
14. Buuren S, Groothuis-Oudshoorn K. Mice: multivariate imputation by chained equations in R. J Stat Softw. 2011;45:1–67.
15. Znaor A, Lortet-Tieulent J, Laversanne M, et al. International variations and trends in renal cell carcinoma incidence and mortality. Eur Urol.2015;67:519–30. https://doi.org/10.1016/j.eururo.2014.10.002.
16. Stafford HS, Saltzstein SL, Shimasaki S, et al. Racial/ethnic and gender disparities in renal cell carcinoma incidence and survival. J Urol. 2008;179: 1704–8 https://doi.org/10.1016/j.juro.2008.01.027.
17. Frank I, Blute ML, Cheville JC, et al. Solid renal tumors: an analysis of pathological features related to tumor size. J Urol. 2003;170:2217–20 https://doi.org/10.1097/01.ju.0000095475.12515.5e.
18. Snyder ME, Bach A, Kattan MW, et al. Incidence of benign lesions for clinically localized renal masses smaller than 7 cm in radiological diameter: influence of sex. J Urol. 2006;176:2391–6 https://doi.org/10.1016/j.juro.2006.08.013.
19. Jeon HG, Lee SR, Kim KH, et al. Benign lesions after partial nephrectomy for presumed renal cell carcinoma in masses 4 cm or less: prevalence and predictors in Korean patients. Urology. 2010;76:574–9 https://doi.org/10.1016/j.urology.2009.11.082.
20. Rodríguez-Covarrubias F, Rivera-Ramirez JA, Gabilondo-Pliego B, et al. Tratamiento quirúrgico del carcinoma de células renales en personas de edad avanzada. Actas Urol Esp. 2016;40:395–9 https://doi.org/10.1016/j.acuro.2016.01.009.
21. Secin FP, Castillo OA, Rozanec JJ, et al. American Confederation of Urology (CAU) experience in minimally invasive partial nephrectomy. World J Urol. 2017;35:57–65 https://doi.org/10.1007/s00345-016-1837-z.
22. Sun M, Abdollah F, Bianchi M, et al. Treatment Management of Small Renal Masses in the 21st century: a paradigm shift. Ann Surg Oncol. 2012;19:2380–7 https://doi.org/10.1245/s10434-012-2247-0.
23. Hollingsworth JM, Miller DC, Daignault S, Hollenbeck BK. Rising incidence of small renal masses: a need to reassess treatment effect. J Natl Cancer Inst. 2006;98:1331–4 https://doi.org/10.1093/jnci/djj362.
24. Lau WKO, Blute ML, Weaver AL, et al. Matched comparison of radical nephrectomy vs nephron-sparing surgery in patients with unilateral renal cell carcinoma and a normal contralateral kidney. Mayo Clin Proc. 2000;75: 1236–42 https://doi.org/10.4065/75.12.1236.
25. Russell DH, Wachtel MS, de Riese HW, et al. Implications on clinical management of the small renal mass in patients 80 years of age and older based on a retrospective review of the SEER database. Int Urol Nephrol. 2015;47:1503–8 https://doi.org/10.1007/s11255-015-1058-1.
26. Thompson RH, Boorjian SA, Lohse CM, et al. Radical nephrectomy for pT1a renal masses may be associated with decreased overall survival compared with partial nephrectomy. J Urol. 2008;179:468–71 https://doi.org/10.1016/j.juro.2007.09.077.
27. Krabbe LM, Kunath F, Schmidt S, et al. Partial nephrectomy versus radical nephrectomy for clinically localized renal masses. Cochrane Database Syst Rev. 2016;Issue 2. Art. No.: CD012045. https://doi.org/10.1002/14651858.CD012045
28. Bandini M, Marchioni M, Pompe RS, et al. The effect of age on cancer-specific mortality in patients with small renal masses : a population-based analysis. Can Urol Assoc J. 2018;12:325–30.
29. Marchioni M, Bandini M, Pompe RS, et al. The impact of lymph node dissection and positive lymph nodes on cancer-specific mortality in contemporary pT2-3 non-metastatic renal cell carcinoma treated with radical nephrectomy. BJU Int. 2018;121:383–92 https://doi.org/10.1111/bju.14024.
30. Ball MW, Gorin MA, Bhayani SB, et al. Preoperative predictors of malignancy and unfavorable pathology for clinical T1a tumors treated with partial nephrectomy: a multi-institutional analysis. Urol Oncol Semin Orig Investig. 2015;33:112 e9-112.e14. https://doi.org/10.1016/j.urolonc.2014.11.003.
31. Daugherty M, Sedaghatpour D, Shapiro O, et al. The metastatic potential of renal tumors: influence of histologic subtypes on definition of small renal masses, risk stratification, and future active surveillance protocols. Urol Oncol Semin Orig Investig. 2017;35:153 e15-153.e20. https://doi.org/10.1016/j.urolonc.2016.11.009.
32. De Cássio ZS, De Campos ECR, Guimarães GC, et al. The use of the american society of anesthesiology classification as a prognostic factor in patients with renal cell carcinoma. Urol Int. 2010;84:67–72 https://doi.org/10.1159/000273469.
33. Ferreira DB, Zequi S de C, Costa WH da, et al (2013) Use of the American Society of Anesthesiologists Classification as an additional planning tool for renal cell carcinoma assessment. J Cancer Ther 04:7–14. https://doi.org/10.4236/jct.2013.49A2002.

17

Myxoma of the renal pelvis masquerading pelviureteric stenosis: conservative limited resection with renal preservation

Najla Aldaoud[1*], Amer Hallak[2], Liqa A. Rousan[3], Omar Halalsheh[4], Bashar Darayseh[1] and Mousa A. Al-Abbadi[5]

Abstract

Background: Myxoma is a relatively rare mesenchymal tumor seen mainly in the heart and skin. Renal myxomas in particular are exceptionally rare where only 17 cases were previously reported in the English Language literature. Only 2 of the 17 reported cases were located in the renal sinus/pelvis.

Case presentation: This is a case of an 18-year-old male patient who complained of right, colicky flank pain associated with abdominal pain and discomfort. Imaging findings revealed right kidney hydronephrosis with a provisional diagnosis of pelviureteric junction (PUJ) stenosis. On computed tomography, there was a very faint thin walled mass abutting the calyces, camouflaged within the dilated renal pelvis. During surgery, a polypoid mass was found at the pelviureteric junction, causing the obstruction. Histological examination showed a hypocellular, paucivascular myxoid neoplasm, with few spindle cells displaying serpentine nuclei and inconspicuous nucleoli. The tumor cells expressed immunoreactivity for vimentin, but not for S100, CD34, actin, or desmin. This will qualify as the third case of renal pelvis myxoma.

Conclusion: Myxomas in the renal pelvis/sinus are extremely rare and can present with hydronephrosis and subtle radiological findings mimicking a PUJ stenosis. Being aware of this entity can save the patient unnecessary nephrectomy with possible preservation of the kidney.

Keywords: Myxoma, Renal pelvis, Sinus, Hydronephrosis

Background

Tumors in the renal pelvis account for around 5–10% of all renal tumors. Urothelial cell carcinoma contributes to around 90% of these cases [1]. Mesenchymal neoplasms are relatively infrequent, but mostly originate from vascular or smooth muscle tissue. Mesenchymal renal neoplasms in the renal pelvis tend to be benign, while in the ureter they are more frequently malignant [2].

Myxomas are unusual soft tissue neoplasms with predilection for the heart, soft tissues, skin, and bone. Large skeletal muscles of the thigh and buttocks have been frequently involved [3]. Nevertheless, only 17 reported cases of pure myxomas have been previously identified within the renal system in the English Language literature [3–20]. Renal myxomas do not have specific radiological findings, and they are usually misdiagnosed as malignant neoplasms. Most of these renal myxomas are located in the renal parenchyma, while those encountered in the renal sinus or capsule are extremely rare.

* Correspondence: naglaadaoud@yahoo.com
[1]Department of Pathology and Microbiology, Jordan University of Science and Technology, P.O. Box 3030, Irbid 22110, Jordan
Full list of author information is available at the end of the article

It is crucial to distinguish between this benign entity and malignant tumors that may show secondary myxoid changes in order to avoid overtreatment; especially with small lesions that can be treated with limited and minimally invasive surgery.

Case presentation

An 18-year-old male patient presented with right, colicky flank pain associated with abdominal pain and discomfort for a few weeks prior to admission. Symptoms were not accompanied by fever, chills, rigors, or any lower urinary tract complaints. His physical examination was normal, apart from slight right flank tenderness with no evidence of palpable masses. All laboratory investigations were within normal limits.

A computed tomography urography scan showed an enlarged right kidney with severe hydronephrosis and ballooning of the renal pelvis, associated with thinning of the overlying renal cortex. The right ureter was not dilated. The density of the ballooned renal pelvis was similar to that of urine, however, there was a thin, faint curvilinear wall abutting the dilated calyces. This was suggestive of the presence of a mass occupying the renal pelvis, a finding which was overlooked during the initial imaging evaluation. Therefore, the diagnosis was suggestive of PUJ obstruction (Fig. 1).

A double J stent was temporarily inserted into the right kidney and pyeloplastic surgical intervention was deemed appropriate. Intraoperatively, a mass was felt at the PUJ which was resected and sent for frozen section evaluation. The specimen contained a portion of the renal pelvis measuring 5.5 × 2.0 × 1.0 cm. A polypoid mass was identified and measured 2 × 1.8 × 1.8 cm. The mass was 1 cm away from the proximal margin and 2 cm from the distal margin. On serial sectioning, an ill-defined mass with white, soft, gelatinous cut surface was observed. Frozen section examination showed an unremarkable urothelial lining with a subepithelial hypocellular myxoid lesion with sparse blood vessels and few spindle cells with serpentine nuclei and inconspicuous nucleoli. There was no evidence of necrosis or increased mitotic activity, therefore, a frozen section interpretation of "myxoid lesion" was given to the surgical team. Consequently, the surgical team decided to proceed with conservative resection of the mass, and save the patient unnecessary nephrectomy. The permanent histological examination revealed an ill-defined mass similar to the frozen section appearance. The tumor involved the muscularis propria but not the urothelial mucosa. No extension beyond the renal pelvis was identified (Fig. 1). By well-controlled, routine immunohistochemical stains, the tumor cells were immunoreactive for vimentin (Fig. 1), while they were negative for actin, desmin, S-100 and CD34 antibodies. Based on the tumor morphology and the immunoprofile, the final diagnosis of renal pelvis myxoma was rendered. The patient was discharged two days after surgery with no immediate complications, and he has been doing well for the past 16 months.

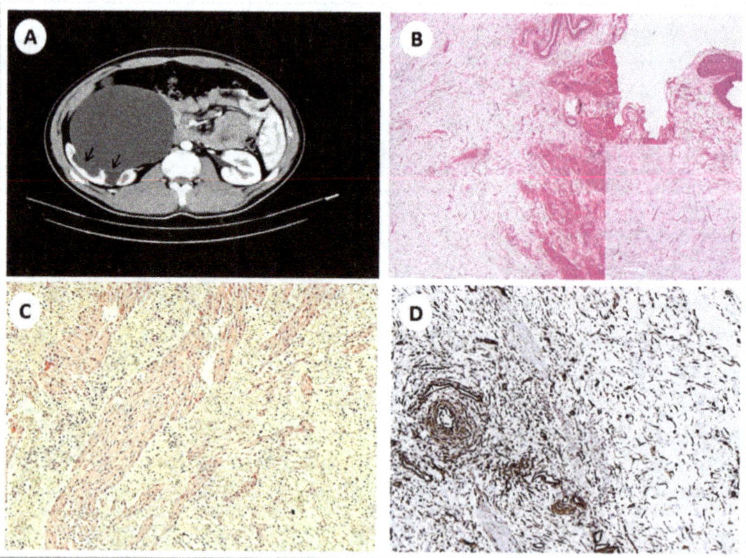

Fig. 1 Radiological and histopathological images for the myxoma case. **a** Enhanced computed tomography scan shows severe right sided hydronephrosis with ballooning of the renal pelvis and thinning of the renal cortex, a faint thin curvilinear wall seen abutting the dilated calyces (arrows). **b** Low power view of an ill-defined myxoid lesion with overlying unremarkable urothelium at the upper right (Hematoxylin and eosin 40X); the insert shows a medium power of spindle / stellate cells with no atypia and a myxoid background. **c** Low power view showing infiltration of the tumor into the muscularis propria (Hematoxylin and eosin 40X). **d** Medium power view showing positive staining of the tumor cells for vimentin immunostain (200X)

Table 1 Clinicopathologic data of the 3 cases of renal sinus/pelvis myxoma in the English language literature

Authors	Age/Sex	Site/location	Presenting symptom	Tumor size	Treatment
Appel and Schoenberg [5]	No/No	Right parapelvic	Hematuria for 2 months	8 cm	Enucleation of mass
Yildirim et al. [6]	82/Male	Left renal sinus	Dysuria, flank pain, urinary obstruction for two years	9 cm	Nephrectomy
Our case	18/Male	Right renal sinus	Right colicky flank pain, abdominal pain, discomfort for weeks	2 × 1.8 × 1.8 cm	Resection of mass

Discussion and conclusions

The first myxoma to be reported in the capsule of the kidney was in 1887 by Hulk [14]. Myxoma cells are thought to originate from fibroblast-like, primitive mesenchymal cells that lack the ability to polymerize collagen [6]. The characteristic gelatinous texture on gross examination is a result of disproportionate amounts of glycosaminoglycans [6, 8].

In most of the previously reported renal cases, myxomas were incidentally detected. However, the most common symptom reported is flank pain. Hematuria, renal colic, urinary tract infection, and obstructive uropathy have also been described [3, 8]. Unfortunately, renal myxomas lack any specific radiological findings and are often mistaken for other malignant lesions, especially renal cell carcinoma. Radiologically, they present as cystic or solid masses with variable degrees of enhancement, and are more commonly located within the renal parenchyma [4, 12]. In our case, there was an ill-defined mass where a faint, thin wall was overlooked on initial imaging studies. We can only speculate that this may be due to the fact that the mass was cystic in nature; its contents had the same density of urine, so the lesion was camouflaged within the fluid attenuated, dilated renal pelvis. Unfortunately, a preoperative magnetic resonance imaging was not performed, which could have added more necessary imaging features.

Pure renal myxomas have been exceptionally unusual [4]. Only 17 reported cases of pure myxomas have been previously identified in the English language literature [3–20]. Parenchymal involvement seemed to be the most frequent location; however, only 2 of these cases involved the renal sinus and pelvis (Table 1). These two cases, reported by Appel et al. [5] and Yildirim et al. [6], showed a large, radiologically visible, renal pelvic/sinus mass. In contrast to our case, that was a small 2 cm mass with subtle radiological findings. Our case is unique because it is the smallest myxoma tumor reported in the kidney thus far. In comparison, the reported cases in the literature had a range from 4 to 28 cm [6]. Our patient is also the youngest among all cases reported, as the age range at the time of diagnosis was from 27 to 82 years [6].

A nephrectomy was performed in all cases except Appel et al. [5, 6], where only enucleation of the mass was performed. In our case a limited, conservative resection of the mass was performed, with preservation of the kidney.

It is essential to differentiate renal myxomas from other benign and malignant tumors that can exhibit secondary myxoid changes. These tumors include perineuroma, myxoid neurofibroma, myxoid leiomyoma, myxolipoma, leiomyosarcoma, rhabdomyosarcoma, extraskeletal chondrosarcoma, low-grade fibromyxoid sarcoma, and myxofibrosarcoma [15, 16]. Our case did not show any areas of neural, fibrous, or muscle differentiation. The absence of S-100 expression ruled out neurofibroma, chondrosarcoma, and lipoma. In addition, the tumor cells in our case didn't express actin or desmin which helped in ruling out smooth and skeletal muscle tumors. The lack of atypia and necrosis distinguished it easily from other sarcomas with secondary myxoid changes.

There seems to be no clear consensus on the appropriate treatment of myxomas in the renal sinus. Yildirim et al. [6] stated that the treatment of choice is radical nephrectomy, but enucleation of the tumor as an alternative method has also been reported by Appel and Schoenberg [5], and is preserved for situations where there is no infiltration into renal parenchyma. As for our case, the unique extent of tumor growth and the polypoid nature of the mass at the PUJ made resection possible with preservation of the remaining collecting system.

In conclusion, Myxomas in the renal pelvis/sinus are extremely rare. Our patient presented with non-specific symptoms, hydronephrosis, and an ill-defined, vague mass in the renal pelvis. We highlight the importance of considering this rare, benign tumor and the importance of performing frozen section for suspicious lesions to avoid radical surgery with possible preservation of the kidney.

Abbreviation

PUJ: Pelviureteric junction

Acknowledgments

Not applicable.

Authors' contributions

NA conceived the case presentation and drafted the manuscript. AH drafted the manuscript. LAR interpreted radiology images. OH performed the operation. BD prepared the images. MA edited the manuscript. All authors read and approved the manuscript.

Author details

[1]Department of Pathology and Microbiology, Jordan University of Science and Technology, P.O. Box 3030, Irbid 22110, Jordan. [2]Faculty of Medicine, Jordan University of Science and Technology, Irbid, Jordan. [3]Department of Diagnostic and Interventional Radiology and Nuclear Medicine, Jordan University of Science and Technology, Irbid, Jordan. [4]Department of Surgery and Urology, Jordan University of Science and Technology, Irbid, Jordan. [5]Department of Pathology, Microbiology and Forensic Medicine, School of Medicine, University of Jordan, Amman, Jordan.

References

1. Brady JD, Korman HJ, Civantos F, Soloway MS. Fibroepithelial polyp of the renal pelvis: nephron-sparing surgery after false-positive biopsy for transitional cell carcinoma. Urology. 1997;49(3):460–4.
2. Petersen RO, Sesterhenn IA, Davis CJ. Urologic pathology, 3rd edition edn. Philadelphia: Lippincott Williams & Wilkins; 2009.
3. Suthar KS, Vanikar AV, Patel RD, Kanodia KV. Renal Myxoma- A Rare Variety of Benign Genitourinary Tumour. J Clin Diagn Res. 2015;9(10):Ed11–2.
4. Thakker P, Ramsey T, Navarro F. Renal Myxoma, an Incidental Finding. Urol Case Rep. 2017;13:131–2.
5. Appel SD, Schoenberg HW. Myxoma of the renal sinus. J Urol. 1968;100(3): 254–6.
6. Yildirim U, Erdem H, Kayikci A, Uzunlar AK, Tekin A, Kuzey MA. Myxoma of the renal sinus: case report and literature review. Turk patoloji dergisi. 2012; 28(1):76–9.
7. Koike H, Hayasi Y, Imanishi M. Case of the renal myxoma. Acta Urol Jpn. 2004;50:128–9.
8. Shah A, Sun W, Cao D. Myxoma of the kidney associated with hemorrhage. Indian J Surg. 2013;75(Suppl 1):480–3.
9. Salehipour M, Geramizadeh B, Dastgheib N, Makarem A, Asadollah Poor A, Taheri N. Renal myxoma, a case report and review of the literature. Urol Case Rep. 2019;23:21–2.
10. Val-Bernal JF, Aguilera C, Villagra NT, Correas MA. Myxoma of the renal capsule. Pathol Res Pract. 2005;200(11–12):835–40.
11. Gómez-González C, Moreno-Nieto V, Vicente-Pablos M, Fernandez-Vega I. Renal myxoma: an unexpected differential diagnosis. Pol J Pathol. 2014; 65(2):157–9.
12. Tenkorang S, Kharbach Y, Omana JP, Efared B, Mellas S, Tazi MF, Sekal M, Harmouch T, Khallouk A, El Fassi JM, et al. Myxoma of the kidney - an unusual benign renal tumor: a case report. J Med Case Rep. 2017;11(1):41.
13. Nishimoto K, Sumitomo M, Kakoi N, Asano T, Hayakawa M. Case of renal myxoma. Int J Urol. 2007;14(3):242–4.
14. Hulke J. Large myxoma enclosing the left kidney, extirpated together with this organ by abdominal section, recovery, recurrence of neoplasms, and death, about 12 months after the operation. Lancet. 1887;ii:1065.
15. Hakverdi S, Gorur S, Yaldiz M. Renal myxoma: a case report and review of literature. Turk J Urol. 2010;36(3):318–21.
16. Bolat FTT, Kayaselcuk F, et al. Primary renal myxoma. Turk J Pathol. 2007;23: 160–3.
17. Shenasky JH, Gillenwater JY. Myxoma of the kidney. Urology. 1973;1(3):240–2.
18. Melamed J, Reuter VE, Erlandson RA, Rosai J. Renal myxoma. A report of two cases and review of the literature. Am J Surg Pathol. 1994;18(2):187–94.
19. Owari Y, Konda R, Omori S, Seo T, Suzuki K, Fujioka T. Myxoma of the kidney. Int J Urol. 2006;13(7):987–9.
20. Kundu AK, Chakraborty AK, Chakraborty S, Das S. Myxoma of the kidney. J Indian Med Assoc. 1995;93(12):462 464.

18

Prognostic value of pretreatment neutrophil-to-lymphocyte ratio in renal cell carcinoma

Yuan Shao[1†], Bo Wu[2†], Wei Jia[1], Zikuan Zhang[1], Qian Chen[1] and Dongwen Wang[1,3*]

Abstract

Background: Numerous studies show that the pretreatment neutrophil-to-lymphocyte ratio (NLR) is associated with the prognosis of patients with RCC. However, their findings are inconsistent, urging us to explore the prognostic value of NLR in RCC patients.

Methods: This study was pre-registered in PROSPERO (CRD42020167131). Two reviewers independently performed a systematical search of PubMed, Web of Science, EMBASE, and Cochrane Library databases for prospective or retrospective cohort studies investigating the prognostic value of pretreatment NLR. Hazard ratios with 95% confidence intervals for overall survival (OS), disease-free survival (DFS), progression-free survival (PFS), cancer-specific survival (CSS), and other useful clinicopathological features were extracted and analyzed with fixed or random-effect models by using Review Manager 5.3 and Stata 12.0 software. Heterogeneity was estimated on the basis of Cochran's Q test and I^2 value. Sensitivity analyses and subgroup analyses were also performed to explore the potential sources of heterogeneity. Publication bias was assessed with funnel plots and precisely assessed by Egger's tests. The quality of the evidence was evaluated in accordance with the Grading of Recommendations Assessment, Development, and Evaluation (GRADE).

Results: Overall, 6461 RCC patients from 24 retrospective studies and 1 prospective study were included. In overall population, elevated pretreatment NLR was associated with poorer OS (pooled HR = 1.90, 95% CI = 1.56–2.30, $p < 0.001$; $I^2 = 87\%$), DFS/PFS (pooled HR = 2.09, 95% CI: 1.49–2.94, $p < 0.001$; $I^2 = 99\%$), and CSS (pooled HR = 2.31, 95% CI: 1.61–3.33, $p < 0.001$; $I^2 = 14\%$). Furthermore, this negative association was further confirmed in patients with nonmetastatic and metastatic RCC patients, respectively. We also investigated the predictive role of NLR in metastatic RCC patients treated with immune checkpoint inhibitors (ICIs). The results indicated that the level of NLR was significantly associated with OS (pooled HR = 3.92, 95% CI: 2.00–7.69, $p < 0.001$; $I^2 = 0\%$) and PFS (pooled HR = 2.20, 95% CI: 95% CI: 1.61–3.01, $p < 0.001$; $I^2 = 20\%$).

(Continued on next page)

* Correspondence: urology2007@126.com
†Co-first authors: Yuan Shao and Bo Wu contributed equally to this work.
[1]Shanxi Medical University, Taiyuan 030001, Shanxi, People's Republic of China
[3]National Cancer Center/National Clinical Research Center for Cancer/Cancer Hospital & Shenzhen Hospital, Chinese Academy of Medical Sciences and Peking Union Medical College, Shenzhen 518116, People's Republic of China
Full list of author information is available at the end of the article

(Continued from previous page)

Conclusions: This study demonstrated that elevated pretreatment NLR was significantly associated with poor prognosis of RCC patients. NLR could be helpful as a potential prognostic biomarker to guide clinical decision-making and select individualized treatment strategies for RCC patients.

Keywords: Inflammation, Neutrophil-lymphocyte ratio, Biomarker, Kidney neoplasms, Prognosis, Survival, Meta-analysis

Background

Renal cell carcinoma (RCC) is a common malignant cancer of the urinary system; its morbidity and mortality have been increasing in recent years [1, 2]. When RCC is identified early by imaging conducted for other reasons serendipitously, long-term survival is generally excellent. When RCC is detected with symptoms, the prognosis is poor [3]. However, reliable biomarkers suitable for clinical application remain undiscovered worldwide, and presently except for imaging examination, no method is effective for the early diagnosis and prognosis of RCC. Therefore, in order to improve the prognosis of RCC patients and guide clinical decision-making, it is necessary to identify reliable pretreatment biomarker to diagnose, monitor, and manage this disease.

There is growing evidence indicating that immune response and systemic inflammation is the crucial component of human cancer development and progression [4–6]. Several studies have indicated that pretreatment neutrophil-to-lymphocyte ratio (NLR), as a systemic inflammatory biomarker, was associated with the prognosis of patients with malignancies; thus providing a new perspective for predicting the prognosis of cancer [7–9]. More recently, various studies evaluated the prognostic value of NLR in RCC patients, whereas their conclusions are controversial [10, 11]. In 2019, a meta-analysis reported that NLR is a predictor associated with prognosis in RCC patients. However, this study did not perform sensitivity analysis and subgroup analysis to explore the potential sources of heterogeneity and assess the publication bias [12]. Therefore, the aim of this systematic review and meta-analysis was to provide a systematical and comprehensive perspective clarifying the prognostic value of pretreatment NLR for both non-metastatic and metastatic RCC patients.

Methods

Search strategy

This study was pre-registered in PROSPERO (CRD42020167131) and conducted in accordance with the guidelines of the Preferred Reporting Items for Systematic Review and Meta-Analysis (PRISMA). A comprehensive online literature search was performed to select the potential studies on PubMed, Web of Science, EMBASE and Cochrane Library databases from inception to December 2019. The main terms used in our search strategy included the following: ("renal" or "kidney") and ("carcinoma" or "neoplasms" or "cancer" or "tumor") and ("NLR" or "neutrophil-lymphocyte ratio" or "neutrophil-to-lymphocyte ratio").

Inclusion and exclusion criteria

The enrolled studies should meet the following inclusion criteria: (1) prospective or retrospective cohort studies evaluating the association between the pretreatment NLR and overall survival (OS), disease-free survival (DFS), progression-free survival (PFS), cancer-specific survival (CSS) of the patients with RCC; (2) patients in these studies did not receive any treatment before obtaining samples; (3) NLR was collected within 30 days before treatment; and (4) the study directly provided hazard ratios (HRs) with 95% confidence intervals (CIs) or had sufficient data to calculate these statistics. If the data in the studies were duplicated, only the data from the most recent study were used. The studies were excluded based on the following exclusion criteria: (1) studies without sufficient survival data for further analysis, (2) duplicated studies or publications, and (3) expert opinions, meeting abstracts, editorials, case reports, letters, reviews or meta-analysis.

Date extraction

For each eligible study, two separate authors independently extracted the following items: study characteristics (first author's name, recruitment region, year of publication, type of study, and sample size); patient information (gender, age, and race), pathological characteristics (TNM stage and histology subtype), disease setting (localized or metastatic), NLR cut-off values (the number and/or percentage of patients with high NLR versus those with low NLR), clinical features (treatment strategy, patient's survival outcome, and follow-up duration), OS, DFS, PFS, and CSS outcomes expressed as HRs (and 95% CI) for RCC patients with high pretreatment NLR versus patients with low pretreatment NLR. In the case of disagreements between individual judgments, the consensus was achieved by discussion with the third investigator.

Quality assessment

The quality of each enrolled study was assessed using the Newcastle-Ottawa Scale (NOS), which consists of three factors: selection, comparability and exposure [13].

The highest score is 9 points and studies with scores 7 or more, 4–6, and lower than 4 were respectively considered to have a low, moderate, and high risk of bias. Any disagreement was resolved by discussion with the third reviewer.

Statistical analysis

Coprimary end-points of the present meta-analysis were OS, DFS, PFS, and CSS in all patients and in patients with nonmetastatic or metastatic RCC. When the included studies directly reported the survival analysis, the HRs and 95% CIs were extracted and used to calculate pooled HRs; otherwise, the Engauge Digitizer software (version 4.1) was used to compute and estimate these data from the Kaplan-Meier survival curves [14, 15].

Cochran's Q test and I^2 statistic were used to assess the heterogeneity among the included studies. If significant heterogeneity existed ($I^2 > 50\%$ and/or $P < 0.10$), the pooled HRs and 95% CIs were calculated by a random-effect model; otherwise, the fixed-effect model was performed ($I^2 < 50\%$ and/or $P > 0.10$) [16]. Sensitivity analyses were conducted to assess the stability of the results by sequentially omitting a single study at a time. Subgroup analyses were conducted to explore the potential sources of heterogeneity. In addition, funnel plots and Egger's tests were used to assess the risk of publication bias. Egger's test and the trim and fill method were performed with Stata 12.0 software (STATA Corporation, College Station, TX, USA). Other statistical analyses were conducted using Review Manager 5.3 software (Cochrane Collaboration, Copenhagen, Denmark). All p-values were two-sided, and a statistically significant difference was defined as $p < 0.05$.

Quality of evidence

The quality of the evidence of the predictive value of pretreatment NLR for the prognosis in RCC patients was assessed according to the Grading of Recommendations Assessment, Development, and Evaluation (GRADE) [17].

Results

Included literature

Based on our search strategies, we identified 1039 potentially relevant studies. After removing duplicates, we viewed the titles and abstracts of the remaining 942 records. Subsequently, we assessed the full text for 76 articles. Finally, 25 studies were enrolled in the present meta-analysis [10, 11, 18–40]. The study selection process is presented as a flowchart in Fig. 1.

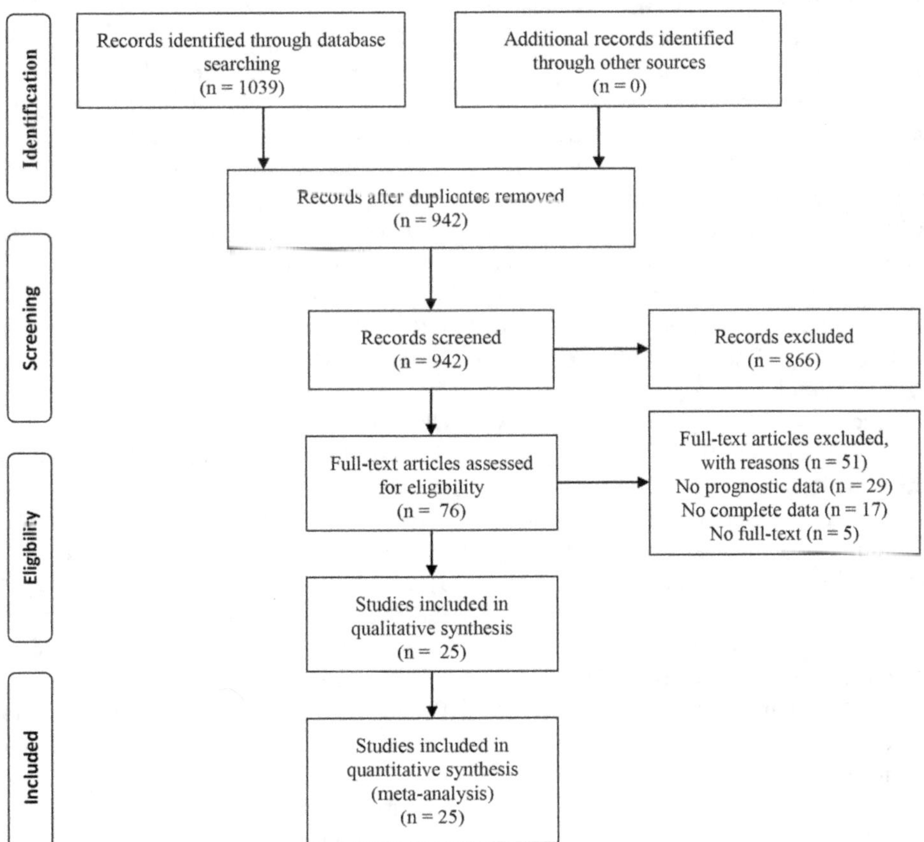

Fig. 1 Flowchart of the eligible studies in the current meta-analysis

Study characteristics

Overall, 6461 patients with RCC were included. Table 1 showed the main characteristics of the 25 enrolled studies. For the study design, 24 were retrospective cohort studies and published between 2010 and 2019. Twelve studies reported localized/non-metastatic RCC, and 13 reported metastatic RCC. Among the 25 studies, OS was reported in 19 studies, DFS or PFS in 18 studies, and CSS in 4 studies. Histology type includes clear cell RCC, papillary RCC, non-clear cell RCC, and mixed type. Cut-off values of NLR ranged from 2.0 to 5.0. The HR and 95% CI data were extracted from the multivariate Cox regression analysis in 25 studies and univariate analysis in two studies. The mean age ranged from 56.3 to 69 years and the mean follow-ups ranged from 7.6 to 107.6 months. The NOS scores ranged from 6 to 8, showing a moderate to high quality of the included studies (Table S1).

NLR and OS in RCC

Nineteen studies, comprising 5768 patients, evaluated the association of NLR with OS in RCC patients. Because of significant heterogeneity ($I^2 = 87\%$, $p < 0.001$), a random-effect model was applied to investigate the prognostic role of NLR. The forest plot indicated that elevated pretreatment NLR was significantly associated with shorter OS in the overall population (pooled HR: 1.90, 95% CI: 1.56–2.30, $p < 0.001$, Fig. 2).

When we evaluated the relationship between pretreatment NLR and OS in nonmetastatic (localized) RCC, we investigated 8 studies, including 4113 patients, while the same relationship was possible in 11 studies including 1420 patients with metastatic RCC. Meta-analysis showed that elevated NLR was significantly associated with worse OS in patients with nonmetastatic and metastatic RCC (pooled HR = 1.78, 95% CI: 1.24–2.56, $p < 0.001$; pooled HR = 2.04, 95% CI: 1.58–2.64, $p < 0.001$, respectively). Of note, heterogeneity was still obvious in nonmetastatic ($I^2 = 85\%$, $p < 0.001$) and metastatic populations ($I^2 = 72\%$, $p < 0.001$) (Fig. 3).

To explore whether a single study affected heterogeneity and conclusions, we performed a sensitivity analysis by sequentially excluding each single study in turn. After removing Viers' study, heterogeneity among studies was reduced ($I^2 = 48\%$, $p = 0.07$) in nonmetastatic RCC. Similarly, after removing Silagy's study, heterogeneity was reduced ($I^2 = 46\%$, $p = 0.05$) in metastatic RCC. Overall, the results of sensitivity analyses did not affect the conclusions described above and validated the robustness of our findings.

NLR and DFS, PFS in RCC

When we investigated the association between NLR and DFS/PFS, 18 studies with 2735 patients were selected. The forest plot revealed that a high pretreatment NLR resulted in worse DFS/PFS in overall population (pooled HR = 2.09, 95% CI: 1.49–2.94, $p < 0.001$; $I^2 = 99\%$; Fig. 2).

When we further evaluated the relationship between NLR and DFS in nonmetastatic RCC patients, we included 9 studies with 3602 patients. The forest plot revealed that elevated NLR showed a significant association with worse DFS (pooled HR = 1.45, 95% CI: 1.19–1.78, $p < 0.001$; $I^2 = 81\%$; Fig. 3). As for the relationship between NLR and PFS in metastatic RCC patients, meta-analyses based on 9 studies indicated that high pretreatment NLR was significantly associated with poorer PFS (pooled HR = 2.99, 95% CI: 2.82–3.18, $p < 0.001$; $I^2 = 18\%$; Fig. 3).

Consequently, sensitivity analyses were also performed in nonmetastatic RCC patients. The results showed that the omission of any one study, except Viers' study, did not significantly affect heterogeneity. However, heterogeneity was still relatively significant after the removal of Viers' study. Since different study features were involved, we further performed subgroup analyses to explore the source of heterogeneity (Table 2). In the subgroup analysis based on sample sizes, elevated pretreatment NLR was significantly associated with poorer DFS in both sample sizes ≥200 (pooled HR = 1.57, 95% CI: 1.09–2.26, $p = 0.02$; $I^2 = 69\%$) and sample sizes < 200 (pooled HR = 1.85, 95% CI: 1.17–2.92, $p = 0.008$; $I^2 = 60\%$). Moreover, histology type, mean age, cut-off value of NLR, treatment strategy, the mean follow-up months, and other study features did not affect the relationship between NLR and DFS in nonmetastatic RCC patients. Interestingly, when stratified by race of patients, heterogeneity was significantly reduced and results demonstrated that elevated NLR was significantly associated with pooer DFS in both Asian and Caucasian RCC patients (pooled HR = 2.31; 95% CI: 1.70–3.14, $p < 0.001$; $I^2 = 0\%$; pooled HR = 1.21, 95% CI: 1.08–1.36, $p = 0.001$; $I^2 = 0\%$, respectively).

NLR and CSS in RCC

Four studies, comprising 2314 patients, provided data on the association of NLR with CSS. The forest plot indicated that higher pretreatment NLR was significantly associated with worse CSS (pooled HR = 2.31, 95% CI: 1.61–3.33, $p < 0.001$, $I^2 = 14\%$; Fig. 2). Considering that the patients enrolled in these four studies were nonmetastatic RCC, we did not further investigated the association between NLR and CSS in metastatic RCC patients. Furthermore, a sensitivity analysis was performed to explore whether a single study affected heterogeneity and conclusions. After removing Zheng's study, heterogeneity among studies was markedly changed ($I^2 = 0\%$, $p = 0.47$) in nonmetastatic RCC. However, the pooled HR recalculated did not affect the conclusion described above, which validated the strength of our results.

Table 1 Characteristics of the studies included in the meta-analysis

Authors and year	Country	Sample size	Histology type	Stage	Mean age (years)	Treatment	Cut-off value and determined method		Outcome	Follow-up (Mean, months)	NOS score
Chen 2019 [18]	China	414	Clear	Non-metastatic	56.3	Radical or partial nephrectomy	2.17	Based on X-tile	OS, CSS	69.2	8
Huszno 2019 [19]	Poland	141	Clear	Metastatic	62	Tyrosine kinase inhibitors or IFN-α	3.68	ROC curve	OS, PFS	NA	7
Ishihara 2019 [20]	Japan	58	Mixed	Metastatic	NA	Nivolumab	3	Based on previous study	OS, PFS	13.1	7
Shirotake 2019 [11]	Japan	54	Clear	Metastatic	69	Nivolumab	2.89	Median value of NLR	PFS	10.6	7
Silagy 2019 [21]	USA	100	Non-clear	Metastatic	61	Cytoreductive nephrectomy	4.0	Median value of NLR	OS	13.3	7
Suzuki 2019 [22]	Japan	65	Mixed	Metastatic	68	Nivolumab	5	ROC curve	OS, PFS	9.5	6
Takagi 2019 [23]	Japan	71	Clear	Metastatic	66	Tyrosine Kinase Inhibitor Therapy	3	Mean value of NLR	OS	NA	7
Tu 2019 [24]	China	76	Papillary	Non-metastatic	57.5	Radical or partial nephrectomy	2.5	ROC curve	DFS	28.0	6
Widz 2019 [25]	Poland	196	Mixed	Non-metastatic	61	Radical or partial nephrectomy	2.69	ROC curve	OS	68	7
Zheng 2019 [26]	China	662	Mixed	Non-metastatic	61.7	Nephrectomy	3.2	Based on X-tile	OS, MFS	50.35	7
Kim 2018 [27]	Korea	190	Mixed	Metastatic	NA	Immunotherapy or/and VEGF	2.56	Median value of NLR	OS	107.6	7
Zahoor 2018 [28]	Austria	90	Clear	Metastatic	65	Nivolumab	4.2	NA	PFS	7.6	7
Zheng 2018 [29]	China	635	Mixed	Non-metastatic	61.71	Radical or partial nephrectomy	3.5	Based on X-tile	OS, CSS	48.40	7
Chang 2017 [30]	China	185	Clear	Localized	NA	Radiofrequency ablation	2.79	ROC curve	DFS, RFS	81	7
Dalpiaz 2017 [10]	USA	587	Clear	Non-metastatic	65	Radical or partial nephrectomy	2.0	Based on previous study	OS, CSS, MFS	NA	8
Jeyakumar 2017 [31]	USA	42	Mixed	Metastatic	61	VEGF and ICIs	3	Based on previous study	OS, PFS	NA	7
Grivas 2014 [32]	Greece	114	Mixed	Non-metastatic	64	Radical nephrectomy	2.7	Based on previous study	OS, DFS	69	7
Viers 2014 [33]	USA	827	Clear	Localized	65	Radical nephrectomy	4.0	NA	OS, DFS	111	7
Cetin 2013 [34]	Turkey	100	Mixed	Metastatic	58	IFN-α + VEGF	3.04	NA	OS, PFS	15	7
de Martino 2013 [35]	Austria	281	Non-clear	Localized	63	Radical or partial nephrectomy	3.6	ROC curve	DFS	37	7
Fox 2013 [36]	Australia	362	Mixed	Locally advanced/ metastatic	62	lapatinib vs. antiangiogenic	3	Median value of NLR	OS	NA	7

Table 1 Characteristics of the studies included in the meta-analysis *(Continued)*

Authors and year	Country	Sample size	Histology type	Stage	Mean age (years)	Treatment	Cut-off value and determined method		Outcome	Follow-up (Mean, months)	NOS score
Chen 2019 [18]	China	414	Clear	Non-metastatic	56.3	Radical or partial nephrectomy	2.17	Based on X-tile	OS, CSS	69.2	8
Keizman 2013 [37]	Israel	244	Mixed	Metastatic	63	Sunitinib	3	Regression tree analysis	OS, PFS	55	6
Pichler 2013 [38]	Austria	678	Clear	Non-metastatic	NA	Radical or partial nephrectomy	3.3	Based on previous study	OS, CSS, MFS	44	7
Santoni 2013 [39]	Italy	97	Clear	Metastatic	64	Everolimus	3	Statistical method	OS, PFS	46.9	7
Ohno 2010 [40]	Japan	192	NA	Non-metastatic	60	Nephrectomy	2.7	Statistical method	RFS	93	7

Abbreviations: *OS* overall survival, *DFS* disease-free survival, *RFS* recurrence-free survival, *PFS* progression-free survival, *MFS* metastasis-free survival, *CSS* cancer-specific survival, *ICIs* immnue checkpoint inhibitors, *ROC* curve receiver operating characteristic curve, *NA* not available, *NOS* score Newcastle-Ottawa Scale score

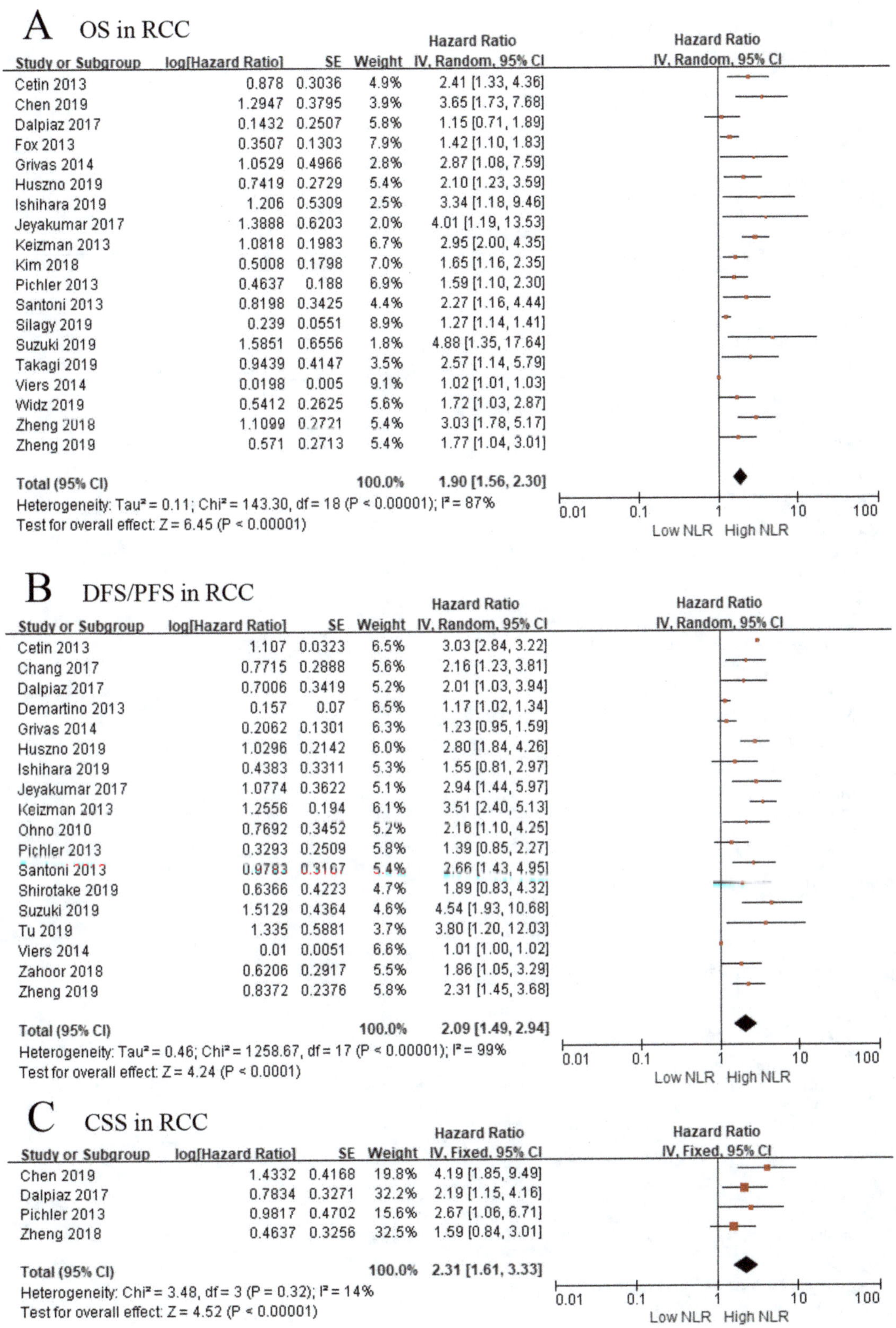

Fig. 2 **a** Effect of the NLR on overall survival, **b** effect of the NLR on disease-free survival/progression-free survival, **c** effect of the NLR on cancer-specific survival

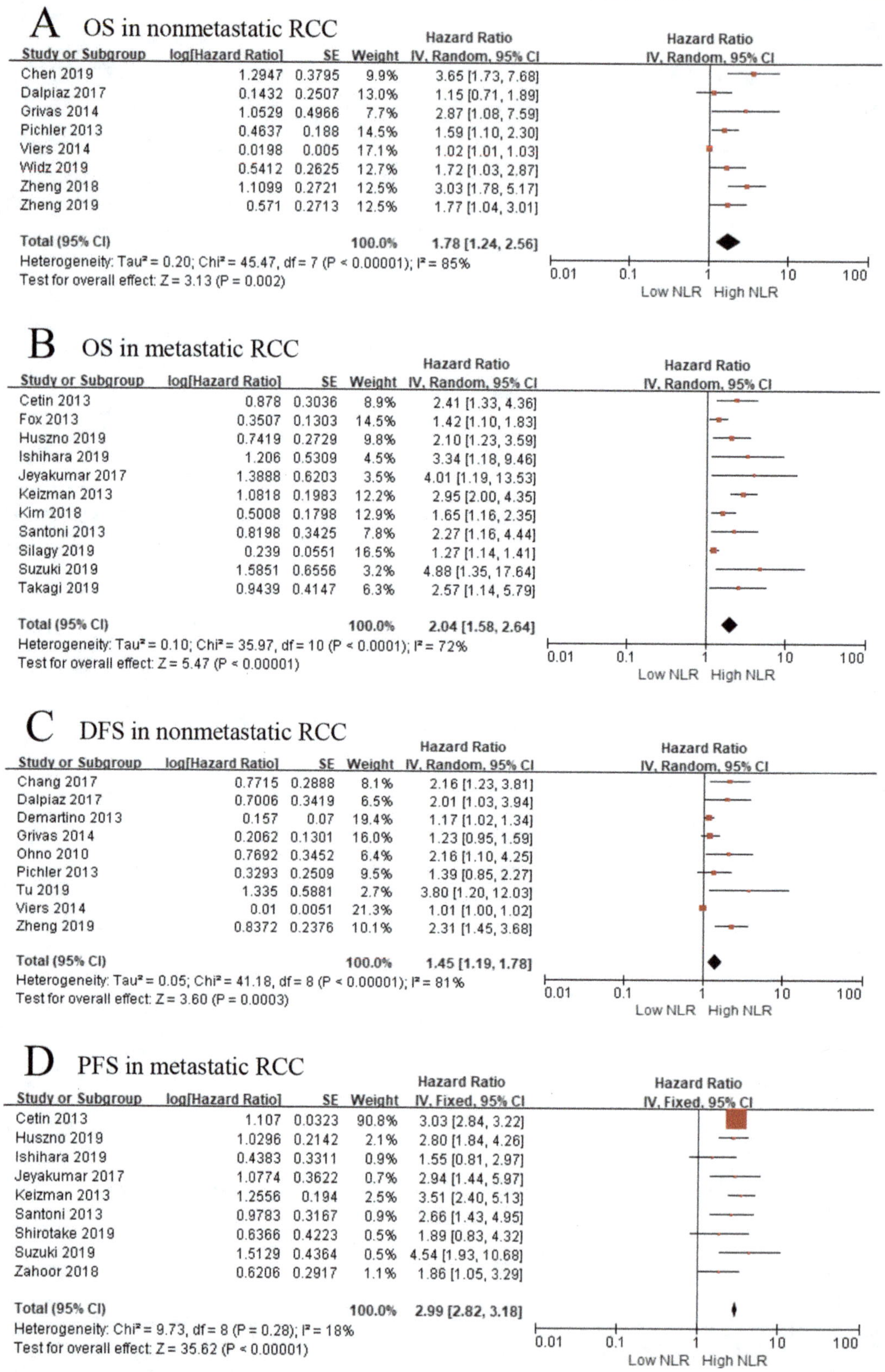

Fig. 3 **a** Effect of the NLR on OS in nonmetastatic RCC, **b** effect of the NLR on OS in metastatic RCC, **c** effect of the NLR on DFS in nonmetastatic RCC, **d** effect of the NLR on PFS in metastatic RCC

Table 2 Subgroup analysis for DFS in non-metastatic RCC patients

Subgroup	No. of studies	No. of patients	HR (95% CI)	*P* value	Heterogeneity	
					I^2 (%)	Ph
Overall	9	3602	1.45 (1.19–1.78)	< 0.001	81	< 0.001
Study for subgroup analysis	8	2775	1.63 (1.27–2.07)	< 0.001	62	0.01
Race						
Caucasian	4	1660	1.21 (1.08–1.36)	0.001	0	0.43
Asian	4	1115	2.31 (1.70–3.14)	< 0.001	0	0.85
Sample size						
≥ 200	4	567	1.57 (1.09–2.26)	0.02	69	0.02
< 200	4	2208	1.85 (1.17–2.92)	0.008	60	0.06
Histology type						
Clear cell carcinoma	3	1450	1.75 (1.27–2.43)	< 0.001	0	0.46
Others	5	1325	1.58 (1.16–2.15)	0.004	71	0.009
Mean age (years)						
≥ 65	1	587	–	–	–	–
< 65	7	2188	1.59 (1.24–2.06)	< 0.001	65	0.009
Treatment						
Nephrectomy	7	2590	1.56 (1.22–2.00)	0.001	61	0.02
Radiofrequency ablation	1	185	–	–	–	–
Cut-off value of NLR						
≥ 2.75	4	1806	1.61 (1.10–2.35)	0.01	73	0.01
< 2.75	4	969	1.79 (1.14–2.81)	0.01	54	0.09
Mean time of follow-up (months)						
≥ 60	3	491	1.65 (1.07–2.55)	0.02	59	0.09
< 60	4	1697	1.66 (1.07–2.56)	0.02	73	0.01

Subgroup analyses based on histology type

Considering that histology type may be the source of heterogeneity, we especially performed subgroup analyses based on histology types of RCC patients. The results revealed that histology types could change heterogeneity significantly. As shown in Table 3, pretreatment NLR could predict the outcome of clear cell RCC patients, including OS in nonmetastatic RCC (HR = 1.75, 95%CI: 1.03–2.99, $p = 0.04$; $I^2 = 69\%$), OS in metastatic RCC (HR = 2.24, 95%CI: 1.55–3.25, $p < 0.001$; $I^2 = 0\%$), DFS in nonmetastatic RCC (HR = 1.75, 95%CI: 1.27–2.43, $p < 0.001$; $I^2 = 0\%$), PFS in metastatic RCC (HR = 2.40, 95%CI: 1.82–3.18, p < 0.001; $I^2 = 0\%$), and CSS in nonmetastatic RCC (HR = 2.77, 95%CI: 1.78–4.32, p < 0.001; $I^2 = 0\%$).

OS and PFS in patients treated with ICIs

In addition to the above analysis, we also investigated the prognostic role of NLR in metastatic RCC patients treated with immune checkpoint inhibitors (ICIs). The results indicated that the high level of NLR was significantly associated with worse OS (HR = 3.92, 95% CI: 2.00–7.69, $p < 0.001$; $I^2 = 0\%$) and PFS (HR = 2.20, 95% CI: 95% CI: 1.61–3.01, p < 0.001; $I^2 = 20\%$) (Fig. 4).

Publication bias

Publication bias was assessed, respectively for OS, DFS/PFS, and CSS without considering the stage of RCC patients. For both OS and DFS/PFS, the funnel plots were asymmetric (Fig. S1). Disappointingly, the Egger's test also showed some degree of publication bias (both $p < 0.001$). Therefore, the trim and fill method was carried out to examine the funnel plot's asymmetry by using hypothetically non-published studies. The recalculated results indicated that elevated NLR was significantly associated with OS (HR: 1.51, 95%CI: 1.28–1.79, $p < 0.001$) and DFS/PFS (HR: 1.96, 95%CI: 1.42–2.72, $p < 0.001$), indicating the stability of the results (Fig. S2). For CSS, the funnel plot was relatively symmetric (Fig. S1). Moreover, the Egger's test showed that there was no obvious publication bias ($p = 0.285$).

Quality of evidence

The assessment of the quality of evidence was performed for OS, DFS/PFS, and CSS which were critical in

Table 3 Subgroup analyses based on histology type

Subgroup	No. of studies	No. of patients	HR (95% CI)	*P* value	Heterogeneity	
					I^2 (%)	Ph
OS in nonmetastatic RCC						
Overall	8	4113	1.78 (1.24–2.56)	< 0.001	85	0.002
Clear cell RCC	4	2506	1.75 (1.03–2.99)	0.04	69	0.04
Others	4	1607	2.15 (1.61–2.87)	< 0.001	6	0.36
OS in metastatic RCC						
Overall	11	1420	2.04 (1.58–2.64)	< 0.001	72	< 0.001
Clear cell carcinoma	3	309	2.24 (1.55–3.25)	< 0.001	0	0.92
Others	8	1111	1.99 (1.47–2.68)	< 0.001	77	< 0.001
DFS in nonmetastatic RCC						
Overall	8	3602	1.45 (1.19–1.78)	< 0.001	81	< 0.001
Clear cell carcinoma	3	1450	1.75 (1.27–2.43)	< 0.001	0	0.46
Others	5	1325	1.58 (1.16–2.15)	0.004	71	0.009
PFS in metastatic RCC						
Overall	9	891	2.99 (2.82–3.18)	< 0.001	18	0.28
Clear cell carcinoma	4	382	2.40 (1.82–3.18)	< 0.001	0	0.64
Others	5	509	3.02 (2.84–3.22)	< 0.001	28	0.24
CSS in nonmetastatic RCC						
Overall	4	2314	2.31 (1.61–3.33)	< 0.001	14	0.32
Clear cell carcinoma	3	1679	2.77 (1.78–4.32)	< 0.001	0	0.47
Others	1	635	–	–	–	–

evaluating the prognosis of RCC patients. The results showed that the quality of evidence of OS and DFS/PFS was both "very low" because of observational studies, some degree of publication bias, and significant heterogeneity. However, the quality of evidence of CSS was "low" due to observational studies (Table S2).

Discussion

Prognostic markers have multiple applications in the diagnosis, treatment, and prediction of clinical outcome and can contribute to choosing the best treatment strategy. Pretreatment NLR, as a prognostic predictor for RCC, has been evaluated by numerous studies, but they

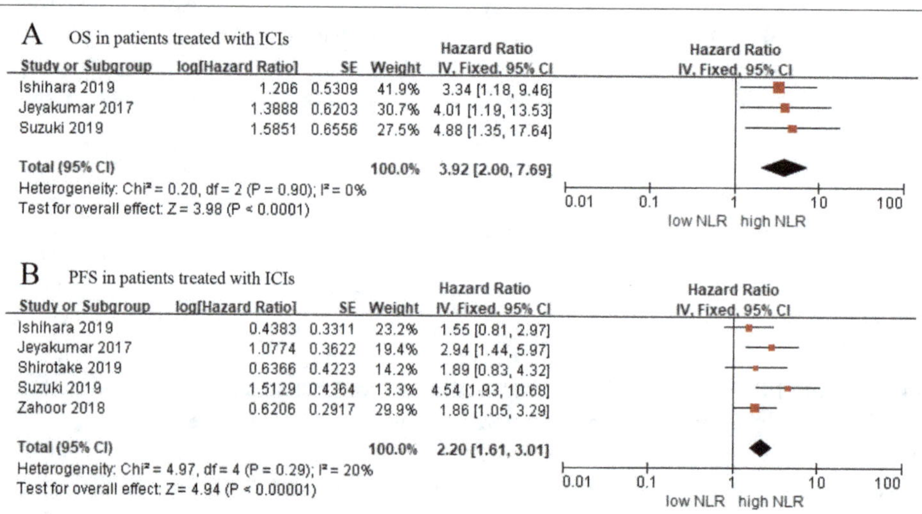

Fig. 4 a OS in RCC patients treated with ICIs, **b** PFS in RCC patients treated with ICIs

reported controversial results. Thus, the aim of this systematic review and meta-analysis of 6461 RCC patients was to clarify the prognostic value of pretreatment NLR in RCC patients. The results indicated that elevated pretreatment NLR was significantly associated with poorer OS, DFS, and CSS in nonmetastatic RCC patients. Similarly, high pretreatment NLR also showed significant association with worse OS and PFS in metastatic RCC patients. To further explore the source of heterogeneity, we performed subgroup analyses according to the features of enrolled studies, which also demonstrated the stability and reliability of our results. Collectively, the pooled data from the present systematic review and meta-analysis demonstrated that NLR may serve as a prognostic indicator in RCC patients and would be helpful in guiding clinical decision-making and selecting individualized treatment strategies.

It is largely recognized that systemic inflammatory response and tumor microenvironment are essential in the development and progression of cancer [5, 41]. Some researchers have shown cancer-related inflammatory response consists of cytokines, chemokines, transcription factors, and inflammatory cells, which play decisive roles at different stages of tumor development including initiation, promotion, malignant conversion, invasion, and metastasis [42, 43]. Hence, several inflammatory biomarkers, such as platelet-to-lymphocyte ratio (PLR) [44], lymphocyte-to-monocyte ratio (LMR) [45], C-reavtive protein to albumin ratio (CAR) [46], C-reactive protein (CRP) [47] and modified Glasgow Prognostic Score (mGPS) [48] are the potential prognostic biomarkers in RCC patients.

Recently, various studies investigated the prognostic value of NLR in RCC patients and the function of neutrophils and lymphocytes may be responsible for the underlying mechanisms. Neutrophils are usually regarded as an important part in the acute phase of inflammation and confer resistance against microbes. Some studies showed that neutrophils were involved in cancer development. Neutrophils could directly affect tumor cells to promote cancer progression. Moreover, neutrophils may indirectly change the tumor microenvironment to promote cancer metastasis [49]. In addition, neutrophils could release tumor growth promoters or immunoregulatory mediators, including vascular endothelial growth factor (VEGF) to affect cancer progression, which is generally regarded as an important part in tumor angiogenesis and has been indicated by the inhibitory effects of anti-VEGF antibodies on tumor growth in vivo [50–52]. By contrast, lymphocytes reflect on cell-mediated immunity and are essential in anti-tumor immune responses. Increased infiltration of lymphocytes in the tumor region has been associated with better responsiveness to therapy and better prognosis in patients with solid tumors [53]. Moreover, lymphopenia, with a decrease in CD4 + T-cells, which are often observed in cancer patients, compromises the anti-tumor response mediated by lymphocytes [54]. In other words, NLR not only reflects the inflammatory response in patients, but it also represents the decline of anti-tumor immunity, thus bringing a new perspective in determining the outcome of RCC patients.

Several meta-analyses have discussed the relationship between NLR and prognosis in RCC patients [55, 56]. Their results were similar to our results, but these meta-analyses did not perform sensitivity analysis and subgroup analysis to evaluate the source of heterogeneity and assess the publication bias. Furthermore, the advent of ICIs has changed the management of metastatic RCC. In particular, we investigated OS and PFS in metastatic RCC patients treated with ICIs, and the negative association was also confirmed in these RCC patients. Additionally, in this analysis, we found that heterogeneity was significantly reduced by dividing the study population according to the race of patients, namely, Caucasian and Asian RCC patients. Besides, we also noted that heterogeneity was significantly reduced by limiting the histology type to clear cell RCC. Therefore, when we explore the clinical role of NLR, it would be better to understand the histology type of patients. Moreover, there were several different defined methods about NLR in our studies. Some studies regarded NLR as a continuous variable, whereas some studies divided it into two groups based on ROC curve, median value, X-tile, and other methods. These different defined methods could potentially lead to heterogeneity. Of note, our study mainly evaluated the prognostic value of the pretreatment NLR. Several studies have shown that the post-treatment NLR was also an effective prognostic biomarker in RCC patients [44, 57, 58]. Therefore, the dynamic detection of the peripheral blood NLR level during treatment could play a more important prognostic role for RCC patients.

This study has several limitations that should be acknowledged. First, most of the included studies were retrospective and some of these studies had small sample sizes. Second, heterogeneity in some subgroup analyses was moderate or high. The possibility of selection biases or other unidentified confounders could not be completely avoided. Third, a certain degree of publication bias in our study may weaken the quality of evidence. Thus, the trim and fill method was performed and the adjusted results validated the stability of our results. Finally, there was no established cut-off value of NLR. Most scholars selected a cut-off value based on the highest sensitivity and specificity or used predefined cut-off values from other studies. Therefore, more large-scale prospective studies are needed to establish the standard cut-off value of NLR and provide more evidence.

Conclusions

Our meta-analysis demonstrated that elevated pretreatment NLR is an indicator associated with poor prognosis in RCC patients. As a potential prognostic biomarker, urologists could combine NLR with TNM stage, Fuhrman nuclear grade, histological subtype and other widely accepted prognostic indicators to more precisely predict the outcome of RCC patients.

Supplementary information

Additional file 1: Figure S1. (a) Funnel plot of NLR and OS, (b) funnel plot of NLR and DFS/PFS, (c) funnel plot of NLR and CSS

Additional file 2: Figure S2. (a) Funnel plot adjusted with trim and fill method for OS, (b) for DFS/PFS.

Additional file 3: Table S1. Newcastle-Ottawa scale score of the reviewed studies

Additional file 4: Table S2. Evaluation of the quality of evidence according to GRADE system

Abbreviations

CAR: C-reactive protein to albumin ratio; CI: Confidence intervals; CRP: C-reactive protein; CSS: Cancer-specific survival; DFS: Disease-free survival; GRADE: Grading of Recommendations Assessment, Development, and Evaluation; HR: Hazard ratio; ICIs: Immune checkpoint inhibitors; LMR: Lymphocyte-to-monocyte ratio; mGPS: Modified Glasgow Prognostic Score; NLR: Neutrophil-to-lymphocyte ratio; OS: Overall survival; PLR: Platelet-to-lymphocyte ratio; PFS: Progression-free survival; RCC: Renal cell carcinoma; ROC curve: Receiver operating characteristic curve

Acknowledgements

We thank two reviewers for providing very useful and professional comments during the revision of this study.

Authors' contributions

YS, BW, and DW conceived and designed the research. YS, QC and WJ performed data acquisition, data analysis and statistical analysis. BW and ZZ assisted with data acquisition, data analysis and manuscript preparation. YS, BW, and DW contributed in writing the manuscript. All authors read and approved the final manuscript.

Author details

[1]Shanxi Medical University, Taiyuan 030001, Shanxi, People's Republic of China. [2]Department of Urology, First Hospital of Shanxi Medical University, Taiyuan 030001, Shanxi, People's Republic of China. [3]National Cancer Center/National Clinical Research Center for Cancer/Cancer Hospital & Shenzhen Hospital, Chinese Academy of Medical Sciences and Peking Union Medical College, Shenzhen 518116, People's Republic of China.

References

1. Siegel RL, Miller KD, Jemal A. Cancer statistics, 2019. CA Cancer J Clin. 2019; 69(1):7–34.
2. Capitanio U, Bensalah K, Bex A, Boorjian SA, Bray F, Coleman J, Gore JL, Sun M, Wood C, Russo P. Epidemiology of renal cell carcinoma. Eur Urol. 2019; 75(1):74–84.
3. Moch H, Cubilla A, Humphrey P, Reuter V, Ulbright T. The 2016 WHO classification of Tumours of the urinary system and male genital organs-part a: renal, penile, and testicular Tumours. Eur Urol. 2016;70(1):93–105.
4. Grivennikov SI, Greten FR, Karin M. Immunity, inflammation, and Cancer. Cell. 2010;140(6):883–99.
5. Khandia R, Munjal A. Interplay between inflammation and cancer. Adv Protein Chem Struct Biol. 2020;119:199–245.
6. McMillan DC. Systemic inflammation, nutritional status and survival in patients with cancer. Curr Opin Clin Nutr Metab Care. 2009;12(3):223–6.
7. Bagley SJ, Kothari S, Aggarwal C, Bauml JM, Alley EW, Evans TL, Kosteva JA, Ciunci CA, Gabriel PE, Thompson JC. Pretreatment neutrophil-to-lymphocyte ratio as a marker of outcomes in nivolumab-treated patients with advanced non-small-cell lung cancer. Lung Cancer. 2017;7(1):13–20.
8. Wu Y, Li C, Zhao J, Yang L, Liu F, Zheng H, Wang Z, Xu Y. Neutrophil-to-lymphocyte and platelet-to-lymphocyte ratios predict chemotherapy outcomes and prognosis in patients with colorectal cancer and synchronous liver metastasis. World J Surg Oncol. 2016;14(1):289–93.
9. Cho HB, Hur HW, Kim SW, Kim SH, Kim JH, Kim YT, Lee K. Pre-treatment neutrophil to lymphocyte ratio is elevated in epithelial ovarian cancer and predicts survival after treatment. Cancer Immunol Immunother. 2009;58(1):15–23.
10. Dalpiaz O, Luef T, Seles M, Stotz M, Stojakovic T, Rummer K, Zigeuner R, Hutterer GC, Pichler M. Critical evaluation of the potential prognostic value of the pretreatment-derived neutrophil-lymphocyte ratio under consideration of C-reactive protein levels in clear cell renal cell carcinoma. Br J Cancer. 2017;116(1):85–90.
11. Shirotake S, Takamatsu K, Mizuno R, Kaneko GO, Nishimoto K, Oya M, Oyama M. Serum lactate dehydrogenase before Nivolumab treatment could be a therapeutic prognostic biomarker for patients with metastatic clear cell renal cell carcinoma. Anticancer Res. 2019;39(8):4371–7.
12. Nunno VD, Mollica V, Gatto L, Santoni M, Cosmai L, Porta C, Massari F. Prognostic impact of neutrophil-to-lymphocyte ratio in renal cell carcinoma: a systematic review and meta-analysis. Immunotherapy. 2019;11(7):631–43.
13. Stang A. Critical evaluation of the Newcastle-Ottawa scale for the assessment of the quality of nonrandomized studies in meta-analyses. Eur J Epidemiol. 2010;25(9):603–5.
14. Tierney JF, Stewart LA, Ghersi D, Burdett S, Sydes MR. Practical methods for incorporating summary time-to-event data into meta-analysis. Trials. 2007; 8(1):16.
15. Parmar MK, Torri V, Stewart L. Extracting summary statistics to perform meta-analyses of the published literature for survival endpoints. Stat Med. 1998;17(24):2815–34.
16. Dersimonian R, Nan L. Meta-analysis in clinical trials. Control Clin Trials. 1986; 7(3):177–88.
17. Guyatt G, Oxman A, Akl E, Kunz R, Vist G, Brozek J, Norris S, Falck-Ytter Y, Glasziou P, DeBeer H, et al. GRADE guidelines: 1. Introduction-GRADE evidence profiles and summary of findings tables. J Clin Epidemiol. 2011; 64(4):383–94.
18. Chen Z, Wang K, Lu H, Xue D, Fan M, Zhuang Q, Yin S, He X, Xu R. Systemic inflammation response index predicts prognosis in patients with clear cell renal cell carcinoma: a propensity score-matched analysis. Cancer Manag Res. 2019;11:909–19.
19. Huszno J, Kolosza Z, Mrochem-Kwarciak J, Rutkowski T, Skladowski K. The role of neutrophil-lymphocyte ratio, platelet-lymphocyte ratio, and platelets in the prognosis of metastatic renal cell carcinoma. Oncology. 2019;97(1):7–17.
20. Ishihara H, Tachibana H, Takagi T, Kondo T, Fukuda H, Yoshida K, Iizuka J, Kobayashi H, Okumi M, Ishida H, et al. Predictive impact of peripheral blood markers and C-reactive protein in Nivolumab therapy for metastatic renal cell carcinoma. Target Oncol. 2019;14(4):453–63.
21. Silagy A, Flynn J, Mano R, Blum K, Marcon J, DiNatale R, Sanchez A, Carlo M, Motzer R, Coleman J, et al. Clinicopathologic features associated with survival after cytoreductive nephrectomy for nonclear cell renal cell carcinoma. Urol Oncol. 2019;37(11):9–16.
22. Suzuki K, Terakawa T, Furukawa J, Harada K, Hinata N, Nakano Y, Fujisawa M. C-reactive protein and the neutrophil-to-lymphocyte ratio are prognostic biomarkers in metastatic renal cell carcinoma patients treated with nivolumab. Int J Clin Oncol. 2019;25(1):135–44.
23. Takagi T, Fukuda H, Kondo T, Ishihara H, Yoshida K, Kobayashi H, Iizuka J, Okumi M, Ishida H, Tanabe K. Prognostic markers for refined stratification of IMDC intermediate-risk metastatic clear cell renal cell carcinoma treated with first-line tyrosine kinase inhibitor therapy. Target Oncol. 2019;14(2):179–86.

24. Tu X, Wang F, Chang T, Zhang C, Zhang M, Liu Z, Qiu S, Yang L, Wei Q. Predictive value of preoperative neutrophil-to-lymphocyte ratio in non-metastatic papillary renal cell carcinoma patients after receiving curative surgery. Cancer Manag Res. 2019;11:7515–24.
25. Widz D, Mitura P, Buraczynski P, Plaza P, Bar M, Cabanek M, Nowak G, Ostrowska A, Bar K. Preoperative neutrophil-lymphocyte ratio as a predictor of overall survival in patients with localized renal cell carcinoma. Urol J. 2020;17(1):30–5.
26. Zheng Y, Bao LM, Ye J, Pan Y, Wang Q, Gao X. Impact of diabetes mellitus on the prognostic value of the neutrophil-lymphocyte ratio in renal cell carcinoma. Exp Ther Med. 2019;17(2):1268–75.
27. Kim SH, Kwon WA, Kim S, Joung JY, Seo HK, Lee KH, Chung J. The neutrophil-to-lymphocyte ratio makes the Heng risk model improve better the prediction of overall survival in metastatic renal cell cancer patients. Jpn J Clin Oncol. 2018;48(9):835–40.
28. Zahoor H, Barata PC, Jia X, Martin A, Allman KD, Wood LS, Gilligan TD, Grivas P, Ornstein MC, Garcia JA, et al. Patterns, predictors and subsequent outcomes of disease progression in metastatic renal cell carcinoma patients treated with nivolumab. J Immunother Cancer. 2018;6(1):107.
29. Zheng Y, Bao L, Wang W, Wang Q, Pan Y, Gao X. Prognostic impact of the controlling nutritional status score following curative nephrectomy for patients with renal cell carcinoma. Medicine. 2018;97(49):e13409.
30. Chang X, Zhang F, Liu T, Wang W, Guo H. Neutrophil-to-lymphocyte ratio as an independent predictor for survival in patients with localized clear cell renal cell carcinoma after radiofrequency ablation: a propensity score matching analysis. Int Urol Nephrol. 2017;49(6):967–74.
31. Jeyakumar G, Kim S, Bumma N, Landry C, Silski C, Suisham S, Dickow B, Heath E, Fontana J, Vaishampayan U. Neutrophil lymphocyte ratio and duration of prior anti-angiogenic therapy as biomarkers in metastatic RCC receiving immune checkpoint inhibitor therapy. J Immunother Cancer. 2017; 5(1):82.
32. Grivas N, Kafarakis V, Tsimaris I, Raptis P, Hastazeris K, Stavropoulos NE. Clinico-pathological prognostic factors of renal cell carcinoma: a 15-year review from a single center in Greece. Urol Ann. 2014;6(2):116–21.
33. Viers BR, Houston Thompson R, Boorjian SA, Lohse CM, Leibovich BC, Tollefson MK. Preoperative neutrophil-lymphocyte ratio predicts death among patients with localized clear cell renal carcinoma undergoing nephrectomy. Urol Oncol. 2014;32(8):1277–84.
34. Cetin B, Berk V, Kaplan MA, Afsar B, Tufan G, Ozkan M, Isikdogan A, Benekli M, Coskun U, Buyukberber S. Is the pretreatment neutrophil to lymphocyte ratio an important prognostic parameter in patients with metastatic renal cell carcinoma? Clin Genitour cancer. 2013;11(2):141–8.
35. de Martino M, Pantuck AJ, Hofbauer S, Waldert M, Shariat SF, Belldegrun AS, Klatte T. Prognostic impact of preoperative neutrophil-to-lymphocyte ratio in localized nonclear cell renal cell carcinoma. J Urol. 2013;190(6):1999–2004.
36. Fox P, Hudson M, Brown C, Lord S, Gebski V, De Souza P, Lee CK. Markers of systemic inflammation predict survival in patients with advanced renal cell cancer. Br J Cancer. 2013;109(1):147–53.
37. Keizman D, Gottfried M, Ish-Shalom M, Maimon N, Peer A, Neumann A, Hammers H, Eisenberger MA, Sinibaldi V, Pili R, et al. Active smoking may negatively affect response rate, progression-free survival, and overall survival of patients with metastatic renal cell carcinoma treated with sunitinib. Oncologist. 2014;19(1):51–60.
38. Pichler M, Hutterer GC, Stoeckigt C, Chromecki TF, Stojakovic T, Golbeck S, Eberhard K, Gerger A, Mannweiler S, Pummer K, et al. Validation of the pre-treatment neutrophil-lymphocyte ratio as a prognostic factor in a large European cohort of renal cell carcinoma patients. Br J Cancer. 2013;108(4):901–7.
39. Santoni M, De Giorgi U, Iacovelli R, Conti A, Burattini L, Rossi L, Luca Burgio S, Berardi R, Muzzonigro G, Cortesi E, et al. Pre-treatment neutrophil-to-lymphocyte ratio may be associated with the outcome in patients treated with everolimus for metastatic renal cell carcinoma. Br J Cancer. 2013;109(7): 1755–9.
40. Ohno Y, Nakashima J, Ohori M, Hatano T, Tachibana M. Pretreatment neutrophil-to-lymphocyte ratio as an independent predictor of recurrence in patients with nonmetastatic renal cell carcinoma. J Urol. 2010;184(3):873–8.
41. Hanahan D, Weinberg RA. Hallmarks of cancer: the next generation. Cell. 2011;144(5):646–74.
42. Diakos CI, Charles KA, McMillan DC, Clarke S. Cancer-related inflammation and treatment effectiveness. Lancet Oncol. 2014;15(11):e493–503.
43. Balkwill F, Mantovani A. Inflammation and cancer: back to Virchow? Lancet Oncol. 2001;357(9255):539–45.
44. Kim TW, Lee JH, Shim KH, Choo SH, Choi JB, Ahn HS, Kim SJ, Kim SI. Prognostic significance of preoperative and follow-up neutrophil-to-lymphocyte ratio and platelet-to-lymphocyte ratio in patients with non-metastatic clear cell renal cell carcinoma. Invest Clin Urol. 2019;60(1):14–20.
45. Yamamoto Y, Matsuyama H, Matsumoto H, Sakano S, Fuji N, Oba K, Yamamoto M, Kamiryo Y, Hiragino T, Nagao K, et al. Prognostic value of risk stratification using blood parameters for nivolumab in Japanese patients with metastatic renal-cell carcinoma. Jpn J Clin Oncol. 2020; 50(2):214–20.
46. Zhou W, Zhang GL. C-reactive protein to albumin ratio predicts the outcome in renal cell carcinoma: a meta-analysis. PLoS One. 2019;14(10): e0224266.
47. Tsujino T, Komura K, Hashimoto T, Muraoka R, Satake N, Matsunaga T, Tsutsumi T, Yoshikawa Y, Takai T, Minami K, et al. C-reactive protein-albumin ratio as a prognostic factor in renal cell carcinoma - a data from multi-institutional study in Japan. Urol Oncol. 2019;37(11):e811–8.
48. Ohmura H, Uchino K, Kajitani T, Sakamoto N, Baba E. Predictive value of the modified Glasgow prognostic score for the therapeutic effects of molecular-targeted drugs on advanced renal cell carcinoma. Mol Clin Oncol. 2017;6(5): 669–75.
49. Shaul M, Fridlender Z. Tumour-associated neutrophils in patients with cancer. Nat Rev Clin Oncol. 2019;16(10):601–20.
50. Templeton AJ, McNamara MG, Šeruga B, Vera-Badillo FE, Aneja P, Ocaña A, Leibowitz-Amit R, Sonpavde G, Knox JJ, Tran B, et al. Prognostic role of neutrophil-to-lymphocyte ratio in solid tumors: a systematic review and meta-analysis. J Natl Cancer Inst. 2014;106(6):2.
51. Masucci MT, Minopoli M, Carriero MV. Tumor Associated Neutrophils. Their Role in Tumorigenesis, Metastasis, Prognosis and Therapy. Front Oncol. 2019;9:1146.
52. Kusumanto YH, Dam WA, Hospers GAP, Meijer C, Mulder NH. Platelets and granulocytes, in particular the neutrophils, form important compartments for circulating vascular endothelial growth factor. Angiogenesis. 2003;6(4):283–7.
53. Gooden MJM, de Bock GH, Leffers N, Daemen T, Nijman HW. The prognostic influence of tumour-infiltrating lymphocytes in cancer: a systematic review with meta-analysis. Br J Cancer. 2011;105(1):93–103.
54. Wang BH, Gu WJ, Wan FN, Shi GH, Ye DW. Prognostic significance of the dynamic changes of systemic inflammatory response in metastatic renal cell carcinoma. Int Braz J Urol. 2019;45(1):89–99.
55. Boissier R, Campagna J, Branger N, Karsenty G, Lechevallier E. The prognostic value of the neutrophil-lymphocyte ratio in renal oncology: a review. Urol Oncol. 2017;35(4):135–41.
56. Jiang T, Qiao M, Zhao C, Li XF, Gao GH, Su CX, Ren SY, Zhou CC. Pretreatment neutrophil-to-lymphocyte ratio is associated with outcome of advanced-stage cancer patients treated with immunotherapy: a meta-analysis. Cancer Immunol Immunother. 2018;67(5):713–27.
57. Ohno Y, Nakashima J, Ohori M, Gondo T, Hatano T, Tachibana M. Followup of neutrophil-to-lymphocyte ratio and recurrence of clear cell renal cell carcinoma. J Urol. 2012;187(2):411–7.
58. Ito K, Masunaga A, Tanaka N, Mizuno R, Shirotake S, Yasumizu Y, Ito Y, Miyazaki Y, Hagiwara M, Kanao K, et al. Impact of inflammatory marker levels one month after the first-line targeted therapy initiation on progression-free survival prediction in patients with metastatic clear cell renal cell carcinoma. Jpn J Clin Oncol. 2019;49(1):69–76.

19

Renal cystic tumoural calcinosis with ossification and bone marrow formation

Mancheng Xia[1], Chun Liu[2], Haosen Yang[1], Keqiang Yin[1], Yusheng Wang[1], Xunan Tong[3], Siyu Zhang[4] and Weibing Shuang[2*]

Abstract

Background: Tumoural calcinosis (TC) is a rare disorder characterized by nonneoplastic amorphous calcium deposition that tends to occur in soft tissues around the large joint. Here, we report a case of cystic TC with ossification and bone marrow formation in the kidney.

Case presentation: We report a 63-year-old woman who presented with a complaint of intermittent right lumbar pain for 2 months. Computed tomography (CT) revealed a large cystic lesion on the lateral side of the right kidney, with a circular calcified wall around the lesion, which compressed, deformed and displaced the right kidney. To relieve the symptoms of right lumbar pain, the patient underwent surgical resection of this cystic lesion without partial removal of the renal parenchyma. The pathological results further confirmed the diagnosis of cystic TC with ossification and bone marrow formation in the right kidney. No recurrence was detected 1 year after surgery.

Conclusions: The main differential diagnoses of TC in the kidney are kidney stone, renal tuberculosis, renal cyst with a calcified wall, and tumour. Patients are treated mainly by complete surgical resection of the lesion.

Keywords: Cystic tumoural calcinosis, Ossification, Bone marrow formation, Kidney, Lesion resection

Background

Tumoural calcinosis (TC) is a rare benign disease that was first named by Inclan and Leon in 1943 [1]. TC often occurs in the soft tissues around large joints in the hip, shoulder, elbow, and knee, as well as occasionally around small joints in the hand, feet, head, and neck [2–4]; no cases have been reported in the kidney. The disease should be differentiated from primary hyperparathyroidism, hypervitaminosis D, gout, vascular calcification in chronic kidney disease, and dystrophic calcification associated with connective tissue disorders [5]. If TC occurs in the kidney, it needs to be differentiated from kidney stones, renal tuberculosis, renal cysts with calcified walls, and tumours and is treated mainly by complete surgical resection of the lesion. To improve the recognition of renal TC, we report herein a case of cystic TC with ossification and bone marrow formation in the kidney.

* Correspondence: shuangweibing@126.com
[2]Department of Urology, The First Hospital of Shanxi Medical University, No. 85, JieFang South Road, Yingze District, Taiyuan 030001, Shanxi, China
Full list of author information is available at the end of the article

Case presentation

A 63-year-old woman was admitted to the hospital with intermittent right lumbar pain, without other symptoms such as fever, weakness, weight loss, and other joint-related symptoms (swelling, joint stiffness, etc.). The patient had a history of right lumbar trauma 2 years prior and hypertension and multiple lacunar infarcts for 6 months. The patient was treated with rosuvastatin calcium (5 mg once daily), compound Danshen tablets

Table 1 Related laboratory tests of this patient

Laboratory tests	Values	Unit	Reference ranges
Serum phosphate	1.14	mmol/L	0.85–1.51
Total calcium	2.41	mmol/L	2.11–2.52
Ionized calcium	1.16	mmol/L	1.15–1.29
Urea	2.94	mmol/L	2.8–7.6
Creatinine	57.4	umol/L	49–90
Alkaline phosphatase	84	U/L	50–135
Albumin	45.7	g/L	40–55
Uric acid levels	206	umol/L	150–350
Arterial blood gas analysis			
PaO_2	99.9	mmHg	80–100
SaO_2	97.5	%	95–99
$PaCO_2$	35.1	mmHg	35–45
PH	7.44		7.35–7.45
ABE	−0.8	mmol/L	−3 - + 3
SBE	−0.9	mmol/L	−3 - + 3
SBC	23.8	mmol/L	22–27
HCO_3^-	23.2	mmol/L	21–28
Anion gap	10.1	mmol/L	8–16

ABE Actual base excess, *SBE* Standard base excess, *SBC* Standard bicarbonate radical

(0.96 g once daily), and benazepril hydrochloride (2.5 mg once daily). The patient denied a history of tuberculosis and a related family or consanguinity history of tumoural calcification. Clinical examination revealed no swelling, tenderness and percussive pain in the right lumbar region and no nodules or masses on each joint. Serum phosphate, total calcium, ionized calcium, urea, creatinine, alkaline phosphatase, arterial

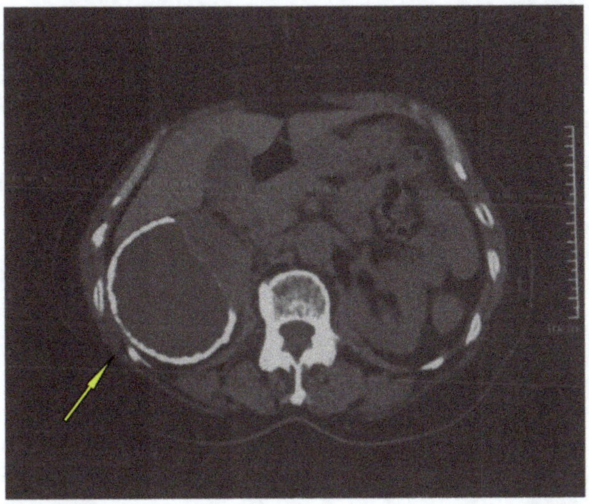

Fig. 1 CT scan showing the annular calcification wall around the right kidney, with a size of 11.5 cm*6.9 cm*5.1 cm

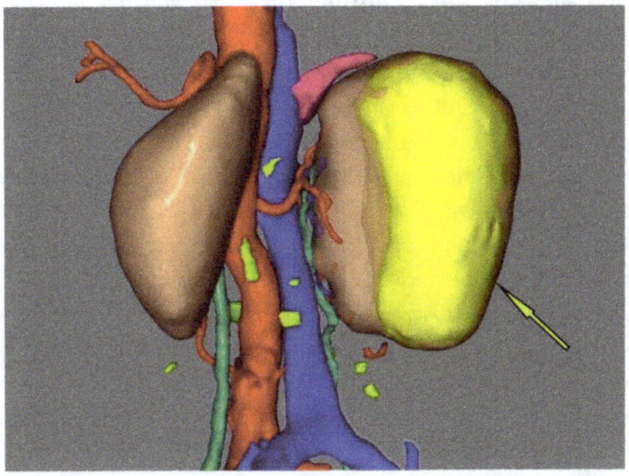

Fig. 2 Spiral CT 3D image showing the annular calcification wall around the right kidney, with a size of 11.5 cm * 6.9 cm * 5.1 cm

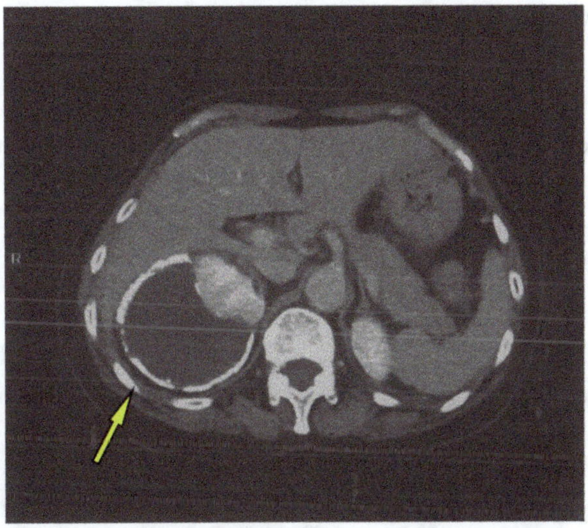

Fig. 3 Enhanced CT scan showing a circular low-density shadow under the annular calcification wall

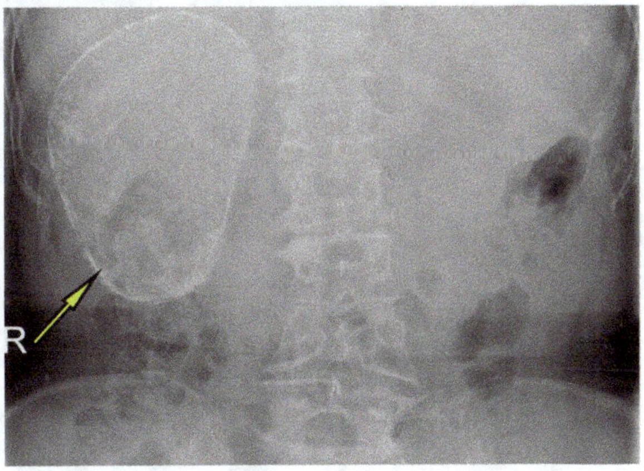

Fig. 4 Plain X-ray image of KUB showing the high-density shadow of the right kidney, approximately 10.2 cm * 7.5 cm in size

blood gas analysis, albumin, and uric acid levels were within the normal range (Table 1), and the tuberculin or purified protein derivative (PPD) test result was negative. Computed tomography (CT) scanning and spiral CT 3-D imaging revealed a large cystic lesion on the lateral side of the right kidney, with the circular calcified wall around the lesion, which compressed, deformed and displaced the right kidney. In the annular calcified wall, a low-density circular mass with a size of 11.5 × 6.9 × 5.1 cm and a CT value of 15 HU were identified (Figs. 1 and 2). The density of the circular lesion did not increase in the enhanced CT scan (Fig. 3). Plain X-ray film of the kidneys, ureters and bladder (KUB) showed a high-density shadow in the right waist area measuring 10.2 × 7.5 cm (Fig. 4). In addition, intravenous urography (IVU) revealed that the size of the right kidney decreased, a large cystic lesion was found on the lateral side of the right kidney, and only a few minor calyces were found (Fig. 5).

To relieve the symptoms of soreness on the right side of the lumbar region, the patient underwent surgical resection of this lesion under general anaesthesia without

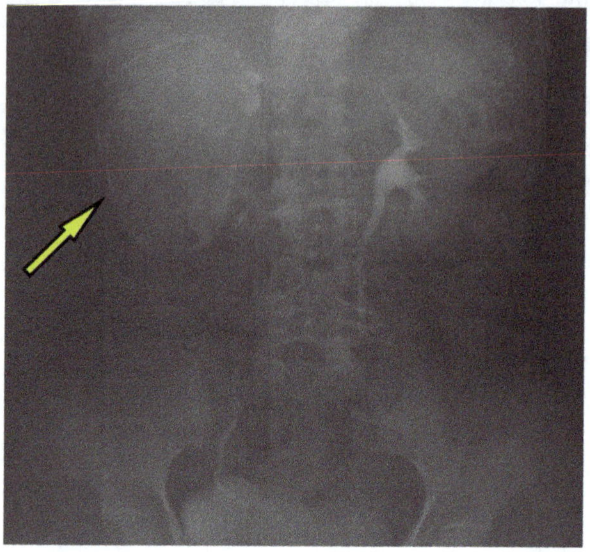

Fig. 5 IVU showing only a few minor calyces in the right kidney

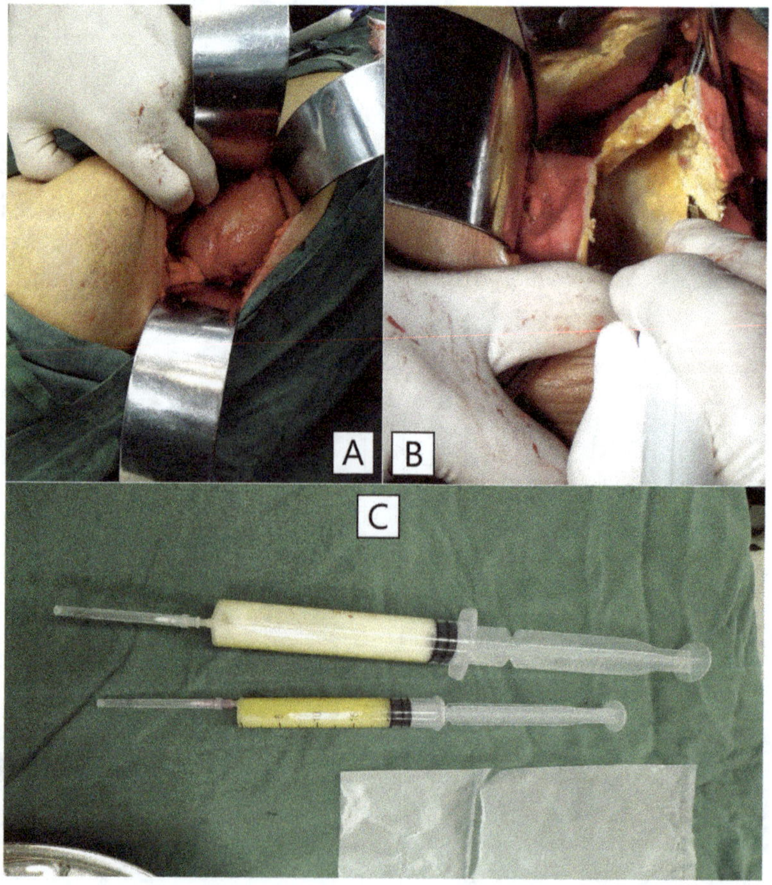

Fig. 6 A chalky white cystic mass containing chalky white cystic fluid that was aspirated using two syringes

partial removal of the renal parenchyma. During the operation, a hard and fluctuant cystic mass measuring 11.5 × 6.9 × 5.1 cm was found on the lateral side of the right kidney, which contained approximately 400 mL of chalky white fluid (Fig. 6). Before incising the renal mass, 70 mL cystic fluid was aspirated using the syringes (Fig. 6) and tested during the operation. No cancer cells or *Mycobacterium tuberculosis* were found in the smear test, which excluded the possibility of tumour and tuberculous abscess and indicated that the lesion was benign. Therefore, the cystic wall was opened by incision, and chalky calcifications were found in the inner layer of the cystic wall. The cystic wall was removed, and the cyst was not connected with the renal collecting system (Fig. 7). Postoperative culture of *M. tuberculosis*, aerobic bacteria and anaerobic bacteria in the cystic fluid was negative. The pathological observation showed the presence of fibrosis, calcification, infiltrated inflammatory cells, ossification and bone marrow formation in the cystic wall, so the patient was diagnosed with right renal cystic TC with ossification and bone marrow formation (Figs. 8 and 9). No recurrence was detected 1 year after surgery, and the patient's quality of life was greatly improved.

Discussion and conclusions

TC is a condition where calcium deposition tends to occur in soft tissues around the large joints, forming tumour-like nodular calcifications. Here, we describe a case of cystic TC with ossification and bone marrow formation that occurred in the kidney. The first symptom was intermittent right lumbar pain, without fever, weakness or weight loss.

TC can be divided into two categories with hyperphosphatemia and without hyperphosphatemia. TC with hyperphosphatemia mainly involves mutations of three genes, namely, GALNT3, FGF23, and KL [2, 5, 6]. Mutations of these three genes would lead to abnormal

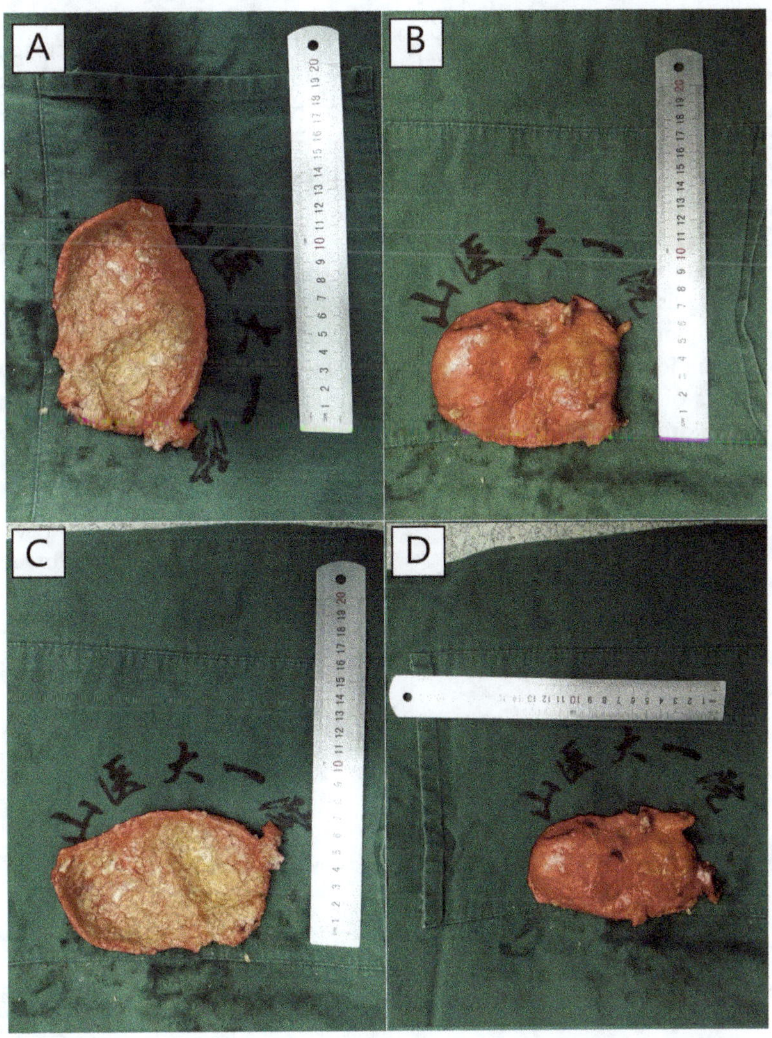

Fig. 7 Chalky white cystic wall

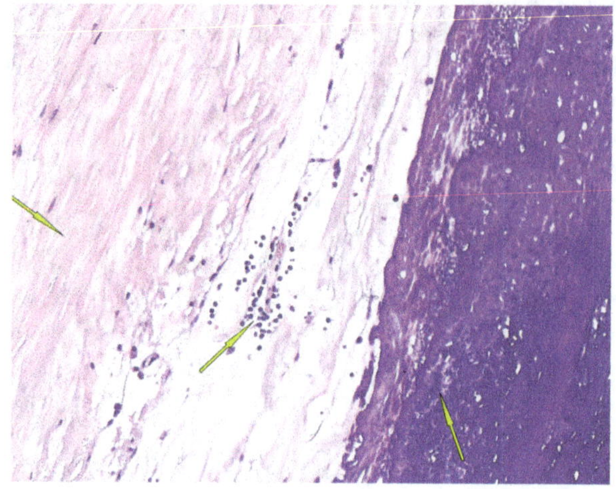

Fig. 8 Representative images of cystic wall fibrosis, calcification and inflammatory cell infiltration (arrows: haematoxylin and eosin staining, magnification X 200)

coding and expression of proteins, resulting in dysfunction of phosphate reabsorption in renal tubules, which would cause TC. TC without hyperphosphatemia mainly involves gene mutations of SMAD9 [7, 8]. SAMD9, an IFN-γ reactive protein, can interact with RGL2 to reduce the expression of EGR1, which is a protein directly related to ectopic calcification and inflammation [7]. Since our patient did not have hyperphosphatemia, this case may be related to a gene mutation of SMAD9, which still needs more research to discuss. In addition, we speculated that the pathophysiological changes might be related to the local inflammation caused by trauma, resulting in excessive synthesis of collagen fibres around the vessels and adipose tissues around the kidney, which could lead to calcium deposition.

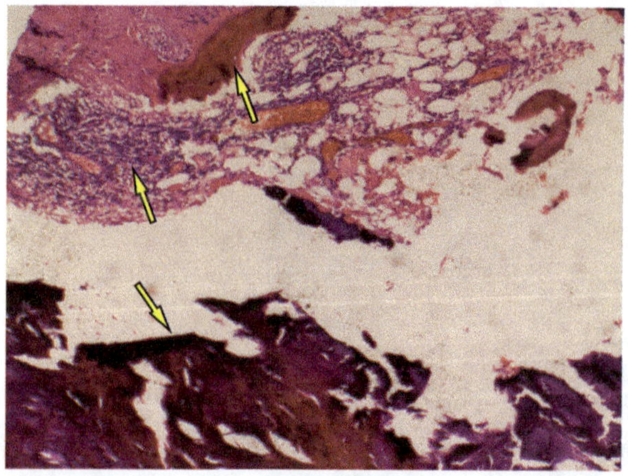

Fig. 9 Representative images of biopsy samples showing the presence of ossification and bone marrow formation in the cyst wall (arrows; haematoxylin and eosin staining, magnification X 40)

Pathologically, TC can be divided into active and inactive phases [9–11], which can occur simultaneously. Amorphous granular calcifications, macrophages, osteoclast-like giant cells, and chronic inflammatory cells were seen at the active stage of TC, while calcifications were surrounded by dense fibrous tissues at the inactive stage. In this case, the pathological examination showed the presence of fibrous tissues, calcium deposition and infiltrated inflammatory cells in the calcified wall around the lesion, and especially the presence of ossification and bone marrow formation in the calcified wall. Chalky cystic fluid and granular calcification is surrounded by the circular calcified wall. These characteristics were distinctly different from the calcification of the simple renal cyst wall. After consultation with the relevant pathologists, this patient was diagnosed with renal cystic TC with ossification and bone marrow formation at the inactive stage. In addition, we only performed surgical resection of the lesion in this case and did not remove part of the renal parenchyma. During the 1-year follow-up, the prognosis for the patient was quite good, and no related complications or recurrence were found. We expect that this case report can provide valuable insights into the diagnosis and treatment of similar diseases to avoid unnecessary large-scale resection and reduce harm to patients. Some types of TC can recur after surgery [2, 10], even causing greater damage to the body; consequently, long-term follow-up is required for patients presenting renal cystic TC with ossification and bone marrow formation.

Renal cystic TC with ossification and bone marrow formation is a rare benign disease that needs to be differentiated from kidney stones, renal tuberculosis, renal cysts with calcified walls, and tumours. Complete surgical resection of the lesion is recommended, and there is no need to remove part of the renal parenchyma. The limitation of this paper is that certain laboratory tests and gene tests were not performed due to the initial lack of understanding of this new disease, and therefore, renal cystic TC still requires more research for further discussion.

Abbreviations

TC: Tumoural calcinosis; CT: Computed tomography; KUB: Plain film of kidney ureters and bladder; IVU: Intravenous urography

Acknowledgements

Not applicable.

Authors' contributions

MX, CL and WS conducted the literature search, performed the surgery, captured clinical photos, and wrote the report. HY, KY, and YW revised the report. XT and SZ performed the histopathological examination and reported the diagnosis. All authors read and approved the final manuscript.

Author details

[1]First Clinical Medical College, Shanxi Medical University, No. 85, JieFang South Road, Yingze District, Taiyuan 030001, Shanxi, China. [2]Department of Urology, The First Hospital of Shanxi Medical University, No. 85, JieFang South Road, Yingze District, Taiyuan 030001, Shanxi, China. [3]Kidney Transplantation Centre, Shanxi Second People's Hospital, Taiyuan, Shanxi, China. [4]Department of Pathology, Shanxi People's Hospital, Taiyuan, Shanxi, China.

References

1. Inclan A, Leon P, Camejo MG. Tumoral calcinosis. JAMA. 1943;121(7):490–5.
2. Hsiao CC, Lee CC, Chen KH. Successful treatment of tumoral calcinosis by lanthanum carbonate. Internal Med. 2018;57(24):3589–91.
3. Lee SY, Lee HG, Kim KS, et al. A rare development of tumoral calcinosis of the ear auricle. Arch Craniofac Surg. 2018;19(4):287–90.
4. Mageau A, Guigonis V, Ratzimbasafy V, et al. Intravenous sodium thiosulfate for treating tumoral calcinosis associated with systemic disorders: report of four cases. Joint Bone Spine. 2017;84(3):341–4.
5. Tiwari V, Goyal A, Nagar M, et al. Hyperphosphataemic tumoral calcinosis. Lancet. 2019;393(10167):168.
6. Chakhtoura M, Ramnitz MS, Khoury N, et al. Hyperphosphatemic familial tumoral calcinosis secondary to fibroblast growth factor 23 (FGF23) mutation: a report of two affected families and review of the literature. Osteoporos Int. 2018;29(9):1987–2009.
7. Hershkovitz D, Gross Y, Nahum S, et al. Functional characterization of SAMD9, a protein deficient in normophosphatemic familial tumoral calcinosis. J Invest Dermatol. 2011;131(3):662–9.
8. Fathi I, Sakr M. Review of tumoral calcinosis: a rare clinico-pathological entity. World J Clin Cases. 2014;2(9):409–14.
9. Aydin A, Tuncer S, Erer M, et al. Tumoral calcinosis infiltrating the biceps brachii tendon - excision and reconstruction with allograft: a case report. J Hand Surg. 2004;29(2):170–2.
10. Megaloikonomos PD, Mavrogenis AF, Panagopoulos GN, et al. Tumoral calcinosis of the shoulder. Lancet Oncol. 2017;18(2):e126.
11. Richardson PH, Yang YM, Nimityongskul P, et al. Tumoral calcinosis in an infant. Skelet Radiol. 1996;25(5):481–4.

20

Squamous cell carcinoma of the renal parenchyma presenting as hydronephrosis

Xirong Zhang[1,2], Yuanfeng Zhang[1], Chengguo Ge[1], Junyong Zhang[1] and Peihe Liang[1*]

Abstract

Background: Primary squamous cell carcinoma of the renal parenchyma is extremely rare, only 5 cases were reported.

Case presentation: We probably report the fifth case of primary Squamous cell carcinoma (SCC) of the renal parenchyma in a 61-year-old female presenting with intermittent distending pain for 2 months. Contrast-enhanced computed tomography (CECT) revealed hydronephrosis of the right kidney, but a tumor cannot be excluded completely. Finally, nephrectomy was performed, and histological analysis determined that the diagnosis was kidney parenchyma squamous cell carcinoma involving perinephric adipose tissue.

Conclusions: The present case emphasizes that it is difficult to make an accurate preoperative diagnosis with the presentation of hidden malignancy, such as hydronephrosis.

Keywords: Kidney, Renal parenchyma, Squamous cell carcinoma, Hydronephrosis, Malignancy

Background

Squamous cell carcinoma (SCC) of the renal pelvis is a rare neoplasm, accounting for only 0.5 to 0.8% of malignant renal tumors [1], SCC of the renal parenchyma is even less common. A review of the literature shows that only five cases of primary SCC of the renal parenchyma have been reported to date [2–6]. Here, we are reporting a case of primary SCC of the renal parenchyma, which was post-surgically diagnosed according to tissue pathology. A review of recent related literature is provided as well. The ethics committee of Chongqing Medical University has reviewed and approved the project and the Ethics board approval number is 2016–064.

* Correspondence: lphsubmit@163.com
[1]Department of Urology, The Second Affiliated Hospital of Chongqing Medical University, Yuzhong, Chongqing 400010, China
Full list of author information is available at the end of the article

Case presentation

The patient is a 61-year-old female. After suffering from intermittent pain in the right flank region for 2 months she was referred to the urology department at an outside hospital. The patient was diagnosed with hydronephrosis of the right kidney and underwent a right ureteroscopy with placement of a double J stent. The patient was subsequently discharged. After removal of the double J stent (which occurred 1 month following discharge), the patient presented intermittent colicky pain at the right flank region. Subsequently, the patient was referred to our department for further evaluation and treatment. The patient had reviewed and provided written consent to participate in the study. The ethics committee of Chongqing Medical University has reviewed and approved the project and the Ethics board approval number is 2016–064.

In our department, we asked about her medical history in detail. She denied having symptoms such as frequent micturition, urgent urination, odynuria, hematuria, dysuria, abdominal pain, fever, chills, nausea or vomiting. Her medical history included hypertension with blood pressure up to 160/100 mmHg. She had never taken any medication for hypertension. There was no history of prior radiation exposure or kidney stones. She denied prior smoking and alcohol consumption. Physical examination revealed mild right costovertebral angle tenderness, but was otherwise normal. We performed the following auxiliary checks: Her routine blood tests demonstrated a red blood cell count (RBC) of 4.12×10^{12}/L, white blood cell count (WBC) of 10.75×10^9/L, and a total number of platelets (PLT) of 332×10^9/L. The erythrocyte sedimentation rate (ESR) was 70 mm/h. Procalcitonin (PCT) was 0.949 ng/mL (normal, < 0.50 ng/mL). Tuberculosis T cell detection and the Tuberculin Purified Protein Derivative (PPD) test were within the normal ranges. Her serum chemistry, routine urine tests, renal and liver function were within the normal ranges as well.

Her chest X-ray was within the normal range, but ultrasonography of the urinary system revealed heavy hydronephrosis of the right kidney. Contrast-enhanced computed tomography (CECT) of the abdomen showed marked hydronephrosis of the right kidney (which presented as a cyst-like structure), and some perinephric exudates (Fig. 1a-c). Further CECT (Fig. 1d-f) and CT (coronal and sagittal, Fig. 1g,h) of the abdomen revealed right gross hydronephrosis with a markedly dilated cystic pelvicalyceal system and right perinephric chronic inflammation; a tumor could not be completely ruled out in the lower pole of the right kidney due to uneven renal parenchyma and mild to moderate enhancement in the nephritic phase. Renal radionuclide imaging revealed that the glomerular filtration rate (GFR) of the right kidney was 12.3 mL/min, GFR of the left kidney was 57.9 mL/min and the total GFR was 70.2 mL/min (normal GFR>64.8 mL/min). A careful study of the imaging ruled out the presence of any other systemic involvement. Infectious lesions were considered before surgery, but tumors could not be excluded. The patients and her family members refused to perform other further examinations.

Retroperitoneal laparoscopic radical nephrectomy was performed under general anesthesia. Severe perinephric adhesions were found during the procedure (especially the hilum), therefore lymph nodes were not subjected to lymphadenectomy. It can be seen that the resected kidney specimen presented an irregular and enlarged "skin capsule" shape. The thickness of the capsule wall was uneven, and the thickening was obvious in some areas, especially in the lower pole, but there was no round or oval solid mass with any clear boundary. The resected specimen was submitted to histopathology following surgery. The pathologist evaluated the right kidney (11.0 × 6.0 × 5.0 cm) with the upper ureter (0.8 × 0.6 cm). The bisected right kidney showed a grayish white cut surface and a markedly dilated cystic pelvis, incrassated parenchyma of the lower pole, and incrassated renal capsules. The histological examination revealed well-differentiated squamous cell carcinoma (SCC), displaying typical morphological features of SCC (including: epithelioid cell niche, mild to moderate heterotypic cells, visible keratin pearls and intercellular bridges). Immunohistochemistry results also supported this diagnosis. Normal glomeruli and tubule structures were also observed around the cancerous foci, involving perinephric adipose tissue, but not including the renal pelvis, renal vein, or ipsilateral ureter. There was no distant metastasis. Therefore, a pathological stage of pT3aNxM0 was assigned. Immunohistochemistry showed EMA(−), CK(+++), HCK(+++), CK5/6(++), LCK(++), P63(+++), CK8(−), Ki67(++), 40% P53(+++), CerbB-2(−) (Figs. 2 and 3).

The patient refused additional treatment after surgery. She attended the phone call follow-up for 3 months, after which she was lost to follow-up. Written informed consent was obtained from the patient and her immediate family for the publication of the present study.

Discussion and conclusions

SCC of the kidney is a rare clinical entity representing only 0.5 to 0.8% of malignant renal tumors [1]. SCC of the renal parenchyma is extremely rare when compared to SCC of the renal pelvis. No less than 15 literature references have reported SCC of the renal pelvis in the recent 5 years, and a current review of the literature could identify only 5 literature references concerning SCC of the renal parenchyma [2–7] (Table 1). Until recently, SCC of the renal pelvis was regarded as urothelium metaplasia [7–9], however, the histological origin and mechanism of renal parenchyma SCC remains unknown. It probably originates from convoluted tubules or undifferentiated stem cells of the renal mesenchyme. SCC of the kidney is frequently associated with urolithiasis and hydronephrosis [3, 5, 6]. The present patient had a history of hydronephrosis for 2 months and surgery was performed to relieve the hydronephrosis. Hydronephrosis is a predisposing factor resulting in squamous metaplasia, which may develop into SCC later on.

Due to its nonspecific clinical presentation compared to other kidney tumors, hydronephrosis presents a great challenge for early diagnosis. The main symptoms presented by the five case reports of SCC of the rena parenchyma (Table 1) are hematuria and pain. Image examinations are valuable but are non-specific. Because of the rarity and the short follow-up of the cases, a prognosis is very difficult to predict.

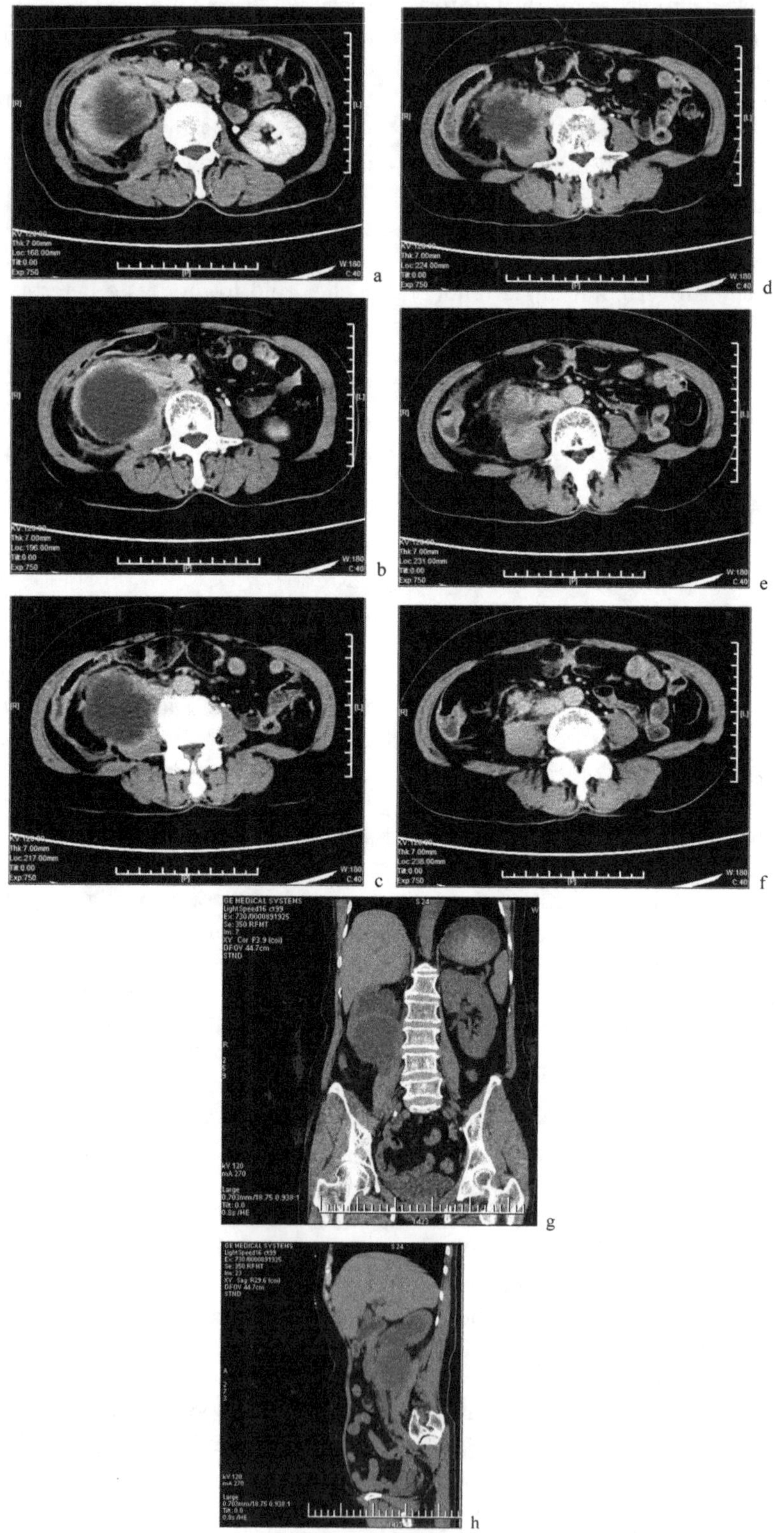

Fig. 1 a-c Contrast-enhanced computed tomography showed marked hydronephrosis of the right kidney and some perinephric exudates. **d-f**. Contrast-enhanced computed tomography revealed right gross hydronephrosis and right perinephric chronic inflammation; in the lower pole of the right kidney, a tumor could not be completely excluded with mild to moderate enhancement. **g,h** Plain scan of coronal and sagittal images

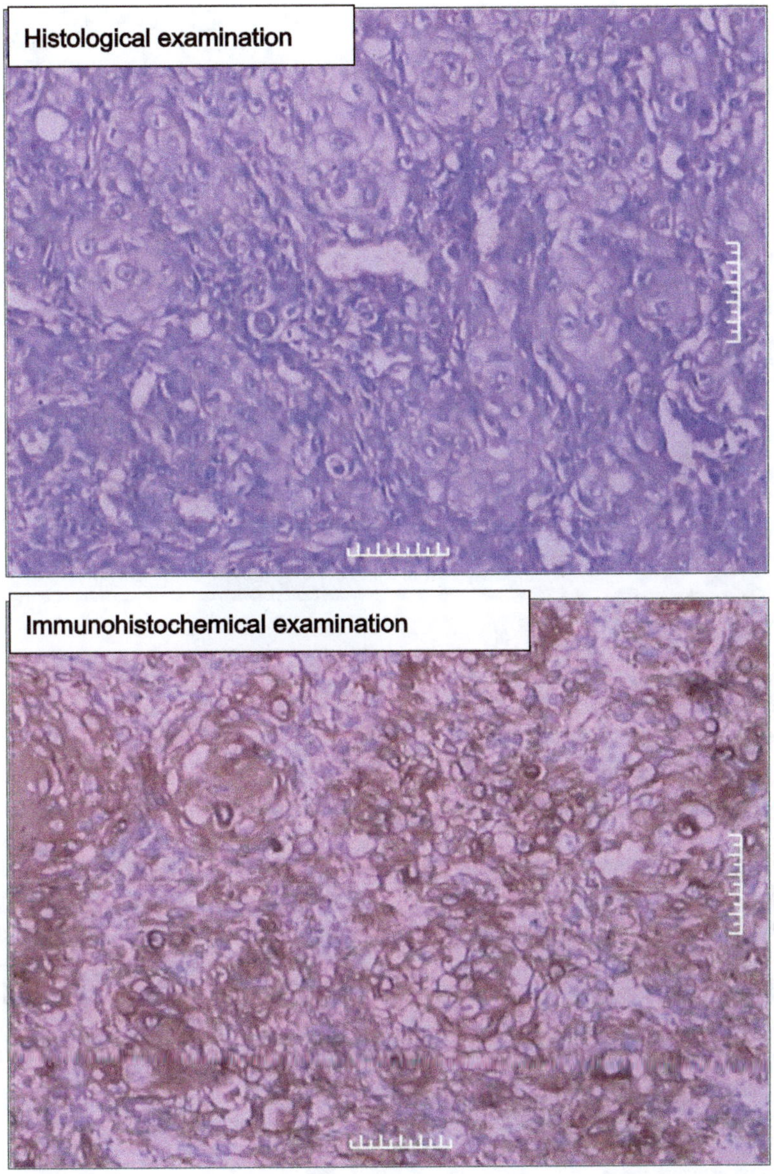

Fig. 2 (upper) Histological examination, showing classical morphology of squamous carcinoma (HE staining, 200×). (Fig. 2 lower) immunohistochemistry, CK5/6 positive (200×)

Ultrasonography typically only reveals only hydronephrosis. Conversely, CT is an important tool and can provide high-resolution imaging to evaluate masses and stages in renal malignancies. In the present case, CECT revealed hydronephrosis with a markedly dilated cystic pelvicalyceal system with perinephric chronic inflammation. This is consistent with the renal specimen seen after resection. Ureteral obstruction is the main cause of the presenting symptoms.

Furthermore, the significance of the case can also be considered as a lesson, which teaches us to consider the possibility of renal malignant tumors when encountering the patients with long-term hydronephrosis, uneven thickness of kidney parenchyma and uneven enhancement of CT scanning.

According to the patient's medical history and primary clinical examinations, tuberculosis and uretero pelvic junction obstruction were rather unlikely. One of the most consistent initial diagnoses is a neoplasm with unknown character. Primary SCC of the kidney should further rule out metastatic SCC with the combination of clinical history, imaging studies, and histopathology [7, 10]. Nevertheless, it is difficult to make a definite diagnosis prior to surgery considering the nonspecific features of this case. FDG-PET/CT has been validated as an effective tool in diagnosis, preoperative evaluation and prognosis of kidney

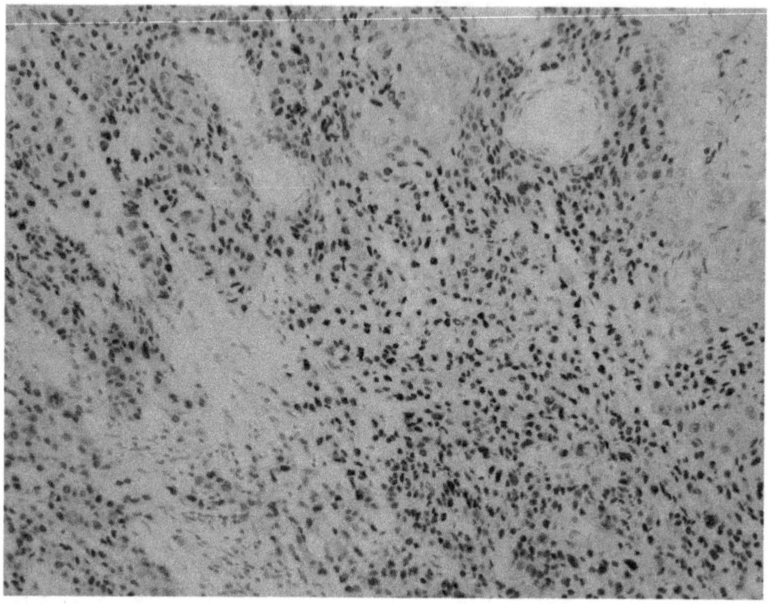

Fig. 3 immunohistochemistry of p63, positive (+++) (200×)

malignancies [11]. However, FDG-PET/CT were ineffective for distinguishing renal inflammation diseases from various types of tumors in some cases [6]. Renal tumors can be biopsied by puncture. Patients with hydroneprosis can be biopsied through ureteroscopy for stenosis. In addition, urocytology is helpful to determine the diagnosis of primary or invading lesions in renal pelvis and calves.

Regrettably, this patient did not undergo any examinations other than those mentioned above. The main reasons for this were as follows: 1) The imagological diagnosis showed dilation of the collecting system and chronic perinephritis, and the judgment of the tumor was not clear. 2) The Double J stent implantation was performed in an outside hospital. Due to the two reasons, it was difficult to make decisions on puncture biopsy, ureteroscopy and biopsy of stenoses. In addition, the ureteroscopy procedure may have introduced an increased the risk of tumor metastasis. 3) The positive rate of urocytology was low and not beneficial in affecting the decision to perform surgery. Meanwhile the double J stent placed in the outside hospital had just been removed before admission. Therefore, infectious lesions were primarily considered, affecting the clinical decision. Afterwards, the tumor did not invade the collective system. 4) The most important factor was the refusal of the patient and her family to undergo further medical examination as we suggested, including FDG-PET/CT because of the cost. They insisted on proceeding directly

Table 1 Characteristics of the reported cases

Author	Sex	Age	Presentation	radiological feature	Treatment	Prognosis
Terada (2010) [2]	M	73	Hematuria and lumbago	A bladder tumor, a left ureter tumor, and a left kidney tumor.	Nephroureterectomy	Alive at 3 months after surgery
Kulshreshtha (2012) [3]	F	60	Significant weight loss of 3 months duration	A mass in the mid and lower pole of left kidney with areas of necrosis are notable, and retroperitoneal lymph nodes (LN) were enlarged	Radical nephrectomy with dissection LN stations	Alive and disease free at 13 months post-surgery.
Ghosh(2014) [5]	M	51	Dull and intermittent pain	A solitary mass in the lower pole of right kidney	Nephrectomy	Asymptomatic with no evidence of recurrent or metastatic disease 12 months after surgery
Tapan Kumar Sahoo (2015) [7]	F	50	pain on the right side of the abdomen for 6 months	mild to moderate enhancing mass of size approximately 6 × 8 cm at upper pole of the right kidney	Radical nephrectomy	on regular follow-up for 6 months without any evidence of disease.
Wang 2016 (et al) [6]	M	61	Lumbago and gross hematuria	Multiloculated cyst-like masses with soft tissues of right kidney and fuzzy perirenal fatty space	Radical nephrectomy	No febrile, gross hematuria or abnormal abdominal signs one month after surgery

to surgery. Therefore, after the informed consent was signed, retroperitoneal laparoscopic radical nephrectomy was performed.

Because renal SCC is insensitive to chemotherapeutics and radiotherapy, the patient did not receive any further treatment. The cost of treatment was also taken into consideration. In addition, the prognosis of renal SCC is generally poor, and more extensive follow-up data is essential to evaluate the prognosis of renal parenchyma SCC.

In conclusion, SCC of the kidney parenchyma is a rare upper tract urothelial carcinoma, which presents a diagnostic challenge to the urologist and which should be considered in the patients with chronic hydronephrosis. According to the recent literature, 5 cases of renal parenchyma SCC have been reported to date (Table 1). As more cases are presented in the literature, urologists will be able to make a quick and accurate diagnosis and provide treatment of this disease by understanding its presentation and natural history.

Abbreviations

SCC: Squamous cell carcinoma; WBC: White blood cell count; PLT: Total number of platelets; ESR: Erythrocyte sedimentation rate; PCT: Procalcitonin; CECT: Contrast-enhanced computed tomography; PPD: Tuberculin purified protein derivative; CT: Computed tomography; GFR: Glomerular filtration rate; FDG-PET/CT: [18F]-fluorodeoxyglucose- positron emission tomography-computed tomography

Acknowledgements

We would like to thank Qing Jiang for general supervision of the research, thank Chuan Liu and Yulong Chen for data collection, thank Lingyu Liang for language polish.

Authors' contributions

Here we state XRZ contribute to acquisition and analysis of the case, draft of the work and interpretation of the data. YFZ, CGG and JYZ contributes to the drafted the work and substantively revised it. PHL made substantial contributions to the conception, design of the work, interpretation of data, provide the funding, drafted the work or substantively revised it. The author (s) read and approved the final manuscript.

Author details

[1]Department of Urology, The Second Affiliated Hospital of Chongqing Medical University, Yuzhong, Chongqing 400010, China. [2]Department of Urology, Jiangmen Central Hospital, Jiangmen 529030, Guangdong, China.

References

1. Li MK, Cheung WL. Squamous cell carcinoma of the renal pelvis. J Urol. 1987;138(2):269–71.
2. Terada T. Synchronous squamous cell carcinoma of the kidney, squamous cell carcinoma of the ureter, and sarcomatoid carcinoma of the urinary bladder: a case report. Pathol Res Pract. 2010;206(6):379–83. https://doi.org/10.1016/j.prp.2009.07.021.
3. Kulshreshtha P, Kannan N, Bhardwaj R, Batra S. Primary squamous cell carcinoma of the renal parenchyma. Indian J Pathol Microbiol. 2012;55(3):370–1. https://doi.org/10.4103/0377-4929.101747.
4. Pusiol T, Zorzi MG, Morini A. Comment on: primary squamous cell carcinoma of the renal parenchyma. Indian J Pathol Microbiol. 2013;56(1):70. https://doi.org/10.4103/0377-4929.116160.
5. Ghosh P, Saha K. Primary Intraparenchymal squamous cell carcinoma of the kidney: a rare and unique entity. Case Rep Pathol. 2014;2014:1–3. https://doi.org/10.1155/2014/256813.
6. Wang Z, Yan B, Wei YB, Hu NA, Shen Q, Li D, Yang JR, Yang X. Primary kidney parenchyma squamous cell carcinoma mimicking xanthogranulomatous pyelonephritis: a case report. Oncol Lett. 2016;11(3):2179–81. https://doi.org/10.3892/ol.2016.4200.
7. Sahoo TK, Das SK, Mishra C, Dhal I, Nayak R, Ali I, Panda D, DasMajumdar SK, Parida DK. Squamous cell carcinoma of kidney and its prognosis: a case report and review of the literature. Case Rep Urol. 2015;2015:469327. https://doi.org/10.1155/2015/469327.
8. Palmer CJ, Atty C, Sekosan M, Hollowell CM, Wille MA. Squamous cell carcinoma of the renal pelvis. Urology. 2014;84(1):8–11. https://doi.org/10.1016/j.urology.2013.11.020.
9. Jiang P, Wang C, Chen S, Li J, Xiang J, Xie L. Primary renal squamous cell carcinoma mimicking the renal cyst: a case report and review of the recent literature. BMC Urol. 2015;15:69. https://doi.org/10.1186/s12894-015-0064-z.
10. Bhaijee F. Squamous cell carcinoma of the renal pelvis. Ann Diagn Pathol. 2012;16(2):124–7. https://doi.org/10.1016/j.anndiagpath.2011.08.009.
11. Ferda J, Ferdova E, Hora M, Hes O, Finek J, Topolcan O, Kreuzberg B. 18F-FDG-PET/CT in potentially advanced renal cell carcinoma: a role in treatment decisions and prognosis estimation. Anticancer Res. 2013;33(6):2665–72.

21

The neutrophil-lymphocyte ratio has a role in predicting the effectiveness of nivolumab in Japanese patients with metastatic renal cell carcinoma: A multi-institutional retrospective study

Naotaka Nishiyama[1*], Megumi hirobe[2], Takuya Kikushima[1], Masahiro Matsuki[2], Atsushi Takahashi[3], Masahiro Yanase[4], Keisuke Ichimatsu[5], Masayuki Egawa[5], Norihiro Hayashi[6], Takahito Negishi[7], Naoya Masumori[2] and Hiroshi Kitamura[1]

Abstract

Background: The neutrophil-lymphocyte ratio (NLR) is a well-known prognostic marker in various cancers. However, its role as a predictive marker for the effectiveness of nivolumab in patients with metastatic RCC (mRCC) remains unclear. We evaluated the relationships between the NLR and progression-free survival (PFS) or overall survival (OS) in mRCC patients treated with nivolumab.

Methods: The data of 52 mRCC patients who received nivolumab therapy were collected from seven institutes and evaluated. The median follow-up period from treatment with nivolumab was 25.2 months (IQR 15.5–33.2).

Results: The median duration of nivolumab therapy was 7.1 months (IQR 2.9–24.4). The objective response rate was 25% and the 1- and 2-year PFS rates were 46.2 and 25.2%, respectively. The median NLR values at baseline and 4 weeks were 3.7 (IQR 2.7–5.1) and 3.3 (IQR 2.4–5.7), respectively. In the multivariate analysis, an NLR of ≥3 at 4 weeks was an independent predictor of PFS ($P = 0.013$) and OS ($P = 0.034$). The 1-year PFS of patients with an NLR of < 3 at 4 weeks was better than that of those with an NLR of ≥3 (75% versus 29%, $P = 0.011$). The 1-year OS of patients with an NLR of < 3 at 4 weeks was also better than that of those with an NLR of ≥3 (95% versus 71%, $P = 0.020$).

Conclusions: Although the baseline NLR was not associated with PFS or OS, an NLR of ≥3 at 4 weeks after the initiation of therapy might be a robust predictor of poor PFS and OS in mRCC patients undergoing sequential treatment with nivolumab.

Keywords: Metastatic renal cell carcinoma, Nivolumab, Neutrophil-lymphocyte ratio

Background

Over the last decade, the treatment of metastatic renal cell carcinoma (mRCC) has dramatically changed. Vascular endothelial growth factor (VEGF) and mammalian target of rapamycin (mTOR)-targeting agents have superseded cytokine therapies. More recently, immune checkpoint inhibitors (ICIs) have emerged as a new treatment option for mRCC. Nivolumab, a programmed cell death protein-1 (PD-1) antibody, induces restoration of the anticancer T cell mediated immune response by

* Correspondence: nishiyan@med.u-toyama.ac.jp
[1]Department of Urology, Faculty of Medicine, University of Toyama, 2630 Sugitani, Toyama 930-0194, Japan
Full list of author information is available at the end of the article

blocking PD-1 [1]. In a global multicenter phase 3 trial (CheckMate 025), nivolumab treatment was associated with longer overall survival (OS) in mRCC patients who were previously treated with tyrosine kinase inhibitors (TKIs), in comparison to everolimus [2]. On the basis of these results, the major guidelines recommend nivolumab as a second-line treatment for mRCC patients [3, 4].

Although ICIs, including nivolumab, have resulted in changes to the treatment strategies for mRCC, there are unmet needs for biomarkers to predict the effectiveness of ICIs. The Memorial Sloan Kettering Cancer Center (MSKCC) risk category and International Metastatic Renal Cell Carcinoma Database Consortium (IMDC) risk category are widely used for predicting the prognosis of patients [5, 6]. However, the MSKCC and IMDC risk categories were developed using data from patients who received cytokine therapy and targeted therapy, respectively. Thus, novel prognostic biomarkers or models are required in the ICI era.

Many studies have reported the role of the systemic inflammation response, including C-reactive protein (CRP), albumin, neutrophil, and related variables, for predicting the prognosis of patients with various cancers [7–9], including mRCC [10]. Recently, the neutrophil-lymphocyte ratio (NLR) has been recognized as a predictive marker for both non-metastatic RCC [11–13] and for mRCC treatment with TKI [14–17]. Although some studies [18, 19] revealed that a lower NLR was a significant predictor of favorable progression-free survival (PFS) and OS in mRCC patients treated with ICIs, these studies analyzed data from various lines and ICIs. Thus, there are no robust data about the NLR as a prognostic factor from studies focused on sequential treatment with nivolumab. The aim of this study was to evaluate whether the NLR is a predictor of poor oncological outcomes in mRCC patients undergoing sequential treatment with nivolumab.

Methods

Patients' characteristics (Table 1)

Data from 52 patients who underwent nivolumab treatment between January 2016 and November 2018 were collected from 7 institutes (Sapporo Medical University Urologic Oncology Consortium and Toyama Urologic Study Group), retrospectively. All patients received one or more prior anti-VEGF therapy. The median follow-up period from the initiation of nivolumab treatment was 25.2 months (IQR: 15.5–33.2). The patients consisted of 36 (69%) men and 16 (31%) women (median age, 67.0 years [IQR, 60.2–71.0]).

Clinical data collected from medical records included demographic information, IMDC risk factors [6], Eastern Cooperative Oncology Group performance status (ECOG PS), treatment line of nivolumab, number of metastatic sites, C-reactive protein at baseline, NLR at baseline and NLR at 4 weeks after the initiation of therapy. Hematological analyses were performed, and the serum chemistry was examined at baseline and at every nivolumab treatment. Response or progression were determined according to the Response Evaluation Criteria in Solid Tumors version 1.1 [20]. The follow-up protocol consisted of computed tomography or magnetic resonance imaging at baseline and every 3 months. This study was approved by the ethics committees of all participating institutions.

Table 1 Patient characteristics ($n = 52$)

Characteristic		N (%)
Sex	Male	36 (69)
	Female	16 (31)
Prior nephrectomy	Yes	45 (87)
	No	7 (13)
Age at start of nivolumab	Median (range)	67.0 (38–86)
ECOG PS	0	35 (67)
	1	15 (29)
	2	2 (4)
Histologic type	Clear cell carcinoma	42 (81)
	Non-clear cell carcinoma	6 (11)
	Unknown	4 (8)
Treatment line of nivolumab	Second	18 (35)
	Third line or later	34 (65)
IMDC risk classification	Favorable	8 (15)
	Intermediate	37 (71)
	Poor	7 (14)
Number of metastatic sites	< 3	31 (60)
	≥3	21 (40)
CRP at baseline	< 10 mg/L	29 (56)
	≥10 mg/L	23 (44)
NLR at baseline	< 3	20 (39)
	≥3	32 (61)
NLR at 4 weeks	< 3	20 (39)
	≥3	31 (59)
	unknown	1 (2)

ECOG Eastern Cooperative Oncology Group; *PS* Performance status; *IMDC* International Metastatic Renal Cell Carcinoma Database Consortium; *CRP* C-reactive protein; *NLR* Neutrophil-to-lymphocyte ratio

Statistical analyses

OS was calculated from the day of the initiation of nivolumab therapy to the date of death from any cause and was censored at the date of the last follow-up for surviving patients. PFS was calculated from the day of the initiation of nivolumab therapy to the date of documented progression or death (in the absence of progression) and was censored at the last date without any events. The treatment line at the start of nivolumab, number of metastatic organ sites and Eastern Cooperative Oncology Group (ECOG) performance status (PS) were compared using Fisher's exact test. The IMDC risk classification was compared using the chi-squared test. The OS and PFS were analyzed by a log-rank test and a Cox regression analysis was performed to estimate HRs. The OS and PFS were estimated using the Kaplan-Meier method. The distribution of the NLR values was compared using a paired *t*-test. All statistical analyses were performed using the SPSS software program (version 25.0 SPSS; Chicago, IL, USA). *P* values of < 0.05 were considered to indicate statistical significance.

Results

The patients' characteristics are shown in Table 1. Of the 52 patients, 18 (35%) and 34 (65%) received one and two or more prior therapeutic treatments, respectively. Eight, 37 and 7 patients had a favorable, intermediate and poor risk IMDC classification, respectively. The median duration of nivolumab therapy was 7.1 months (IQR: 2.9–24.4). The best responses during nivolumab therapy were a complete response in 2 (4%), partial response in 11 (21%), stable disease in 22 (42%) and progressive disease (PD) in 17 (33%) patients. The objective response rate was 25%.

The median NLR at baseline was 3.7 (IQR: 2.7–5.1). At baseline, 32 (61%) had an NLR of ≥3 and 20 (39%) patients had an NLR of < 3. The median NLR at 4 weeks after the initiation of nivolumab treatment was 3.3 (IQR: 2.4–5.7). At 4 weeks, 31 (59%) patients had an NLR of ≥3 and 20 (39%) patients had an NLR of < 3. The NLR at 8 weeks after the initiation of nivolumab treatment could not be analyzed in 11 (21%) of the patients because of discontinuation due to progression disease or adverse events. The median NLR at 8 weeks was 3.2 (IQR: 2.3–5.7). The NLR at baseline and that at 4 weeks did not differ to a statistically significant extent (*P* = 0.351). The NLR at 4 weeks and at 8 weeks did not differ to a significant extent (*P* = 0.688). In non-responders (defined as a best response of PD), the NLR at 4 weeks tended to be higher than that at baseline; however, the difference did not reach statistical significance (Fig. 1). Supplementary Table 1 shows predictive factors for patients with NLR of < 3 and NLR of ≥3 at baseline and at 4 weeks after the initiation of nivolumab treatment. There were no significant difference between the proportion of predictive factors and NLR.

The PFS

The 1-year and 2-year PFS were 46.2 and 25.2%, respectively (Fig. 2a). In the univariate analysis of all 52 patients, prior nephrectomy (*P* = 0.046), ECOG PS (0.026), IMDC poor risk (*P* = 0.045), and an NLR ≥3 at 4 weeks (*P* = 0.013) were identified as significant predictors of a poor PFS. In the multivariate analysis, only an NLR ≥3 at 4 weeks (HR 2.340, 95% CI 1.19–4.59, *P* = 0.013) as independently associated with the PFS (Table 2). The 1-year PFS of patients with an NLR of ≥3 and those with an NLR of < 3 at 4 weeks were 29.0 and 75.0%, respectively (*P* = 0.011). A significant difference in PFS was seen between patients with an NLR of ≥3 and those with an

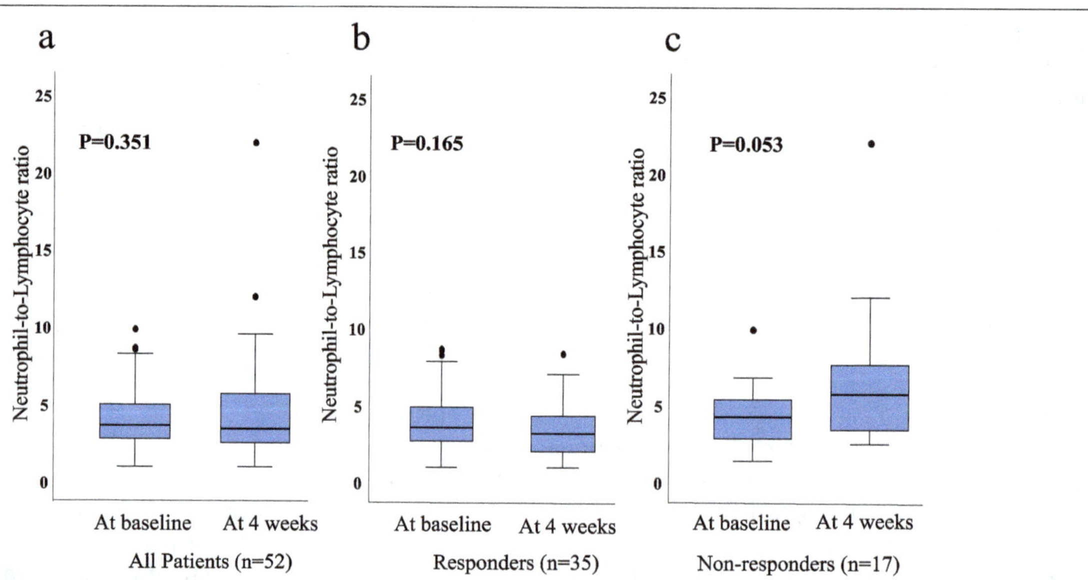

Fig. 1 The neutrophil-lymphocyte ratio (NLR) of all patients (**a**), responders whose best response was a complete response (CR), partial response (PR) or stable disease (SD) (**b**) and non-responders whose best response was progressive disease (PD) (c)

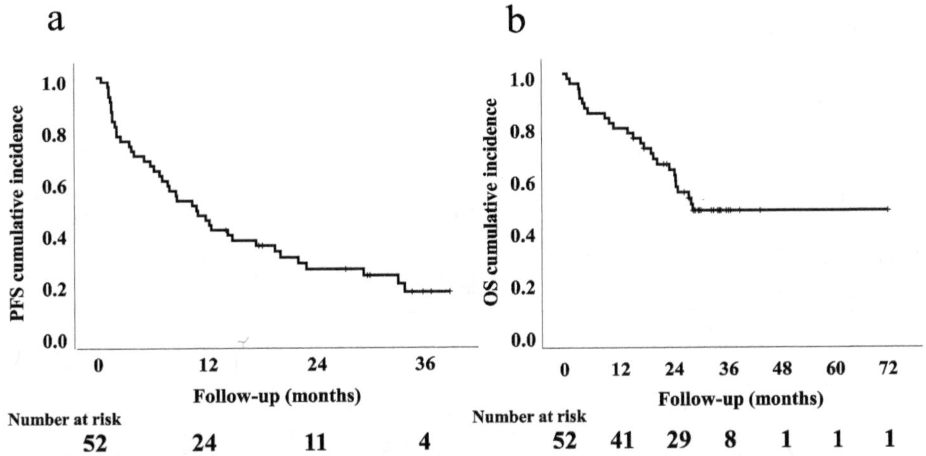

Fig. 2 Kaplan-Meier curves for progression-free survival (PFS) (**a**) and overall survival (OS) (**b**) of mRCC patients receiving nivolumab as a sequential therapy

NLR of < 3 at 4 weeks, but not at baseline (Fig. 3a and b).

The OS

The 1-year and 3-year OS after nivolumab treatment were 78.8 and 47.2%, respectively. The median OS was 27.9 months (Fig. 2b). In the univariate analysis of all 52 patients, sex female ($P = 0.004$), ECOG PS ≥1 ($P = 0.021$) and NLR ≥3 at 4 weeks ($P = 0.026$) were significant predictors for poor OS (Table 3). In the multivariate analysis, female sex (HR 1.679, 95% CI 1.13–2.50, $P = 0.011$) and an NLR ≥3 at 4 weeks after nivolumab treatment (HR 2.734, 95% CI 1.08–6.92, $P = 0.034$) were independent risk factors for the OS (Table 3). The 1-year OS of patients with an NLR of ≥3 and those with an NLR of < 3 at 4 weeks were 71.0 and 95.0%, respectively ($P =$

Table 2 The results of the univariate analyses and Cox multivariate analyses of factors predicting the PFS ($n = 52$)

	Univariate		Multivariate	
Variables	HR (95% CI)	*p* Value*	HR (95% CI)	*p* Value*
Age				
(< 70 years vs. ≥70 years)	1.084 (0.57–2.06)	0.801		
Sex				
(Male vs. Female)	1.281 (0.92–1.76)	0.137		
Prior nephrectomy				
(yes vs. no)	2.341 (1.01–5.04)	0.046		
ECOG PS				
(0 vs. ≥1)	2.072 (1.09–3.94)	0.026		
Treatment line of nivolumab				
(2 vs. ≥3)	1.454 (0.77–2.75)	0.251		
IMDC risk classification				
(Favorable, Intermediate vs. Poor)	2.331 (1.02–5.33)	0.045		
Number of Metastatic Organ site				
(1,2 vs. ≥3)	1.023 (0.55–1.92)	0.944		
CRP at baseline				
(< 10 mg/L vs. ≥10 mg/L)	1.001 (0.53–1.89)	0.997		
NLR at baseline				
(< 3 vs. ≥3)	1.147 (0.60–2.12)	0.676		
NLR at 4 weeks				
(< 3 vs. ≥3)	2.340 (1.19–4.59)	0.013	2.340 (1.19–4.59)	0.013

*Cox proportional hazards model

PFS Progression-free survival; *HR* Hazard ratio; *CI* Confidence interval; *ECOG* Eastern Cooperative Oncology Group; *PS* Performance status; *IMDC* International Metastatic Renal Cell Carcinoma Database Consortium; *CRP* C-reactive protein; *NLR* Neutrophil-to-lymphocyte ratio

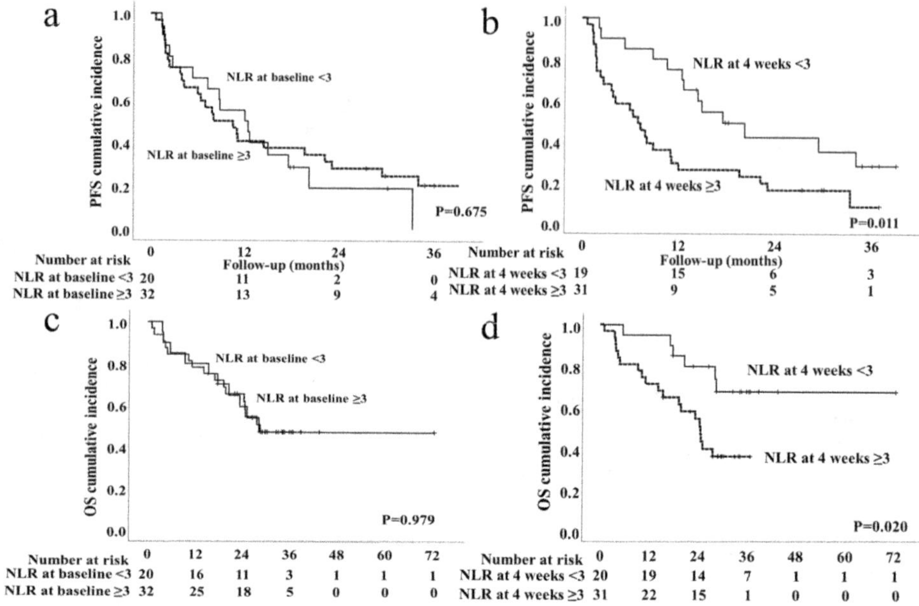

Fig. 3 Kaplan-Meier curves for progression-free survival (PFS) of mRCC patients treated with nivolumab stratified by the neutrophil-lymphocyte ratio (NLR) at baseline (**a**), and the NLR at 4 weeks (**b**). Overall survival (OS) stratified by the NLR at baseline (**c**) and that at 4 weeks (**d**)

Table 3 The results of the univariate analyses and Cox multivariate analyses of factors predicting the OS ($n = 52$)

	Univariate		Multivariate	
Variables	HR (95% CI)	*p* Value*	HR (95% CI)	*p* Value*
Age				
(< 70 years vs. ≥70 years)	2.307 (0.93–5.76)	0.073		
Sex				
(Male vs. Female)	1.773 (1.20–2.61)	0.004	1.679 (1.13–2.50)	0.011
Prior nephrectomy				
(yes vs. no)	1.190 (0.41–3.46)	0.749		
ECOG PS				
(0 vs. ≥1)	2.481 (1.14–5.38)	0.021		
Treatment line of nivolumab				
(2 vs. ≥3)	1.371 (0.62–3.03)	0.434		
IMDC risk classification				
(Favorable, Intermediate vs. Poor)	1.939 (0.73–5.16)	0.185		
Number of Metastatic Organ site				
(1,2 vs. ≥3)	1.799 (0.83–3.89)	0.135		
CRP at baseline				
(< 10 mg/L vs. ≥10 mg/L)	1.025 (0.47–2.23)	0.951		
NLR at baseline				
(< 3 vs. ≥3)	1.011 (0.46–2.23)	0.979		
NLR at 4 weeks				
(< 3 vs. ≥3)	2.857 (1.14–7.18)	0.026	2.734 (1.08–6.92)	0.034

*Cox proportional hazards model

OS Overall survival; *HR* Hazard ratio; *CI* confidence interval; *ECOG* Eastern Cooperative Oncology Group; *PS* Performance status; *IMDC* International Metastatic Renal Cell Carcinoma Database Consortium; *CRP* C-reactive protein; *NLR* Neutrophil-to-lymphocyte ratio

0.020). A significant difference was observed in the OS of patients with an NLRs of ≥3 and < 3 at 4 weeks; however, this difference was not observed between patients with these NLRs at baseline ($P = 0.979$) (Fig. 3c and d). The Kaplan-Meier curves of the patients stratified by sex ($P = 0.002$) are shown in Supplementary Fig. 1.

Discussion

This study showed that the NLRs of non-responders at 4 weeks after the initiation of nivolumab tended to be higher than at baseline. We also found that an NLR of ≥3 at 4 weeks was significantly associated with poor PFS and OS. These results suggested that a decline in the NLR may predict a favorable clinical outcome in mRCC patients treated with nivolumab as a sequential therapy.

Cancer-related inflammation is well recognized to be associated with cancer development and a poor prognosis. Tumor-associated neutrophils (TANs) are key regulators of cancer-related inflammation. TANs have been shown to induce genetic instability through the release of reactive oxygen species (ROS) and to produce tumor necrosis factor, IL-1, IL-6 and VEGF, which contribute to tumor proliferation and immune escape [21, 22]. TANs also activate and form neutrophil extracellular traps (NETs), which play a pro-tumor role in tumor progression. TANs are an important factor in the tumor microenvironment, and an increased number of TANs might play a pivotal role in treatment resistance [23].

Boissier et al. performed a meta-analysis to evaluate the prognostic role of the NLR in RCC and demonstrated that a high NLR was associated with a poor prognosis. In patients with both mRCC and localized RCC, an NLR of < 3 predicted better OS and PFS [14]. In non-metastatic clear cell RCC, recurrence-free survival in patients with an NLR of ≥2.7 was significantly shorter than that in patients with an NLR of < 2.7 [11]. Another study on mRCC showed that an NLR of ≥4.0 was an independent predictor of OS [24]. Kobayashi et al. reported that patients with an NLR of < 3.32 had longer PFS in comparison to those with an NLR of ≥3.32 after 1st-line targeted therapy [22].

Several reports have evaluated the role of NLR in the clinical outcomes of mRCC patients were treated with ICI. Jeyakumar et al. showed that an NLR of ≥3 was a predictor of a poor response, PFS and OS in patients with mRCC who were treated with nivolumab, ipilimumab, avelumab, pembrolizumab, or atezolizumab [18]. Lalani et al. reported that a high NLR at baseline and at 6 weeks after the initiation of therapy were associated with short PFS, short OS and a poor response [19]. In our study, the NLR at baseline was not a significant predictor of the response to nivolumab. This may be because all of the patients had received two or more TKI treatments and 63% of them had received three or more such therapies before the initiation of nivolumab treatment. Kobayashi et al. also reported that the NLR significantly decreased, even after treatment with TKIs, especially after sunitinib [22]. However, the NLR before nivolumab treatment was not a significant factor in this study. These results suggested that a decline in the NLR after ICI treatment—rather than TKI treatment—is useful information for predicting a response to nivolumab treatment.

Numerous studies have investigated different cutoff values for the NLR. In mRCC patients, most studies have used a cutoff value of around 3 [15–19, 22, 24–26]. We adopted NLR ≥3 as a significant predictor of poor PFS and OS in patients undergoing sequential treatment with nivolumab, based on the results of the meta-analysis by Hu et al. [15, 18].

The present study is associated with some limitations. First, this was a multi-institutional retrospective study. The patients' characteristics and treatment strategies might have differed among the institutions. The second limitation was the small number of patients included in this study. Despite these limitations, we believe that these results are clinically informative and will be useful for predicting the clinical outcomes of patients receiving nivolumab as a sequential treatment. However, a prospective study using a larger cohort is needed to confirm this.

Conclusions

Although the NLR at baseline was not associated with PFS or OS, an NLR of ≥3 at 4 weeks after the initiation of nivolumab therapy could predict poor PFS and OS. However, a larger prospective study is needed to validate these results.

Supplementary information

Additional file 1 Supplementary Figure 1. The Kaplan-Meier curve for the overall survival (OS) of patients stratified by sex.

Additional file 2 Supplementary Table 1. Characteristics of patients with an NLR of < 3 or ≥ 3 at baseline and at 4 weeks.

Abbreviations

NLR: Neutrophil-lymphocyte ratio; RCC: Renal cell carcinoma; mRCC: Metastatic renal cell carcinoma; PFS: Progression-free survival; OS: Overall survival; ICI: Immune checkpoint inhibitor; PD-1: Programmed cell death protein-1; TKI: Tyrosine kinase inhibitor; VEGF: Vascular endothelial growth factor; MSKCC: Memorial sloan kettering cancer center; IMDC: International metastatic renal cell carcinoma database consortium; ECOG PS: Eastern cooperative oncology group performance status; CRP: C-reactive protein; TANs: Tumor-associated neutrophils; ROS: Reactive oxygen species; NET: Neutrophil extracellular traps

Authors' contributions

NN and NM designed the study. NN wrote the manuscript. NN and HK analyzed the data. MH data collection and analysis. TK data collection. MM data collection. AT data collection and analysis. MY data collection. KI data collection. ME data collection. NH data collection. NT data collection. HK data collection, supervision and management. All authors read and approved the final manuscript.

Author details

[1]Department of Urology, Faculty of Medicine, University of Toyama, 2630 Sugitani, Toyama 930-0194, Japan. [2]Department of Urology, Sapporo Medical University School of Medicine, Sapporo, Japan. [3]Department of Urology, Hakodate Goryoukaku Hospital, Hakodate, Japan. [4]Department of Urology, Sunagawa City Medical Center, Sunagawa, Japan. [5]Department of Urology, Tonami general hospital, Tonami, Japan. [6]Department of Urology, Takaoka city hospital, Takaoka, Japan. [7]Department of Urology, National Hospital Organization Kyushu Cancer Center, Fukuoka, Hakata, Japan.

References

1. Chen DS, Mellman I. Oncology meets immunology: the cancer-immunity cycle. Immunity. 2013;39:1–10.
2. Motzer RJ, Escudier B, McDermott DF, George S, Hammers HJ, et al. Nivolumab versus Everolimus in advanced renal-cell carcinoma. N Engl J Med. 2015;373:1803–13.
3. NCCN Clinical Practice Guidelines in Oncology, https://www.nccn.org/professionals/physician_gls/pdf/kidney.pdf; [accessed 8 May 2019] 2019.
4. European Association of Urology Renal Cell Carcinoma Guidelines, https://uroweb.org/guideline/renal-cell-carcinoma/#7; [accessed 8 May 2019] 2019.
5. Heng DY, Xie W, Regan MM, Harshman LC, Bjarnason GA, Vaishampayan UN, et al. External validation and comparison with other models of the international metastatic renal-cell carcinoma database consortium prognostic model: a population-based study. Lancet Oncol. 2013;14:141–8.
6. Motzer RJ, Bacik J, Murphy BA, Russo P, Mazumdar M. Interferon-alfa as a comparative treatment for clinical trials of new therapies against advanced renal cell carcinoma. J Clin Oncol. 2002;20:289–96.
7. Templeton AJ, McNamara MG, Šeruga B, Vera-Badillo FE, Aneja P, Ocaña A, et al. Prognostic role of neutrophil-to-lymphocyte ratio in solid tumors: a systematic review and meta-analysis. J Natl Cancer Inst. 2014;106:dju124.
8. Qi Q, Zhuang L, Shen Y, Geng Y, Yu S, Chen H, et al. A novel systemic inflammation response index (SIRI) for predicting the survival of patients with pancreatic cancer after chemotherapy. Cancer. 2016;122:2158–67.
9. Mbeutcha A, Shariat SF, Rieken M, Rink M, Xylinas E, Seitz C, et al. Prognostic significance of markers of systemic inflammatory response in patients with non-muscle-invasive bladder cancer. Urol Oncol. 2016;34:483.e17–24.
10. Ramsey S, Lamb GW, Aitchison M, McMillan DC. Prospective study of the relationship between the systemic inflammatory response, prognostic scoring systems and relapse-free and cancer-specific survival in patients undergoing potentially curative resection for renal cancer. BJU Int. 2008;101:959–63.
11. Ohno Y, Nakashima J, Ohori M, Gondo T, Hatano T, Tachibana M. Followup of neutrophil-to-lymphocyte ratio and recurrence of clear cell renal cell carcinoma. J Urol. 2012;187:411–7.
12. de Martino M, Pantuck AJ, Hofbauer S, Waldert M, Shariat SF, Belldegrun AS, et al. Prognostic impact of preoperative neutrophil-to-lymphocyte ratio in localized nonclear cell renal cell carcinoma. J Urol. 2013;190:1999–2004.
13. Viers BR, Houston Thompson R, Boorjian SA, Lohse CM, Leibovich BC, Tollefson MK. Preoperative neutrophil-lymphocyte ratio predicts death among patients with localized clear cell renal carcinoma undergoing nephrectomy. Urol Oncol. 2014;32:1277–84.
14. Boissier R, Campagna J, Branger N, Karsenty G, Lechevallier E. The prognostic value of the neutrophil-lymphocyte ratio in renal oncology: a review. Urol Oncol. 2017;35:135–41.
15. Hu K, Lou L, Ye J, Zhang S. Prognostic role of the neutrophil-lymphocyte ratio in renal cell carcinoma: a meta-analysis. BMJ Open. 2015;5:e006404.
16. Chrom P, Stec R, Semeniuk-Wojtas A, Bodnar L, Spencer NJ, Szczylik C. Fuhrman grade and neutrophil-to-lymphocyte ratio influence on survival in patients with metastatic renal cell carcinoma treated with first-line tyrosine kinase inhibitors. Clin Genitourin Cancer. 2016;14:457–64.
17. Templeton AJ, Knox JJ, Lin X, Simantov R, Xie W, Lawrence N, et al. Change in neutrophil-to-lymphocyte ratio in response to targeted therapy for metastatic renal cell carcinoma as a prognosticator and biomarker of efficacy. Eur Urol. 2016;70:358–64.
18. Jeyakumar G, Kim S, Bumma N, Landry C, Silski C, Suisham S, et al. Neutrophil lymphocyte ratio and duration of prior anti-angiogenic therapy as biomarkers in metastatic RCC receiving immune checkpoint inhibitor therapy. J Immunother Cancer. 2017;5:82.
19. Lalani AA, Xie W, Martini DJ, Steinharter JA, Norton CK, Krajewski KM, et al. Change in neutrophil-to-lymphocyte ratio (NLR) in response to immune checkpoint blockade for metastatic renal cell carcinoma. J Immunother Cancer. 2018;6:5.
20. Eisenhauer EA, Therasse P, Bogaerts J, Schwartz LH, Sargent D, Ford R, et al. New response evaluation criteria in solid tumours: revised RECIST guideline (version 1.1). Eur J Cancer. 2009;45:228–47.
21. Galdiero MR, Marone G, Mantovani A. Cancer inflammation and cytokines. Cold Spring Harb Perspect Biol. 2018;10. pii: a028662.
22. Kobayashi M, Kubo T, Komatsu K, Fujisaki A, Terauchi F, Natsui S, et al. Changes in peripheral blood immune cells: their prognostic significance in metastatic renal cell carcinoma patients treated with molecular targeted therapy. Med Oncol. 2013;30:556.
23. Lingyun Wu, Sugandha Saxena, Mohammad Awaji and Rakesh K. Singh. Tumor-associated neutrophils in cancer: going pro. Cancers (Basel). 2019;11: pii: E564.
24. Ohno Y, Nakashima J, Ohori M, Tanaka A, Hashimoto T, Gondo T, et al. Clinical variables for predicting metastatic renal cell carcinoma patients who might not benefit from cytoreductive nephrectomy: neutrophil-to-lymphocyte ratio and performance status. Int J Clin Oncol. 2014;19:139–45.
25. Cetin B, Berk V, Kaplan MA, Afsar B, Tufan G, Ozkan M, et al. Is the pretreatment neutrophil to lymphocyte ratio an important prognostic parameter in patients with metastatic renal cell carcinoma? Clin Genitourin Cancer. 2013;11:141–8.
26. Fox P, Hudson M, Brown C, Lord S, Gebski V, De Souza P, Lee CK. Markers of systemic inflammation predict survival in patients with advanced renal cell cancer. Br J Cancer. 2013;109:147–53.

Sharing the initial experience of pan-cancer panel analysis in high-risk renal cell carcinoma in the Korean population

Jungyo Suh[1,2†], Chang Wook Jeong[1†], Seongmin Choi[3], Ja Hyeon Ku[1], Hyeon Hoe Kim[1], Kwangsoo Kim[4] and Cheol Kwak[1*]

Abstract

Background: This study aimed to assess the feasibility of a pan-cancer panel assay for high-risk renal cell carcinoma (RCC) in the Korean population. We also analyzed the clinical and genetic factors contributing to metastasis in clear cell RCC.

Methods: Thirty-one patients with advanced RCC who underwent radical nephrectomy were analyzed. A 1.8 Mb multi-cancer panel (including 25 RCC-related genes, such as VHL, PBRM1, SETD2, and MET), comprising 181 target genes, 23 fusion genes, and 45 drug target lesions developed by Seoul National University Hospital, was used for this study.

Results: We extracted DNA from 30 of the 31 (96.7%) RCC specimens. Twenty-one patients (average age 63.3 ± 11.3 years) with clear cell RCC, 5 with papillary RCC, 3 with chromophobe RCC, and one patient, each with MiT family translocation carcinoma RCC and succinate dehydrogenase deficiency RCC, were analyzed. The sequencing depth was 430.8 ± 206.6 and 97 mutations (7.3 ± 2.7 mutations per patient) were detected. The most commonly mutated genes were *VHL* (46%), *PBRM1* (30%), and *BAP1*, *NOTCH4*, and *POLQ* (23.33% each). Compared with TNM stage matched data from TCGA of clear cell RCC, *VHL* and *PBRM1* are most common in both cohorts. Univariate and multivariate analyses revealed that tumor size (Hazard ratio = 2.47, $p = 0.04$) and *PBRM1* (Hazard ratio = 28.69, $p = 0.05$) were related to metastasis in clear cell RCC.

Conclusion: The pan-cancer panel comprised of RCC-related genes is a feasible and promising tool to evaluate genetic alterations in advanced RCC. However, large-scale studies and a focus on the clinical utility of this cancer panels is needed.

Keywords: Kidney cancer, Genes, VHL gene, PBRM1 mutation, Metastasis, Pan-cancer panel, Next-generation sequencing

Background

Renal cell carcinoma (RCC) is a malignancy that arises in the nephron tubules and has very heterogeneous histologic and clinical manifestations, accounting for approximately 90% of all cases of kidney cancer and 2.4% of all adult tumors [1]. The incidence of RCC continues to increase [2]. As of 216, there are more than 15 RCC subtypes classified by the World Health Organization [2], based on histologic and molecular criteria. Clear cell RCC (ccRCC) is the most common subtype, accounting for 75% of RCC cases, followed by papillary RCC (pRCC) and chromophobe RCC (chrRCC) [3]. The MiT family of translocation carcinomas (tRCC) and succinate dehydrogenase deficiency RCC (SDHD RCC) are rare subtypes, which are diagnosed based on molecular alterations.

Recent advances in next-generation sequencing (NGS) technology have revealed numerous genetic alterations

* Correspondence: mdrafael@snu.ac.kr
†Jungyo Suh and Chang Wook Jeong contributed equally to this work.
[1]Department of Urology, Seoul National University College of Medicine, Seoul, South Korea
Full list of author information is available at the end of the article

that are important in RCC pathogenesis and prognosis [4–6]. For instance, the driver mutation of each subtype, such as von Hippel-Lindau (VHL), PBRM1, and BRCA-1 associated tumor protein 1 (BAP1) in ccRCC; MET and fumarate hydratase (FH) in pRCC; and phosphatase and tensin homolog (PTEN) or TP53 in chrRCC; as well as the mutations related to prognosis, such as BAP1, PBRM1, or SET domain-containing 2 (SETD2) in ccRCC and cyclin-dependent kinase inhibitor 2A (CDKN2A) in pRCC have been identified in numerous NGS studies [7]. In the era of precision medicine, determining the molecular alteration in each RCC by NGS analysis is essential for diagnosis and treatment planning. However, Asian data have been limited in previously conducted large-scale NGS studies [8] and the histologic subtype and clinical behavior of RCC can differ among races [9]. Thus, Korean NGS data are essential for precision medicine.

We developed a pan-cancer panel to screen for important genetic alterations in various solid tumors, including major urological cancers, such as prostate, kidney, and bladder cancers. We assessed the feasibility of the pan-cancer panel assay for high-risk RCC in the Korean population. We also analyzed the clinical and genetic factors contributing to metastasis in ccRCC to determine the clinical utility of the pan-cancer panel assay for high-risk ccRCC.

Methods

Patient selection

All patients were selected from the Seoul National University Prospectively Enrolled Registry for Renal Cell Carcinoma – Nephrectomy (SUPER-RCC-Nx). This is a prospective, multidisciplinary, and biobank lined cohort that was established in March 2016 [10]. This prospective cohort collects patients' preoperative information, pathologic reports, surgical procedure details, and information on postoperative complications functional outcomes, and oncological outcomes. We selected 31 advanced RCC patients who were pathologically T3–4 or N1 or M1. The patients had undergone radical nephrectomy surgery from March 2016 to June 2016. The tumor and normal tissues that were collected in the operating room or frozen biopsy room were immediately stored in a – 195 °C liquid nitrogen tank at the SNUH Cancer Tissue Bank.

Cancer panel

The FIRST-panel version 3 and 3.1 SNUH cancer panel was used for this analysis. The panel was developed by SNUH. It includes all exons of 183 genes, specific introns of 23 fusion genes, the telomerase reverse transcriptase promoter region, 8 microsatellite instability (MSI) markers, and 45 drug target lesions. The total length captured was approximately 1.949 Mbp. The FIRST-panel was designed to screen for the important genetic alterations in major urological malignancies, including prostate, bladder, and kidney cancers [11]. We selected RCC-related mutations by reviewing landmark studies, and finally selected 25 renal cell carcinoma-related genes, including VHL, PBRM1, SETD2, and MET mutations, in the FIRST-panel version 3.x.

DNA extraction from fresh frozen tissue

Fresh frozen tumor tissues were homogenized and lysed with proteinase K. Total DNA was isolated from each target using the Maxwell® 16 CSC DNA Blood kit (Promega Corp., Madison, WI, USA). Extracted DNA was quantitated using a Quantus fluorometer (Promega Corp.) and TapeStation4200 (Agilent Technologies, Santa Clara, CA, USA).

Capture library preparation and sequencing

The quality of functional genomic DNA was assessed using the 2200 TapeStation System (Agilent Technologies) before preparation of the library. The input DNA (200 ng ~ 1 μg) was sheared using an S220 Focused-ultrasonicator (Covaris, Inc., Woburn, MA, USA). Paired-end libraries were prepared with the SureSelectXT Target Enrichment System Kit (Agilent Technologies) for the Illumina paired-end sequencing library protocol using SNUH FIRST Cancer Panel v3.0 and v.3.1, according to the manufacturer's instructions. The quality of the DNA library was evaluated using a Bioanalyzer 2100 and DNA 1000 chips (Agilent Technologies). The final libraries were sequenced on the Illumina Hiseq 2500 platform (2× 100 bp and 1000× coverage).

Next-generation sequencing

Targeted NGS was performed using the Illumina Hiseq 2500 platform. Sequencing data were transformed as FASTQ files and quality control (QC) by FASTQC and Trimmomatic (0.33). Binary alignment/map (BAM) formation was performed after alignment based on the reference genome (GRCh 37) by BWA (0.7.12) and Picard (1.134). QC of BAM files was performed using SAMtools (v1.2) and GATK (v3.3). Single nucleotide polymorphism (SNP) discovery was performed using MuTect (1.1.7) and SAMtools (v1.2). Indel and copy number variation (CNV) discovery were performed by IndelGeontyper (0.36.3336) and CoNIFER (0.2.2), respectively. The fusion search was conducted using Delly (0.7.2). All data were converted to VCF format and annotated using ANNOVAR.

Variant prevalence comparison of SNUH pan-cancer data and TCGA prostate cancer data

Three RCC databases were downloaded from The Cancer Genome Atlas (TCGA; TCGA-KIRC, TCGA-

KIRP, TCGA-KICH) variant MAF files, belonging to the NCI GDC data portal. We extracted the variants of interest from the MAF files: *VHL, PBRM1, BAP1, SETD2, KMT2D, MET, TP53, FH, BRCA2, TSC1, TSC2, KMT2D, NOTCH3, NOTCH4*, DNA polymerase theta (*POLQ*), Franconi anemia complementation group A (*FANCA*), and ataxia telangiectasia and Rad3-related (ATR). Four MAF files were provided for their corresponding variant callers: MuSE, Mutect2, VarScan2, and SomaticSniper. We selected variants that were present in at least two of these files. According to the "Variant_Classification" column of the MAF files, the data were categorized as missense mutation, truncating mutation (frameshift indels, splice site variants, and nonsense mutations), and in-frame indels. After matching pathologic TNM staging (T3 over or N1 or M1) of TCGA data with SNUH data, the prevalence of the mutations was compared with our SNUH pan-cancer data.

Integrative statistical analyses of clinical and genomic data

The clinical and demographic variables of three of the major subtypes of RCC were compared. As the tRCC and SDHD RCC groups contained one patient each, only described characteristics were compared, without statistical analysis. The continuous variables are summarized as the median value, and categorical variables are reported as actual numbers and percentages. A one-way ANOVA test was performed for three of the major groups (ccRCC, pRCC, and chrRCC).

We performed univariate and multivariate analyses of clinical and genomic data from 20 ccRCC patients. The factors associated with the presence of metastasis (both synchronous and metachronous) were compared using Student's t-test, Pearson Chi-square test, or Fischer's exact test. Univariate and multivariate logistic regression analyses were then performed for the presence of metastasis. All statistical analyses were conducted using SPSS Statistics 22 (IBM, Armonk, NY, USA). A p-value < 0.05 was considered significant.

Results

Patient characteristics

The demographic and clinical characteristics of the enrolled patients are presented in Table 1. The 31 patients were categorized into the following subclasses of RCC: ccRCC (n = 21), pRCC (n = 5), chrRCC (n = 3), tRCC (n = 1), and SDHD RCC (n = 1). Our data only contained type 2 subtypes of pRCC. The mean follow-up period

Table 1 Baseline characteristics of five types of RCC evaluated by this study

Characteristics	Clear cell N = 20	Papillary N = 5	Chromophobe N = 3	P-value	tRCC N = 1	SDHD N = 1
Age (range) - yr	63.6 ± 11.3	67.6 ± 10.2	63.0 ± 8.66	0.752	60	39
Sex – male (%)	13 (65)	4 (80)	2 (66.7)	0.830	1 (100)	0 (0)
BMI (kg/m^2)	24.9 ± 5.1	25.2 ± 3.4	24.6 ± 2.4	0.985	22.60	24.20
DM	6 (30)	2 (40)	0 (0)	0.495	1 (100)	0 (0)
HTN	12 (60)	3 (60)	2 (66.7)	0.978	1 (100)	0 (0)
Mass size	7.04 ± 3.1	7.08 ± 4.3	7.67 ± 4.0	0.434	10.9	2.5
Pathologic T stage – N (%)				0.927		
< T2	2 (10)	1 (20)	0 (0)		0 (0)	0 (0)
T3	17 (85)	4 (80)	3 (100)		1 (100)	1 (100)
T4	1 (5)	0 (0)	0 (0)		0 (0)	0 (0)
Tumor thrombus level– N (%)				0.354		
Level 1	3 (15)	0 (0)	I (33.3)		0 (0)	0 (0)
Level 2	1 (5)	1 (25)	0 (0)		1 (100)	0 (0)
Fuhrman grade				0.830		
2	0 (0)	0 (0)	0 (0)		0 (0)	1 (100)
3	19 (95)	5 (100)	3 (100)		1 (100)	0 (0)
4	1 (5)	0 (0)	0 (0)		0 (0)	0 (0)
Pathologic N stage – N (%)				–		
N1	0 (0)	0 (0)	0 (0)		1 (100)	0 (0)
Pathologic M stage – N (%)				0.642		
M1	4 (20)	1 (20)	0 (0)		1 (16.7)	0 (0)

was 19.0 months. Twelve patients presented with metastatic lesions within the follow-up period, including 6 synchronous and 6 metachronous metastases. There were no deaths in the follow-up period.

Sequencing QC

DNA was successfully extracted from the 30 fresh frozen tissue samples (96.8%) for library preparation. DNA could not be extracted from a sample with 90% necrotic lesion (ccRCC) in the library preparation step. The total read number ranged from 22,704,326 to 35,508,848, and the average size of FASTQ data was 2084.7 ± 265.3 Mb in the cancer panel analysis of the 30 patients. The average sequencing depth was 430.8 ± 206.6, ranging from 152 to 971. Average values of coverage above 50 and 100 were 98.6 ± 3.5% and 96.4 ± 5.8%, respectively.

Pan-cancer panel report

A total of 97 mutations were detected in the pan-cancer panel analysis. *VHL* was the most commonly mutated gene (46.67%). This observation was evident only in ccRCC. Genetic alterations in *PBRM1* (30%), *NOTCH4*, *POLQ*, and *BAP1* (23.3% each) were also frequently detected. An average of 7 SNPs was detected per patient. However, no fusion or CNVs were noted (Fig. 1). Integrative analysis of the pan-cancer panel data are presented in Fig. 2. We detected *SDHB* mutation in the specimen obtained from the SDHD RCC patient. The *TFE3* mutation was detected in the specimen of a tRCC patient. None of the mutations detected was exclusive to a particular subtype of RCC. No mutation common to all mutational profiles was detected.

Comparison with TCGA database

We compared the SNUH database with 110 TNM stage matched advanced RCC data from TCGA (TCGA-advance KIRC). The 17 mutations of interest (*VHL, PBRM1, BAP1, SETD2, KMT2D, MET, TP53, FH, BRCA2, TSC1, TSC2, KMT2D, NOTCH3, NOTCH4, POLQ, FANCA*, and *ATR*) were compared between the two groups. *VHL* (70.0% vs. 59.0%) and *PBRM1* (35.0% vs. 52.0%) were prevalent in both groups. *KMT2D, TSC1, TSC2, NOTCH3, NOTCH4, BRCA2, FANCA*, and *ATR* were more frequently mutated in the FIRST-panel analysis of RCC, compared to the TCGA-advance KIRC database. However, mutations in *PBRM1, SETD2*, and *BAP1* were more common in the TCGA-advance KIRC database. No mutations were detected in *POLQ, BAP1, MET, TP53*, and *FH* genes in the FIRST-panel analysis for ccRCC (Fig. 3).

The FIRST-panel results revealed that *PBRM1, POLQ, TSC1*, and *SETD2* genes were commonly mutated in papillary RCC. The MET mutation was frequently detected in the TCGA-KIRP database. However, no mutation or CNVs were observed in the FIRST-panel analysis of RCC patients. The type 1 and 2 pRCC displayed different

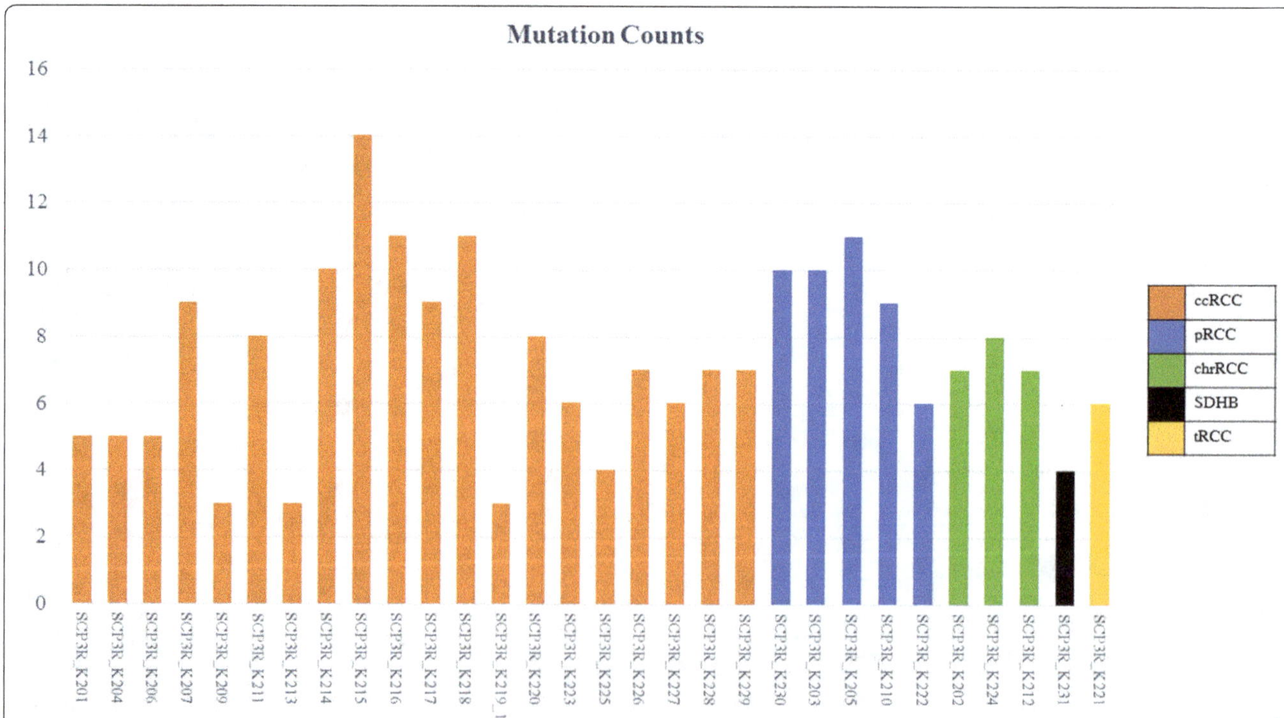

Fig. 1 Specific genetic alteration counts of each RCC patient. Minimum 3 to maximum 14 mutations per each patient was founded by pan-cancer panel analysis. Each bar shows SNP or INDEL mutations. There were no structural variations

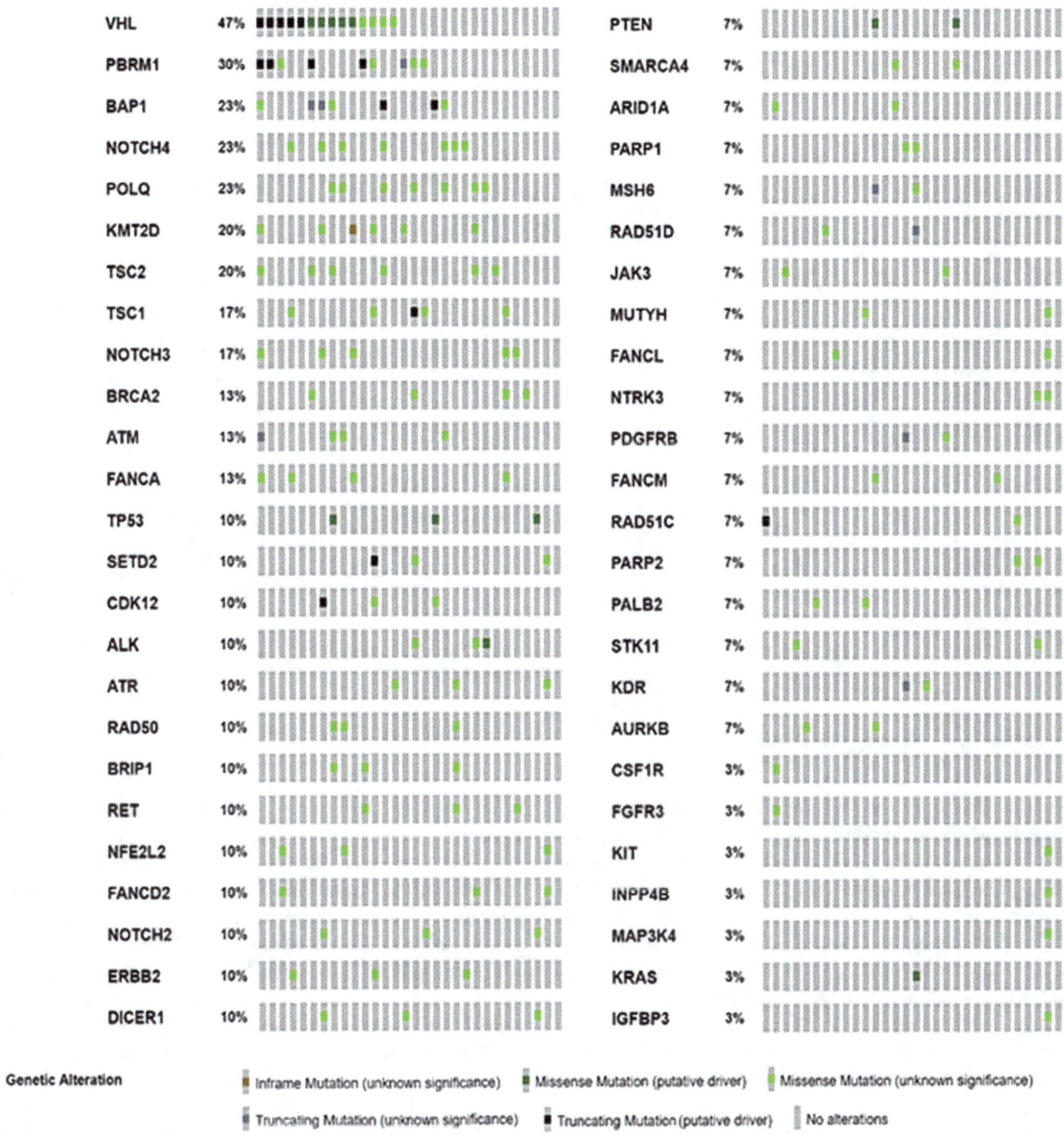

Fig. 2 Integrative analysis of pan-cancer panel analysis of 30 RCC patients. Each grey column represented a specific 30 patient data in order. This oncoprint obtained by The cBioPortal for Cancer Genomics (http://cbioportal.org) graphic visualization tool

molecular signatures, and MET mutations were more frequently found in the type 1 subtype. All five patients were the type 2 subtype, featuring commonly altered *CDKN2A, SETD2, BAP1,* and *PBRM1* mutations, consistent with our data. In the chromophobe subtype, the TP53 mutation was common in TCGA-KICH database. However, FIRST-panel analysis did not reveal any mutations in the TP53 gene in this subtype. A detailed comparison of the FIRST-panel and TCGA database was performed for papillary RCC and chromophobe RCC (Supplementary Table 1). Owing to the limited number of mutations included in the FIRST-panel, we could not examine some of the important mutations of RCC (*TTN, MUC4,* and *MUC16*), which are relatively common in the TCGA database.

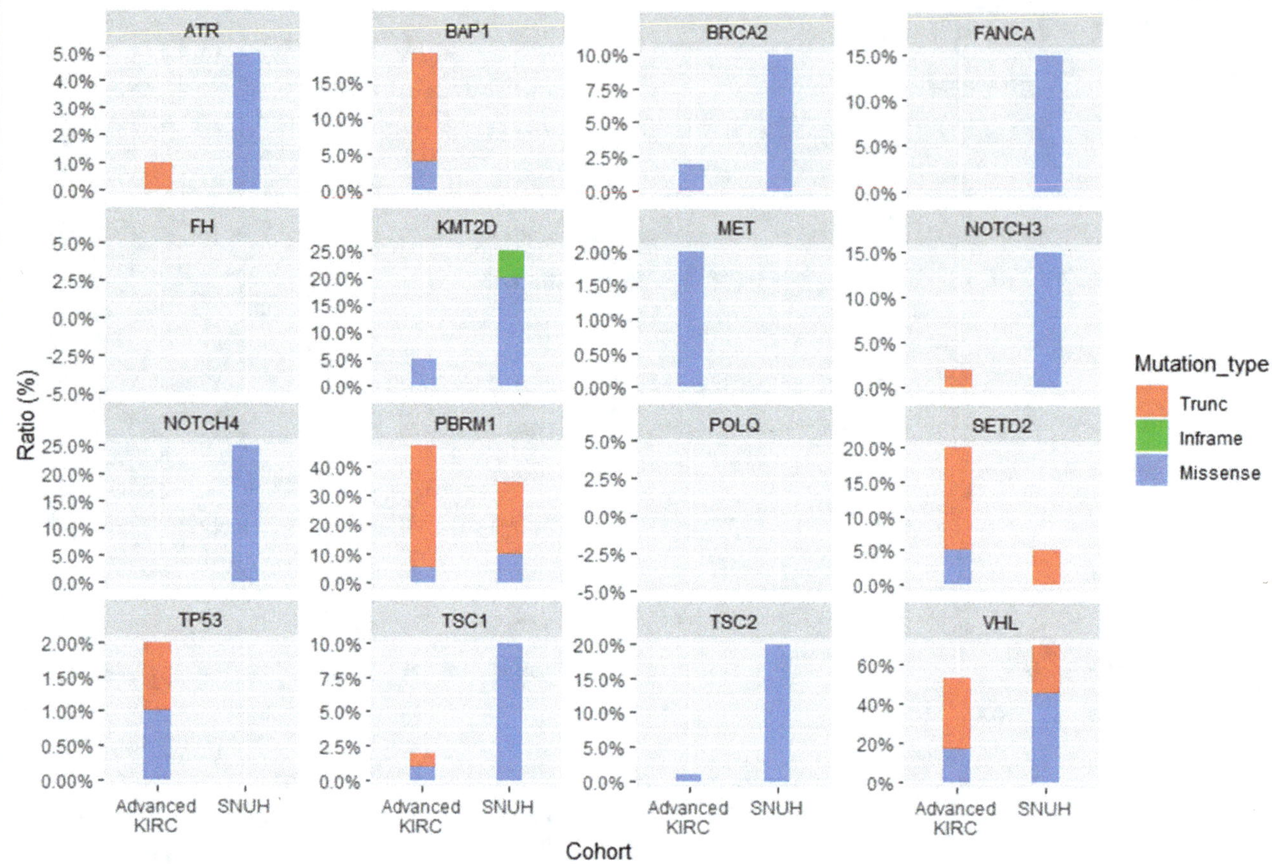

Fig. 3 The comparison of FIRST panel result to TNM stage matched TCGA cohort for clear cell RCC

Univariate and multivariate analyses of metastatic events

Clinical and pathologic information concerning the presence of a metastatic event was compared (Table 2). Mass size ($p = 0.008$) was significantly different between metastatic and localized RCC. In the mutation profile data, only *PBRM1* showed a possible relationship with metastasis. ($p = 0.062$). Univariate and multivariate logistic regression analyses data for metastasis are presented in Table 3. Among the clinicopathologic information and mutation data, only tumor size ($p = 0.042$) and *PBRM1* ($p = 0.046$) mutations were statistically correlated with metastasis.

Discussion

In this study, we successfully identified 97 genomic alterations in various subtypes of RCC. DNA was extracted from 30 of the 31 patients' samples. All 30 DNA samples were successfully analyzed using the pan-cancer panel. DNA could not be extracted from the fresh frozen tissue of one patient, which consisted mostly of necrotized tissue. Using univariate and multivariate analyses, we assessed the risk factors contributing to metastasis in ccRCC patients.

Most of the mutational signatures of ccRCC detected by this pan-cancer panel analysis were similar to those in the TCGA database and previous genetic studies. For example, in this study, *VHL* mutation was the most common mutation (70.0%) in ccRCC samples, followed by the PBRM1 mutation (35.0%). Genetic or epigenetic alterations in chromatin remodeling genes, which include *VHL*, *BAP1*, *PBRM1*, and *SETD2*, are the most prevalent events in the development of ccRCC [12, 13]. Similar to our findings, alterations in the *VHL* gene are reported to be the most frequent (60–70%), while those in *PBRM1*, *BAP1*, and *SETD2* were reported as 40, 10, and 10%, respectively, in previous genetic studies [4, 13, 14]. We also found *TP53* and *PTEN* mutations in chrRCC patients. These are important driver mutations of chrRCC [6, 15]. However because all the patients were papillary type 2, we did not detect MET mutations in pRCC patients in the pan-cancer analysis, which are more important driver mutation of type 1 pRCC than type 2 pRCC [15, 16].

Important driver mutations of uncommon RCC subtypes (tRCC and SDHD RCC) were also detected by the pan-cancer panel analysis. MiT family translocation carcinomas (tRCC) are characterized by translocations involving breakpoint lesions at Xp11.2 and are frequently fused with the *TFE3* gene [17, 18]. SDHD RCC is a

Table 2 Compare of clinicopathologic features and mutational profile by the presence of metastasis in clear cell RCC

	Localized N = 12	Metastatic N = 8	*p*-value
Age	61.4 ± 12.7	66.9 ± 8.6	0.303
Sex – male (%)	8 (66.7%)	5 (62.5%)	1.000‡
BMI (kg/m²)	25.7 ± 4.3	23.8 ± 6.3	0.439
DM	8 (66.7%)	6 (75.0%)	1.000‡
HTN	5 (41.7%)	3 (37.5%)	1.000‡
Mass size (cm)	5.8 ± 2.0	8.8 ± 2.4	**0.008**
Pathologic T stage – N (%)			0.071※
<T2	0 (0%)	2 (25.0%)	
T3	12 (100%)	5 (62.5%)	
T4	0 (0%)	1 (12.55)	
Tumor thrombus level– N (%)			0.225※
Level 0	10 (83.3%)	5 (62.5%)	
Level 1	1 (8.3%)	3 (37.5%)	
Level 2	1 (8.3%)	0 (0%)	
Fuhrman grade			0.400‡
3	12 (100%)	4 (87.5%)	
4	0 (0%)	1 (12.5%)	
Lymphovascular invasion	2 (16.7%)	4 (50.0%)	0.161‡
Mutation Counts	7.0 ± 3.2	7.1 ± 2.9	0.930
VHL	9 (75.0%)	5 (62.5%)	0.642‡
PBRM1	2 (16.7%)	5 (62.5%)	0.062‡
NOTCH4	4 (33.3%)	1 (12.5%)	0.603‡
KMT2D	1 (8.3%)	1 (12.5%)	1.000‡
NOTCH3	2 (16.7%)	1 (12.5%)	1.000‡
TSC1	3 (25.0%)	1 (12.5%)	0.619
BAP1	5 (41.7%)	2 (25.0%)	0.642‡
BRCA2	2 (16.7%)	0 (0%)	0.495‡
SETD2	0 (0%)	1 (12.5%)	0.400‡

※for Pearson Chi-square, ‡ for Fisher's Exact Test

newly classified subtype that was first announced in the 2016 WHO classification [2]. This subtype is characterized by genetic alterations in the Krebs cycle enzymes (SDHB/C/D) that result in the Warburg effect in ccRCC with the accumulation of hypoxia-inducible factor [19]. SDHD RCC can be diagnosed by distinguishing histologic features, such as vacuolated eosinophil or clear cells. However, detecting SDHB alteration by immunohistochemistry is more effective [2]. We successfully detected SDHB and TFE3 mutations in tissues specimens from SDHD RCC and tRCC patients using the pan-cancer panel analysis.

Although the mutational profile revealed by our pan-cancer panel analysis was mostly similar to the TCGA database, some discrepancies were evident. In this study, *NOTCH* family genes (*NOTCH3/4*), *TSC1*, *TSC2*, and *KMT2D* showed a relatively higher incidence of mutations than TNM matched data from TCGA-KIRC [4]. *BRCA* and *FANCA* is well known mutation of DNA repair pathway and is more common in FIRST panel analysis than TCGA-advanced KIRC. Owing to the small number of Asian patients included in the TGCA database [4–6], these differences may provide clues regarding the prevailing racial differences. However, owing to small number of study population, we cannot made concrete conclusion. More large-scale data are needed before any definitive conclusions can be made.

We conducted univariate and multivariate analyses using genetic alterations and clinicopathologic features in ccRCC. The multivariable analysis showed that the PBRM1 mutation and primary tumor size were significantly associated with metastasis in ccRCC. Primary tumor size is a well-established prognostic factor of metastasis [20, 21]. Eric et al. [21] retrospectively analyzed data from 2651 RCC patients, including 182 cases of synchronous metastasis, and found that the primary tumor size was significantly associated with metastasis. In general, PBRM1 mutations mutually exclusive from

Table 3 Univariate and multivariable analysis of clinco-pathologic feature and mutational profile for metastasis in clear cell RCC

	Univariate OR (95% CIs)	*p*-value	multivariable OR (95% CIs)	*p*-value
Age	1.048 (0.961–1.142)	0.288		
Sex	1.200 (0.185–7.770)	0.848		
Mass size (continuous)	1.952 (1.052–3.622)	**0.034**	2.47 (1.03–5.92)	**0.042**
Pathologic T-stage		1.000		
Thrombus level		0.374		
Fuhrman Grade		1.000		
Mutation count	1.015 (0.748–1.377)	0.925		
VHL mutation	0.556 (0.080–3.858)	0.552		
PBRM1 mutation	8.333 (1.034–67.142)	**0.046**	28.39 (1.06–758.79)	**0.046**
BAP1 mutation	0.467 (0.065–3.344)	0.448		

BAP1 mutations, [3] and both genes harbor a higher number of alterations in cases with metastatic lesions. Eckel-Passow et al. [22] analyzed paired tissue of primary and metastatic ccRCC and found that both BAP1 and PBRM1 were highly altered in metastatic lesions (98 and 90%, respectively), compared to the primary lesions (20 and 57%, respectively). The PBRM1 mutation alone is considered more favorable than the BAP1 mutation, but alterations in both lesions correlate with worst survival [23]. We could not analyze the expression pattern of BAP1 with PBRM1 or study their prognostic impact on survival, as no BAP1 mutations were detected. This observation might be attributed to the small sample size of our study.

With the advancement of NGS technology, there have been several attempts to use genetic analysis in clinical practice. Memorial Sloan Kettering-integrated mutation profiling of actionable cancer targets (MSK-IMPACT) [24] is a well-known pan-cancer NGS panel that targets more than 341 cancer associated genes. The MSK-IMPACT panel was successfully applied for a multi-institutional, diverse primary tumor prospective cohort including more than 12,670 tumor samples in 2017 [25]. These were promising results. However, the clinical application of NGS cancer panels in routine practice is not a reality yet, due to several issues of low matching yield in clinical trials [26, 27], high cost [28], and racial differences [26, 28]. The present study represents only a first step towards oncology precision medicine for clinical practice in advanced RCC. More data from global studies are required for further progress.

This study has several limitations. RCC is a highly heterogeneous disease, and the statistical power of our study (owing to the small sample size) may not be enough to concretely support our findings. In addition, because we used targeted sequencing to detect alterations in RCC, we did not determine the whole mutational profile of the RCC patients who were screened. Despite these limitations, we successfully conducted a pan-cancer panel analysis with good sequencing depth (> 400). The data shed light on the feasibility of using the pan-cancer panel for the diagnosis of RCC, and the possibility of deriving meaningful prognostic information from the mutational profiles.

Conclusion

The pan-cancer panel comprised of RCC-related genes is a feasible and promising tool to evaluate genetic alterations in advanced RCC. However, the limited information on genetic analysis necessitates large-scale studies and a focus on the clinical utility of cancer panels to further explore the routine use of the panel.

Supplementary information

Additional file 1: Supplementary Table 1. Comparison of SNUH pan-cancer panel result with TCGA database of papillary RCC and chromophobe RCC.

Abbreviations

RCC: Renal cell carcinoma; ccRCC: Clear cell renal cell carcinoma; pRCC: Papillary renal cell carcinoma; chrRCC: Chromophobe renal cell carcinoma; tRCC: MiT family translocation renal cell carcinoma; SDHD: Succinate dehydrogenase deficiency; NGS: Next-generation sequencing; SNUH: Seoul National University Hospital; IRB: Institutional review board; SUPER-RCC-Nx: Seoul National University Prospectively Enrolled Registry for Renal cell carcinoma – Nephrectomy; TCGA: The Cancer Genome Atlas

Acknowledgments

The bio-specimens for this study were provided by the Seoul National University Hospital Cancer Tissue Bank. All samples were obtained with the informed consent of patients under institutional review board-approved protocols.

Authors' contributions

CWJ and JS design the study. JS, CWJ and SC collect and analyze the data. SC and KK visualizing the data. JS draft the manuscript. CWJ, JHK, HHK and CK revise the manuscript. CWJ obtain funding. The authors read and approved the final manuscript.

Author details

[1]Department of Urology, Seoul National University College of Medicine, Seoul, South Korea. [2]Hospital Medicine Center, Seoul National University Hospital, Seoul, South Korea. [3]Department of Medicine, Seoul National University College of Medicine, Seoul, South Korea. [4]Transdisciplinary Department of Medicine & Advanced Technology, Seoul National University Hospital, Seoul, South Korea.

References

1. Scelo G, Larose TL. Epidemiology and risk factors for kidney cancer. J Clin Oncol. 2018;36:3574–81.
2. Moch H, Cubilla AL, Humphrey PA, Reuter VE, Ulbright TM. The 2016 WHO classification of Tumours of the urinary system and male genital organs—part a: renal, penile, and testicular Tumours. Eur Urol. 2016;70:93–105. https://doi.org/10.1016/j.eururo.2016.02.029.
3. D'Avella C, Abbosh P, Pal SK, Geynisman DM. Mutations in renal cell carcinoma. Urol Oncol Semin Orig Investig. 2018;000. https://doi.org/10.1016/j.urolonc.2018.10.027.
4. Creighton CJ, Morgan M, Gunaratne PH, Wheeler DA, Gibbs RA, Gordon Robertson A, et al. Comprehensive molecular characterization of clear cell renal cell carcinoma. Nature. 2013;499:43–9. https://doi.org/10.1038/nature12222.
5. The Cancer Genome Atlas Research Network. Comprehensive molecular characterization of papillary renal-cell carcinoma. N Engl J Med. 2016;374:135–45. https://doi.org/10.1056/NEJMoa1505917.
6. Davis CF, Ricketts CJ, Wang M, Yang L, Cherniack AD, Shen H, et al. The somatic genomic landscape of Chromophobe renal cell carcinoma. Cancer Cell. 2014;26:319–30.
7. Puente J, Suárez C, Pérez-Valderrama B, Arranz JÁ, González-Billalabeitia E, Méndez-Vidal MJ, et al. Recent advances in genitourinary tumors: a review focused on biology and systemic treatment. Crit Rev Oncol Hematol. 2017;113:171–90.
8. Spratt DE, Chan T, Waldron L, Speers C, Feng FY, Ogunwobi O, et al. Racial/ethnic disparities in genomic sequencing. JAMA Oncol. 2016;2:1070–4.

9. Batai K, Harb-De la Rosa A, Lwin A, Chaus F, Gachupin FC, Price E, et al. Racial and ethnic disparities in renal cell carcinoma: an analysis of clinical characteristics. Clin Genitourin Cancer. 2019;17:e195–202. https://doi.org/10.1016/j.clgc.2018.10.012.
10. Jeong CW, Suh J, Yuk HD, Tae BS, Kim M, Keam B, et al. Establishment of the Seoul National University prospectively enrolled registry for genitourinary cancer (SUPER-GUC): a prospective, multidisciplinary, bio-bank linked cohort and research platform. Investig Clin Urol. 2019;60. https://doi.org/10.4111/icu.2019.60.e32.
11. Suh J, Jeong CW, Choi S, Ku JH, Kim HH, Kim KS, et al. Targeted next-generation sequencing for locally advanced prostate cancer in the Korean population. Investig Clin Urol. 2020;61:127–35.
12. Riazalhosseini Y, Lathrop M. Precision medicine from the renal cancer genome. Nat Rev Nephrol. 2016;12:655–66. https://doi.org/10.1038/nrneph.2016.133.
13. Mitchell TJ, Turajlic S, Rowan A, Nicol D, Farmery JHR, O'Brien T, et al. Timing the landmark events in the evolution of clear cell renal cell cancer: TRACERx renal. Cell. 2018;173:611–623.e17.
14. Gerlinger M, Horswell S, Larkin J, Rowan AJ, Salm MP, Varela I, et al. Genomic architecture and evolution of clear cell renal cell carcinomas defined by multiregion sequencing. Nat Genet. 2014;46:225–33. https://doi.org/10.1038/ng.2891.
15. Durinck S, Stawiski EW, Pavía-Jiménez A, Modrusan Z, Kapur P, Jaiswal BS, et al. Spectrum of diverse genomic alterations define non-clear cell renal carcinoma subtypes. Nat Genet. 2015;47:13–21.
16. Article O. Comprehensive molecular characterization of papillary renal-cell carcinoma. N Engl J Med. 2016;374:135–45. https://doi.org/10.1056/NEJMoa1505917.
17. Pflueger D, Sboner A, Storz M, Roth J, Compérat E, Bruder E, et al. Identification of molecular tumor markers in renal cell carcinomas with TFE3 protein expression by RNA sequencing. Neoplasia. 2013;15:1231–40. https://doi.org/10.1593/neo.131544.
18. Ross H, Argani P. Xp11 translocation renal cell carcinoma. Pathology. 2010;42:369–73.
19. Gill AJ, Hes O, Sedivcova M, Tan H, Agaimy A, Andresen PA, et al. Succinate dehydrogenase (SDH) -deficient renal a Clinicopathologic series of 36 tumors from 27 patients. Am J Surg Pathol. 2014;38:1588–602 https://www.ncbi.nlm.nih.gov/pmc/articles/PMC4229399/pdf/pas-38-1588.pdf.
20. Thompson RH, Hill J, Babayev Y, Cronin A, Kundu S, Bernstein M, et al. Risk of metastatic renal cell carcinoma according to tumor size. J Urol. 2009;182:41–5.
21. Umbreit EC, Shimko MS, Childs MA, Lohse CM, Cheville JC, Leibovich BC, et al. Metastatic potential of a renal mass according to original tumour size at presentation. Br J Urol Int. 2011;109:190–4.
22. Eckel-Passow JE, Serie DJ, Cheville JC, Ho TH, Kapur P, Brugarolas J, et al. BAP1 and PBRM1 in metastatic clear cell renal cell carcinoma: tumor heterogeneity and concordance with paired primary tumor. BMC Urol. 2017;17:1–7.
23. Pellenz S, Kapur P, Peña-Llopis S, Christie A, Zhrebker L, Pavía-Jiménez A, Rathmell WK, Xie X-J, Brugarolas J. Effects on survival of BAP1 and PBRM1 mutations in sporadic clear-cell renal cell carcinoma: a retrospective analysis with independent validation. Lancet Oncol. 2013;14:159–67.
24. Cheng DT, Mitchell TN, Zehir A, Shah RH, Benayed R, Syed A, et al. Memorial Sloan Kettering-integrated mutation profiling of actionable cancer targets (MSK-IMPACT): a hybridization capture-based next-generation sequencing clinical assay for solid tumor molecular oncology. J Mol Diagn. 2015;17:251–64. https://doi.org/10.1016/j.jmoldx.2014.12.006.
25. Zehir A, Benayed R, Shah RH, Syed A, Middha S, Kim HR, et al. Mutational landscape of metastatic cancer revealed from prospective clinical sequencing of 10,000 patients. Nat Med. 2017;23:703–13.
26. Kato S, Hayashi T, Suehara Y, Hamanoue H, Yamanaka S, Ichikawa Y, et al. Multicenter experience with large panel next-generation sequencing in patients with advanced solid cancers in Japan. Jpn J Clin Oncol. 2019;49:174–82.
27. Stockley TL, Oza AM, Berman HK, Leighl NB, Knox JJ, Shepherd FA, et al. Molecular profiling of advanced solid tumors and patient outcomes with genotype-matched clinical trials: the Princess Margaret IMPACT/COMPACT trial. Genome Med. 2016;8:1–12. https://doi.org/10.1186/s13073-016-0364-2.
28. Zhang S, Wang B, Zhang F, Ye J, Ge L, Ma L. Alterations of renal cell carcinoma and clinical implications in the Chinese population. Med Sci Monit. 2019;25:2959–65.

23

Renal arteriovenous fistula after retrograde ureteroscopic lithotripsy for the lower ureteral stones

Wan-Zhang Liu, Ting Huang, Li Fang and Yue Cheng*

Abstract

Background: Renal arteriovenous fistula was rarely reported in retrograde endoscopic procedure. Up to now, there is still an absence of report on the formation of renal arteriovenous fistula after semi-rigid ureteroscopic lithotripsy for lower ureteral stones.

Case presentation: An 83-year-old man was admitted to our hospital complaining about intermittent left flank pain that had persisted for 1 week. He suffered medium hypertension and nephrolithiasis treated with left open ureterolithotomy and two ureteroscopic lithotripsies. Non-contrast abdominal CT scan revealed two left lower ureteral stones diametered 8 mm and 7 mm respectively with mild hydronephrosis. A retrograde semi-rigid ureteroscopic lithotripsy was performed to remove the stones, after which two Double-J stents were placed for the ureteral stricture. Due to the continuous gross hematuria and hemoglobin droppings 2 days after operation, a variety of conservative therapies, including blood transfusion and bed rest, were adopted. Then, the patient was discharged with a stable hemoglobin. However, he presented himself to our emergency department with aggravating left flank pain and severe gross hematuria as little as 2 days later. Emergent digital subtraction angiography was conducted to reveal an arteriovenous fistula in the left kidney, which was embolized with two platinum coils to stop the bleeding. His hematuria was resolved in 3 days, and two Double-J stents were removed in 4 weeks. The patient was followed up for 1 year, during which no hematuria or flank pain recurred.

Conclusion: This is the first case report on the formation of renal arteriovenous fistula after semi-rigid ureteroscopic lithotripsy. In this case, elevated intrapelvic pressure, historical surgery and hydronephrosis might be associated with the primary risk of the complication.

Keywords: Renal arteriovenous fistula, Severe bleeding, Computed tomography angiography, Digital subtraction angiography, Case report

Background

At present, retrograde semi-rigid URSL has been commonly applied in the observation and treatment of ureteral diseases. It is widely known that, the incidence of postoperative complications is low, mostly manifested as Grade I and II, for example, renal colic, infection, ureteral injury and hematuria [1]. The formation of AVF after retrograde procedure was rarely seen, as a result of which there have been few reports on the retrograde intrarenal lithotripsy for renal stones over the past two decades [2]. Therefore, a patient exhibiting an AVF after semi-rigid URSL in the treatment of the lower ureteral stones is reported in this study, and the relevant literature is reviewed.

* Correspondence: chengyueur@qq.com
Department of Urology, NingBo First Hospital, NingBo Hospital of ZheJiang University, #59 Liuting Street, NingBo City 315000, Zhejiang Province, China

Case presentation

An 83-year-old man was referred to our clinic in May 2019 for the complaint about intermittent left flank pain that had persisted for 1 week. Despite the denial of fevers, dysuria, hematuria, frequency or urgency, he admitted to visiting local clinics and receiving medical therapies. Besides, this patient had medium hypertension and nephrolithiasis treated with left open ureterolithotomy and two URSLs.

Though routine urinalysis revealed 40 WBC/ul and 48 RBC/ul, the result of urine culture was negative. As revealed by non-contrast abdominal CT scan, there were two left lower ureteral stones diametered 8 mm and 7 mm respectively with mild hydronephrosis, as shown in Fig. 1a. In addition, kidney, ureter, bladder (KUB) plain film indicated two lower ureteral stones, as show in Fig. 1b. In spite of this, both preoperative physical examination and laboratory study revealed no abnormality. After the identification of left ureteral stones, semi-rigid URSL with holmium laser was adopted. The surgery was performed by a surgeon with more than 5 years of specialist experience.

As preparation for the operation, the general anesthesia was conducted for 47 min. With the patient was left in the lithotomy position, a 6/7.5-Fr semi-rigid ureteroscope (Storz, Germany) with 220 μm holmium laser was applied to smash the stones. Upon close examination, an ureteral stricture was found beneath the stones, and the semi-rigid ureteroscope passed it carefully with the guidance of a guide wire. For improved visibility, a hand-pump irrigation was carried out by an assistant. The process of smashing stone continued until the visible fragments were ≤ 3 mm in diameter, with most of them extracted into the bladder using a basket. Finally, two 5Fr Double-J stents were placed due to the ureteral stricture and an urethral catheter was indwelled.

The patient displayed slight left flank pain and continuous hematuria after the surgery, which was considered as a complication of Double-J stents. Normal blood tests indicated severe droppings of hemoglobin from 103 g/dL to 61 g/dL 2 days after operation. Low dose abdominal CT-scan revealed mild left hydronephrosis with blood clots, while no remains of stones were observed in the ureter, as shown in Fig. 2a. KUB showed two ureteral stents in the left urinary tract, as shown in Fig. 2b. Due to the continuous gross hematuria and droppings of hemoglobin, various conservative therapies, including blood transfusion (600 ml of red blood cells in total), antibiotics (sulbenicillin) and bed rest, were carried out. After 10 days of observation in hospital, the patient was discharged with a slight hematuria and stable hemoglobin level (84 g/dL). Over the course of observation, creatinine and other laboratory tests invariably showed compliance with the specified limits. Moreover, the patient was instructed to remove his two Double-J stents in 4 weeks.

Two days later, he presented himself to our emergency department with aggravating left flank pain and severe gross hematuria. Four thousand seven hundred eighty-three RBC/ul and 364WBC/ul were detected through urinalysis. Blood test revealed low hemoglobin level at 54 g/dL. According to the multi-detector computed tomography angiography and three-dimensional construction of renal arteries, there was an AVF and contrast leakage into calices in the left kidney, as shown in Fig. 3a and Fig. 3b. Then, the findings were confirmed by emergent digital subtraction angiography, as shown in Fig. 4a. Additionally, the AVF was embolized with two platinum coils to stop bleeding, as shown in Fig. 4b. In the meantime, blood transfusion was conducted until the hemoglobin levels reached 70 g/dL. Hematuria was resolved in 3 days and two Double-J stents were removed

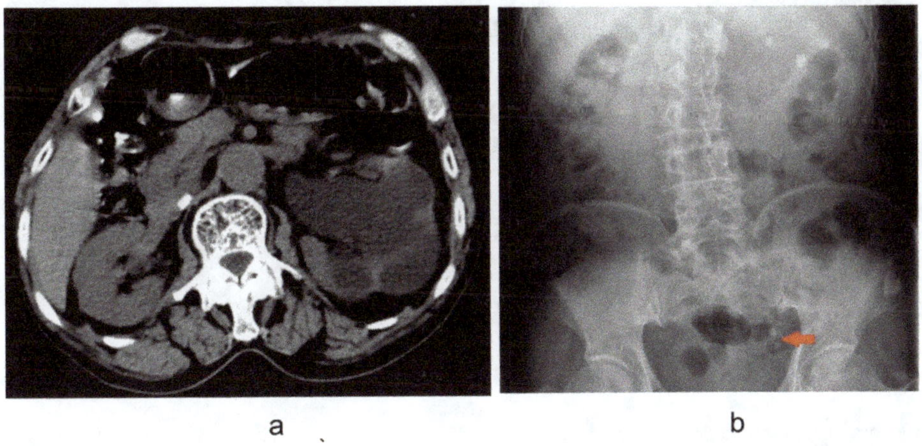

Fig. 1 **a** CT revealed mild hydronephrosis in the left kidney. **b** KUB exhibited two lower ureteral stones

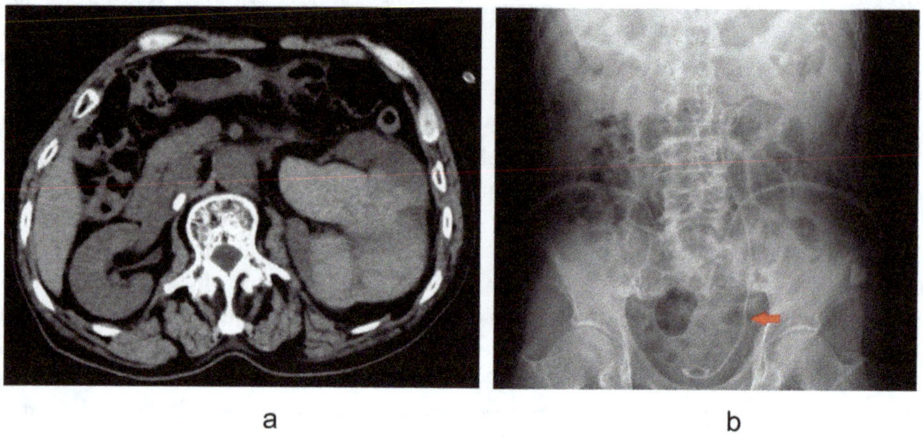

Fig. 2 a CT revealed mild left hydronephrosis with blood clots. **b** KUB showed two ureteral stents in the left ureter

1 month later. During the 12-month follow-up, no hematuria or flank pain recurred.

Discussion and conclusion

Despite renal hemorrhage as a common complication caused by urological endoscopic procedure, it was mostly studied in percutaneous operations, such as PCNL. It might be manifested as pseudoaneurysm, AVF, bleeding spot and combined [3]. Since the kidney is classed as a vascular organ, bleeding might occur as a result of the damage caused to the renal substances, like the introduction of needle, dilatation of tract, fragmentation of stones and elevated intrarenal pressure. In spite of conservative therapies, further digital subtraction angiography and embolization are required to stop bleeding for those with continuous gross hematuria and a severe hemorrhage (hemoglobin dropping>30 g/dL) [4].

Different from PCNL, retrograde ureteroscopic surgery is completely performed through the urinary tract, so as to avoid the potential substantial damage caused to the kidney. Thus, the incidence of renal hemorrhage following retrograde procedures was extremely low (0.15–0.4%) [5–7], and it was mostly manifested as subcapsular and perinephric hematoma. It was believed that the damage caused to pelvicalyceal system by guide wire and the elevated intrarenal pressure leading to the rupture of renal parenchyma might be attributed to bleeding [7]. Kozminski [8] suggested that renal hematoma is associated with such factors as female gender, preoperative hypertension, preoperative ureteral stenting, intraoperative ureteral sheath use, and postoperative ureteral stenting. Tiplitsky [2] presented a case of intrarenal arteriovenous fistula after the flexible ureteroscopic extraction of stone with holmium laser lithotripsy, which led to the finding that the damage caused to interlobar

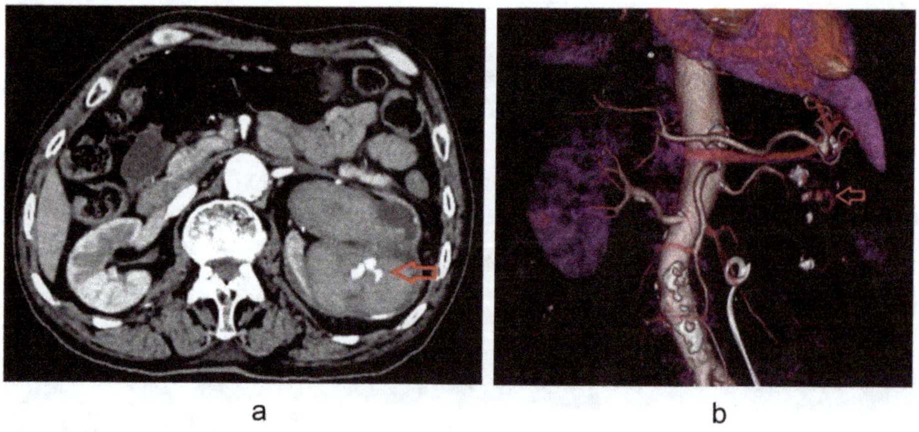

Fig. 3 a multi-detector computed tomography angiography showed mild hydronephrosis with blood clots and AVF in the left kidney. **b** three-dimensional construction of renal arteries found an AVF

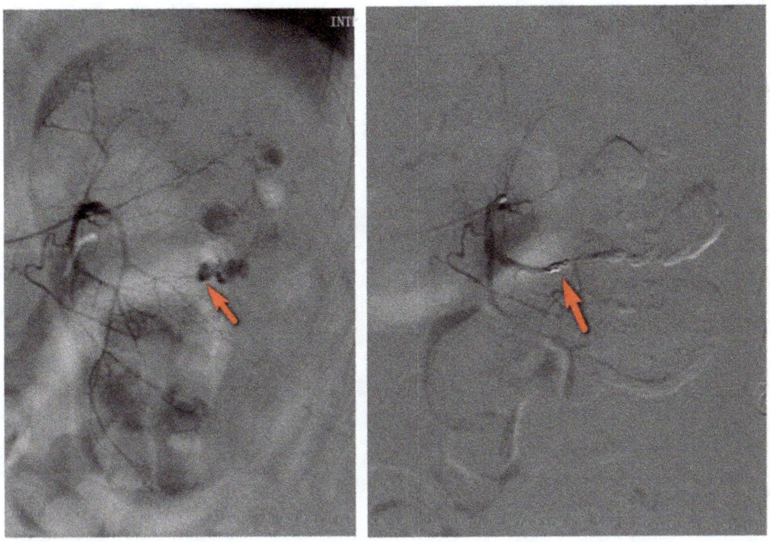

Fig. 4 a digital subtraction angiography revealed an AVF in the left kidney. **b** the AVF was embolized with two platinum coils

arteries by holmium laser was the most likely root cause. As we known, there is still no report on the formation of AVF following semi-rigid ureteroscopic lithotripsy for the lower ureteral stones.

In our case, the elevated intrapelvic pressure during the process of smashing stones is supposed to be the leading cause of AVF and bleeding. On the one hand, the ureteral stricture beneath the stones could reduce not only the gap between the ureteral wall and the ureteroscope, but also the outflow of irrigative fluid as a consequence. Secondly, a hand-pump irrigation, performed by an assistant, provided a high irrigative pressure to ensure the sufficient visibility. In the meantime, however, it caused the intrarenal pressure to increase. But we were not able to measure the exact pressure during the surgery. On the other hand, a long-term hydronephrosis and previous surgery histories could have a detrimental effect on the substantial of kidney, thus leading to the potential formation of AVF.

It marks the first case in relation to the formation of AVF after semi-rigid ureteroscopic procedure, but the exact physiopathology remains unclear. To our knowledge, the elevated intrapelvic pressure that might lead to the rupture of renal parenchyma was mainly responsible for the complication. For the patients with a ureteral stricture beneath the stones, the double-J stent should be placed 2-4 weeks in advance to facilitate the passage of endoscope and the outflow of irrigation while the smashing of stones proceeds. Although the usage of double ipsilateral ureteral stents achieved a higher success rate than single stent in the treatment ureteral strictures after an endoureterotomy [9], the efficiency of two stents placement without an endourological technique in this case is still lack of evidence. Finally, surgeons must be aware of the outflow of irrigative fluid, but not always a good visibility during the smashing of stones.

Abbreviations

AVF: Arteriovenous fistula; URSL: Ureteroscopic lithotripsy; WBC: White blood cell; RBC: Red blood cell; CT: Computed tomography; PCNL: Percutaneous nephrolithotomy

Acknowledgments

None.

Authors' contributions

WZL: Design and drafting of the article, and final approval of the version to be submitted. TH: Data acquisition, drafting of the article, and final approval of the version to be submitted. LF: Data acquisition, critical revision of the article, and final approval of the version to be submitted. YC: Critical revision of the article, and final approval of the version to be submitted.

References

1. Geavlete P, Georgescu D, NiTA G, et al. Complications of 2735 retrograde Semirigid Ureteroscopy procedures: a single-center experience. J Endourol. 2006;20(3):179–85.
2. Tiplitsky SI, Milhoua PM, Patel MB, et al. Case report: Intrarenal Arteriovenous fistula after Ureteroscopic stone extraction with holmium laser lithotripsy. J Endourol. 2007;21(5):530–2.
3. Ganpule AP, Shah DH, Ganpule SA, et al. Role of multi-detector computed tomography (MDCT) in management of post percutaneous nephrolithotomy (PCNL) bleeding. F1000 Res. 2013;2:253.
4. Choi MJ, Kim PH, Shin JH, et al. Angiographic management of percutaneous renal procedure-related bleeding: a single-center experience. Int J Urol. 2019;26(3):406–12.
5. Tao W, Cai CJ, Sun CY, et al. Subcapsular renal hematoma after ureteroscopy with holmium:yttrium-aluminum-garnet laser lithotripsy. Lasers Med Sci. 2015;30(5):1527–32.

6. Chiu KF, Chan CK, Ma WK, et al. Subcapsular hematoma after Ureteroscopy and laser lithotripsy. J Endourol. 2013;27(9):1115–9.
7. Bansal U, Sawant A, Dhabalia J. Subcapsular renal hematoma after ureterorenoscopy: an unknown complication of a known procedure. Urol Ann. 2010;2(3):119–21.
8. Kozminski MA, Kozminski DJ, Roberts WW, et al. Symptomatic subcapsular and Perinephric hematoma following Ureteroscopic lithotripsy for renal calculi. J Endourol. 2015;29(3):277–82.
9. Ibrahim HM, Mohyelden K, Abdel-Bary A, et al. Single versus double ureteral stent placement after laser Endoureterotomy for the Management of Benign Ureteral Strictures: a randomized clinical trial. J Endourol. 2015; 29(10):1204–9.

24

Prevalence of microhematuria in renal colic and urolithiasis

Bruno Minotti[1*], Giorgio Treglia[2], Mariarosa Pascale[3], Samuele Ceruti[4], Laura Cantini[5], Luciano Anselmi[5] and Andrea Saporito[5]

Abstract

Background: This systematic review and meta-analysis aims to investigate the prevalence of microhematuria in patients presenting with suspected acute renal colic and/or confirmed urolithiasis at the emergency department.

Methods: A comprehensive literature search was conducted to find relevant data on prevalence of microhematuria in patients with suspected acute renal colic and/or confirmed urolithiasis. Data from each study regarding study design, patient characteristics and prevalence of microhematuria were retrieved. A random effect-model was used for the pooled analyses.

Results: Forty-nine articles including 15'860 patients were selected through the literature search. The pooled microhematuria prevalence was 77% (95%CI: 73–80%) and 84% (95%CI: 80–87%) for suspected acute renal colic and confirmed urolithiasis, respectively. This proportion was much higher when the dipstick was used as diagnostic test (80 and 90% for acute renal colic and urolithiasis, respectively) compared to the microscopic urinalysis (74 and 78% for acute renal colic and urolithiasis, respectively).

Conclusions: This meta-analysis revealed a high prevalence of microhematuria in patients with acute renal colic (77%), including those with confirmed urolithiasis (84%). Intending this prevalence as sensitivity, we reached moderate values, which make microhematuria alone a poor diagnostic test for acute renal colic or urolithiasis. Microhematuria could possibly still important to assess the risk in patients with renal colic.

Keywords: Renal colic, Urolithiasis, Microhematuria, Stone score

Background

Renal colic is caused by the presence of stones in the urinary tract and it is characterized by sudden onset of severe loin pain, radiating to the flank, groin, and testes or *labia majora* [1]. Incidence amounts to 240 per 100′000 persons [2] with a prevalence up to 10%; men are commonly more affected than women with a ratio of 3–2:1 [3]. Lifetime risk is up to 19% in men and 9% in women [4], varying depending on geographic location and increasing constantly over last years [5]. Guidelines for the diagnostic pathway suggest assessing (micro) hematuria, while the gold standard of imaging is unenhanced multi-detector computed tomography (MDCT) [1]. As diagnostic tool the STONE Score was developed and validated; this score includes parameters as sex, duration of pain prior to presentation, race, nausea, vomiting and microhematuria [6]. Microhematuria prevalence in suspected renal colic has been studied in several trials, ranging from 55% [7] to 93% [8, 9]. In order to better

* Correspondence: bruno.minotti@kssg.ch
[1]Emergency Department, Cantonal Hospital of St. Gallen, Rorschacher Strasse 95, CH-9007 St. Gallen, Switzerland
Full list of author information is available at the end of the article

understand the difference existing in prevalence range, we performed a meta-analysis of studies dealing with microhematuria by suspected acute renal colic and/or confirmed urolithiasis.

Methods

This systematic review and meta-analysis conforms to the statement on Preferred Reporting Items for Systematic reviews and Meta-Analyses [10].

Search strategy

A literature search of the electronic PubMed/MEDLINE database and Cochrane Central Register of Controlled Trials (CENTRAL), without language restriction, was carried out from inception to October 11, 2018. A search algorithm was established using a combination of the following terms: A) renal colic AND urolithiasis (Problem), B) urinalysis (Intervention), C) microhematuria (Outcome). The final search query is reported in Appendix 1. Reference lists of the retrieved articles were also screened for additional studies.

Eligibility criteria

We included in this systematic review and meta-analysis studies which filled the following inclusion criteria: a) original article published in peer-reviewed journal; b) studies including adults only; c) patients presenting with acute renal colic at the emergency department; d) studies reporting data on microhematuria.

Exclusion criteria were: a) articles not within the field of interest of this review; b) review articles, letters or editorials; c) case reports or case series (less than 10 patients included); d) articles with possible patient data overlap.

Study selection

Titles and abstracts of the retrieved studies were independently reviewed by two researchers (MP, GT), applying the inclusion and exclusion criteria mentioned above. Articles were rejected if they were clearly ineligible. The full texts of the potentially eligible articles were reviewed independently by the same researchers to confirm or exclude their eligibility for inclusion. Disagreements were resolved in a consensus meeting.

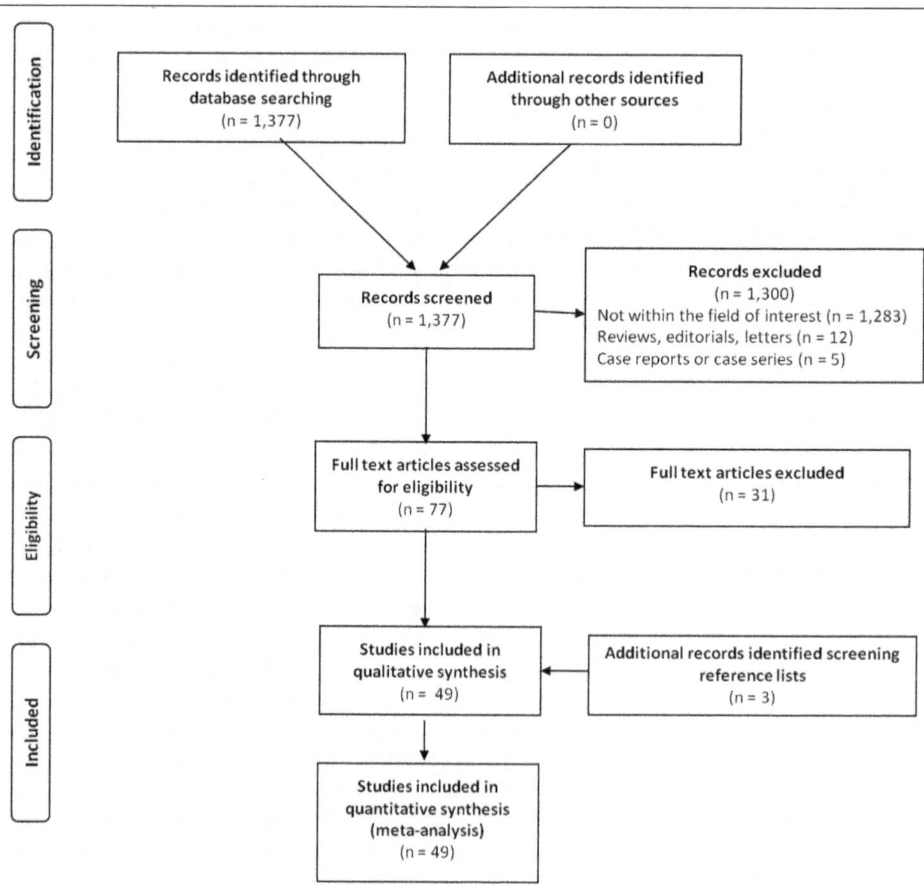

Fig. 1 PRISMA flow chart of the retrieved, excluded and analyzed studies

Table 1 Basic study and patient characteristics. Patients presenting with acute renal colic at the emergency department

Authors	Year	Country	Study design	No. of patients	% Male	Mean age ± SD (years)
Kim et al. [13]	2018	South Korea	Retrospective, observational	798	68.6	48.2 ± 13.3
Desai et al. [14]	2018	USA	Retrospective, observational	350	NR	NR
Türk *and* Ün [15][a]	2017	Turkey	Prospective, observational	516	60.5	37 ± 20.3
Shrestha et al. [16][a]	2017	Nepal	Retrospective, observational	201	55.2	29 ± 13.5
Odoemene et al. [17][a]	2017	Nigeria	Prospective, observational	69	76.8	40.4 ± 2.9
Mefford et al. [18]	2017	USA	Retrospective, observational	393	69	Median 43 (IQR 32–54)
Rapp et al. [19]	2016	USA	Retrospective, observational	613	47	49 ± 0.6
Park et al. [20]	2016	South Korea	Prospective, RCT	103	66	45.6 ± 12.55
Hernandez et al. [21]	2016	USA	Retrospective, observational	536	56	45.9 ± 16.3
Fukuhara et al. [22][a]	2016	Japan	Retrospective, observational	491	70.5	51.8 ± 15
Dorfman et al. [23]	2016	USA	Retrospective, observational	339	55.5	46.8 ± 16.5
Yan et al. [24]	2015	Canada	Prospective cohort study	565	62.8	46.6 ± 14.4
Lee et al. [25]	2015	South Korea	Retrospective, observational	2218	71	43.3 ± 14.2
Hall et al. [26][a]	2015	UK	Retrospective, observational	513	57.1	45 ± 23.3
Zwank et al. [27]	2014	USA	Prospective, observational	93	NR	39 ± NR
Abdel-Gawad et al. [28][a]	2014	UAE	Retrospective, observational	939	87.9	37.9 ± 11
Inci et al. [7]	2013	Turkey	Retrospective, observational	83	42.2	42.1 ± 14.4
Lallas et al. [29]	2011	USA	Prospective, observational	32	NR	NR
Perez et al. [30][a]	2010	Spain	Prospective, multicentre, cross-sectional case-control	146	57.53	51.34 ± NR
Xafis et al. [31][a]	2008	Switzerland	Retrospective, observational	638	NR	44.3 ± 14.6
Serinken et al. [32][a]	2008	Turkey	Retrospective, observational	235	75.7	31.1 ± 7
Cupisti et al. [33]	2008	Italy	Retrospective, observational	696	54	NR
Matani *and* Al-Ghazo [34][a]	2007	Saudi Arabia / Jordan	Retrospective, observational	75	61.3	42.2 ± NR
Kartal et al. [35][a]	2006	Turkey	Prospective, observational	227	64.8	38.4 ± 14
Kirpalani et al. [36]	2005	Canada	Retrospective, observational	299	NR	NR
Gaspari *and* Horst [37]	2005	USA	Prospective, observational	110	NR	NR
Argyropoulos et al. [8]	2004	Greece	Retrospective, observational	609	63.2	49.2 ± 15.9
Unal et al. [38][a]	2003	Turkey	Prospective, observational	137	55	38 ± NR
Tack et al. [39][a]	2003	Belgium	Prospective, observational	106	50	45 ± NR
Kobayashi et al. [40]	2003	Japan	Retrospective, observational	537	78	46.6 ± 14
Eray et al. [41]	2003	Turkey	Prospective, observational	65	60	38.8 ± 13.5
Lucks et al. [42]	2002	USA	Retrospective, observational	587	NR	NR
Hamm et al. [43]	2002	Germany	Prospective, observational	109	69.7	49 ± NR
Li et al. [44][a]	2001	USA	Retrospective, observational	397	73	47 ± 15
Hamm et al. [45]	2001	Germany	Prospective, observational	125	72	55 ± 17
Richards *and* Christman [46]	1999	USA	Retrospective, observational	185	NR	NR
Bove et al. [47]	1999	USA	Retrospective, observational	195	NR	NR
Ooi et al. [9][a]	1998	Singapore	Prospective, observational	122	93	39.7 ± NR
Ghali et al. [48][a]	1998	Saudi Arabia	Prospective, observational	125	80	39.2 ± NR
Eskelinen et al. [49]	1998	Finland	Prospective, observational	57	NR	NR
Gimondo et al. [50][a]	1996	Italy	Retrospective, observational	76	60.5	47 ± NR
Boyd *and* Gray [51]	1996	UK	Prospective, observational	52	NR	NR
Press *and* Smith [52]	1995	USA	Retrospective, observational	109	NR	NR
Chia et al. [53]	1995	Singapore	Prospective, observational	294	72.5	43.5 ± NR
Elton et al. [54][a]	1993	USA	Retrospective / prospective, observational	275	71.2	46.2 ± 15.7
Stewart et al. [55]	1990	USA	Retrospective, observational	160	76.9	NR

Table 1 Basic study and patient characteristics. Patients presenting with acute renal colic at the emergency department *(Continued)*

Authors	Year	Country	Study design	No. of patients	% Male	Mean age ± SD (years)
Freeland [56]	1987	Northern Ireland	Retrospective, observational	134	NR	NR
Dunn et al. [57]	1985	USA	Retrospective, observational	76	NR	42.7 ± NR
Bishop [58]	1980	UK	Prospective, observational	50	NR	NR

Abbreviations (alphabetical order): *IQR* interquartile range, *NR* not reported, *RCT* Randomized controlled study, *SD* standard deviation, *UAE* United Arab Emirates, *UK* United Kingdom, *USA* United States of America
[a]Enrolled also children

Data extraction

For each included study, one author (MP) manually extracted data relevant to the review aims using a customized form. Information regarding basic study data (authors, year of publication, country of origin, type of study), patient characteristics (number of patients, mean age, gender), methods (microhematuria test, microhematuria definition) and outcomes (number of patients with microhematuria, microhematuria prevalence) were retrieved. The number of patients with microhematuria and microhematuria prevalence were also extracted for patients with confirmed urolithiasis, where available. Diagnostic methods for detection of stones were also retrieved. One other author (GT) independently checked all extracted data.

Outcome measures

The primary outcome was the percentage of microhematuria among patients presenting with suspected acute renal colic at the emergency department. The secondary outcome was the percentage of microhematuria among patients presenting with acute renal colic and confirmed urolithiasis at the emergency department.

Quality assessment

The overall quality of the studies included in the systematic review was critically appraised based on the revised "Quality Assessment of Diagnostic Accuracy Studies" tool (QUADAS-2). This tool comprises four domains: patient selection, index test, reference standard, and flow and timing. Each domain was assessed in terms of risk of bias, and the first three domains were also assessed in terms of concerns regarding applicability. Two authors have performed the risk of bias assessment (GT and MP) reaching a consensus.

Statistical analysis

Microhematuria prevalence was defined as the ratio between the number of patients with suspected acute renal colic with microhematuria detected by urinalysis or dipstick and the total number of patients with suspected acute renal colic who underwent the analysis. This proportion was calculated also for patients presenting with acute renal colic and confirmed urolithiasis.

Pooled analyses of the proportion of microhematuria detected by urinalysis or dipstick were performed using data retrieved from the selected studies. When microhematuria was assessed using both urinalysis and dipstick, the test with the better outcome was chosen. Subgroup analyses taking into account the microhematuria test were planned.

A random-effects model was used for statistical pooling of the data, taking into account the heterogeneity between studies. The different weight of each study in the pooled analysis was related to the different sample size. Pooled data were presented with their respective 95% confidence interval (95%CI) values, and data were displayed using plots.

Heterogeneity was estimated by using the I-square index (I^2), which describes the percentage of variation across studies that is due to heterogeneity rather than chance [11] and considered significant if I-square test was higher than 50%.

Publication bias was assessed through the Egger's test [12].

Statistical analyses were performed using the StatsDirect software version 3 (StatsDirect Ltd., Cambridge, UK).

Results

Literature search

The literature search from PubMed/MEDLINE and Cochrane CENTRAL databases yielded a total of 1377 records. After reviewing titles and abstracts, 77 were selected as potentially eligible articles. The full text was retrieved for all. Following eligibility's assessment, 31 articles did not meet the inclusion criteria and were excluded from the systematic review. Within the selected articles, screening of the reference lists allowed to add 3 additional records. Finally, 49 studies [7–9, 13–58] including 15′860 patients were identified as potentially relevant and were selected for the systematic review and meta-analysis. All of the included studies except two [30, 50] were published in English. These studies covered the period from inception to October 11, 2018. Search results and articles' selection are displayed in a PRISMA flow chart (Fig. 1).

Selected studies

The characteristics of selected studies are reported in Table 1. The studies were conducted in different

Table 2 Data on microhematuria in patients presenting with suspected acute renal colic at the emergency department

Authors	Microhematuria test	Type of hematuria	Positive microhematuria definition	No. patients with microhematuria	Microhematuria prevalence
Kim et al. [13]	Urinalysis	Microscopic	Presence of 4 or more RBCs/HPF	750	750/798 (94%)
Desai et al. [14]	Urinalysis	Microscopic or macroscopic	Positive urinalysis for RBCs or for blood	245	245/350 (70%)
Türk *and* Ün [15]	Urinalysis	Microscopic	NR	432	432/516 (83.7%)
Shrestha et al. [16]	Urinalysis	Microscopic	Presence of 3 or more RBCs	70	70/201 (34.8%)
Odoemene et al. [17]	Urinalysis	Microscopic or macroscopic	NR	62	62/69 (89.9%)
Mefford et al. [18]	Urinalysis	Microscopic	Presence of 4 or more RBCs/HPF	321	321/393 (81.7%)
Rapp et al. [19]	Urinalysis	Microscopic or macroscopic	Presence of 4 or more RBCs/HPF	412	412/613 (67.2%)
Park et al. [20]	Urinalysis	Microscopic	NR	90	90/103 (87.4%)
Hernandez et al. [21]	Urine dipstick	Microscopic	Hematuria on urine dipstick	332	332/536 (61.9%)
Fukuhara et al. [22]	Urinalysis or urine dipstick	Microscopic or macroscopic	Occult blood in urine	352	352/491 (71.7%)
Dorfman et al. [23]	Urinalysis	Microscopic	Presence of 5 or more RBCs/HPF	254	254/339 (74.9%)
Yan et al. [24]	Urinalysis	Microscopic	NR	451	451/565 (79.8%)
Lee et al. [25]	Urinalysis	Microscopic	NR	1980	1980/2218 (89.3%)
Hall et al. [26]	Urine dipstick	Microscopic or macroscopic	Scores of 1+ to 3+ on urine dipstick or documented frank hematuria	391	391/513 (76.2%)
Zwank et al. [27]	Urinalysis	Microscopic	RBCs present	66	66/93 (71%)
Abdel-Gawad et al. [28]	Urinalysis	Microscopic	Presence of 4 or more RBCs/HPF	835	835/939 (88.9%)
Inci et al. [7]	Urinalysis	Microscopic	Presence of 5 or more RBCs/HPF	46	46/83 (55.4%)
Lallas et al. [29]	Urinalysis	Microscopic	Presence of 4 or more RBCs/HPF	18	18/32 (56.3%)
	Urine dipstick	Microscopic	Trace or scores of 1+ to 4+ on urine dipstick	21	21/32 (65.6%)
Perez et al. [30]	Urine dipstick	Microscopic	NR	132	132/146 (90.4%)
Xafis et al. [31]	Urinalysis	Microscopic	Presence of 5 or more RBCs/HPF	396	396/638 (62.1%)
Serinken et al. [32]	Urinalysis	Microscopic	Presence of 5 or more RBCs/HPF	194	194/235 (82.6%)
Cupisti et al. [33]	Urine dipstick	Microscopic	NR	592	592/696 (85.1%)
Matani *and* Al-Ghazo [34]	Urinalysis	Microscopic	Presence of 4 or more RBCs/HPF	50	50/75 (66.7%)
Kartal et al. [35]	Urinalysis	Microscopic	Presence of 10 or more RBCs/HPF	146	146/227 (64.3%)
Kirpalani et al. [36]	Urine dipstick	Microscopic	Positive urine dipstick	228	228/299 (76.3%)
Gaspari *and* Horst [37]	Urinalysis	Microscopic	Presence of 5 or more RBCs/HPF	82	82/110 (74.5%)
Argyropoulos et al. [8]	Urine dipstick	Microscopic	Scores of 1+ to 3+ on urine dipstick	566	566/609 (92.9%)
Unal et al. [38]	Urinalysis	Microscopic	Presence of 4 or more RBCs/HPF	100	100/137 (73%)
Tack et al. [39]	Urinalysis or Urine dipstick	Microscopic	Presence of 2 or more RBCs/HPF or positive dipstick	77	77/106 (72.6%)
Kobayashi et al. [40]	Urine dipstick	Microscopic	Scores of 1+ to 3+ on urine dipstick	382	382/537 (71.1%)
	Urinalysis	Microscopic	Presence of 5 or more RBCs/HPF	350	350/537 (65.2%)

Table 2 Data on microhematuria in patients presenting with suspected acute renal colic at the emergency department *(Continued)*

Authors	Microhematuria test	Type of hematuria	Positive microhematuria definition	No. patients with microhematuria	Microhematuria prevalence
Eray et al. [41]	Urinalysis	Microscopic	Presence of 6 or more RBCs/HPF	45	45/20 (69.2%)
Luchs et al. [42]	Urinalysis	Microscopic	Presence of 10 or more RBCs/HPF	492	492/587 (83.8%)
Hamm et al. [45]	Urinalysis	Microscopic	Presence of more than 20 mg/dl hemoglobin	66	66/109 (60.6%)
Li et al. [44]	Urinalysis or Urine dipstick	Microscopic	Presence of any number of RBCs/HPF or trace / scores of 1+ to 3+ on urine dipstick	360	360/397 (90.7%)
Hamm et al. [45]	Urinalysis	Microscopic	Presence of 4 or more RBCs/HPF	99	99/125 (79.2%)
Richards *and* Christman [46]	Urinalysis	Microscopic	Presence of 4 or more RBCs/HPF	156	156/185 (84.3%)
Bove et al. [47]	Urine dipstick	Microscopic	Positive urine dipstick	130	130/180 (72.2%)
	Urinalysis	Microscopic	Presence of 6 or more RBCs/HPF	128	128/195 (65.6%)
	Urinalysis or Urine dipstick	Microscopic	Presence of 2 or more RBCs/HPF or positive urine dipstick	153	153/195 (78.5%)
Ooi et al. [9]	Urine dipstick	Microscopic	Scores of 1+ or more on urine dipstick	114	114/122 (93.4%)
	Urinalysis	Microscopic	Presence of 6 or more RBCs/HPF in males or of 10 or more RBCs/HPF in females	77	77/122 (63.1%)
Ghali et al. [48]	Urinalysis	Microscopic	Presence of 4 or more RBCs/HPF	81	81/125 (64.8%)
Eskelinen et al. [49]	Urinalysis	Microscopic	Presence of 11 or more RBCs/HPF	43	43/57 (75.4%)
Gimondo et al. [50]	Urine dipstick	Microscopic or macroscopic	Positive urine dipstick	56	56/76 (73.7%)
Boyd *and* Gray [51]	Urine dipstick	Microscopic	Positive urine dipstick	45	45/52 (86.5%)
Press *and* Smith [52]	Urinalysis	Microscopic	Presence of 1 or more RBCs/HPF	78	78/109 (71.6%)
Chia et al. [53]	Urinalysis	Microscopic	Presence of 6 or more RBCs/HPF in males or of 10 or more RBCs/HPF in females	181	181/294 (61.6%)
Elton et al. [54]	Urinalysis	Microscopic	Presence of 4 or more RBCs/HPF	194	194/275 (70.5%)
Stewart et al. [55]	Urinalysis	Microscopic	Presence of 3 or more RBCs/HPF	132	132/160 (82.5%)
Freeland [56]	Urine dipstick	Microscopic	Trace or scores of 1+ to 3+ on urine dipstick	102	102/134 (76.1%)
Dunn et al. [57]	Urinalysis	Microscopic	Presence of 3 or more RBCs/HPF	62	62/76 (81.6%)
Bishop [58]	Urine dipstick	Microscopic	Positive urine dipstick	44	44/50 (88%)

Abbreviations (alphabetical order): *NR* not reported, *HPF* High power Field, *RBC* Red Blood Cell

countries worldwide (Europe, North America, Asia, Africa). The sample size of the included trials ranged from 32 to 2218 adults presenting to the emergency department or urology clinic with acute renal colic. Most of the studies were observational with a prospective (19) or retrospective (29) or mixed (1) design.

Microhematuria was tested by urinalysis in 32 studies, urine dipstick in 10 and both methods in 7. Definition of microhematuria was different among the included studies. Six studies included also patients presenting with macroscopic hematuria [14, 17, 19, 22, 26, 50]. Details on the microhematuria test are reported in Table 2.

Quality assessment

Overall quality assessment of the studies included in the systematic review according to QUADAS-2 tool is reported in Supplemental Figure 1.

Microhematuria prevalence and suspected acute renal colic

Primary outcome characteristics on microhematuria prevalence in patients with suspected acute renal colic are summarized in Table 2 and Fig. 2.

Prevalence of microhematuria ranged from 35 to 94%, with a pooled estimate of 77% (95%CI: 73–80%) (Fig. 2). The heterogeneity among the included studies was significant ($I^2 = 96\%$). A publication bias was detected by Egger's test ($p < 0.0001$).

Performing sub-group analyses taking into account different microhematuria tests, the pooled prevalence of microhematuria using urinalysis or urine dipstick was 74% (95%CI: 69–78%) and 80% (95%CI: 74–86%) respectively, without significant difference between two groups.

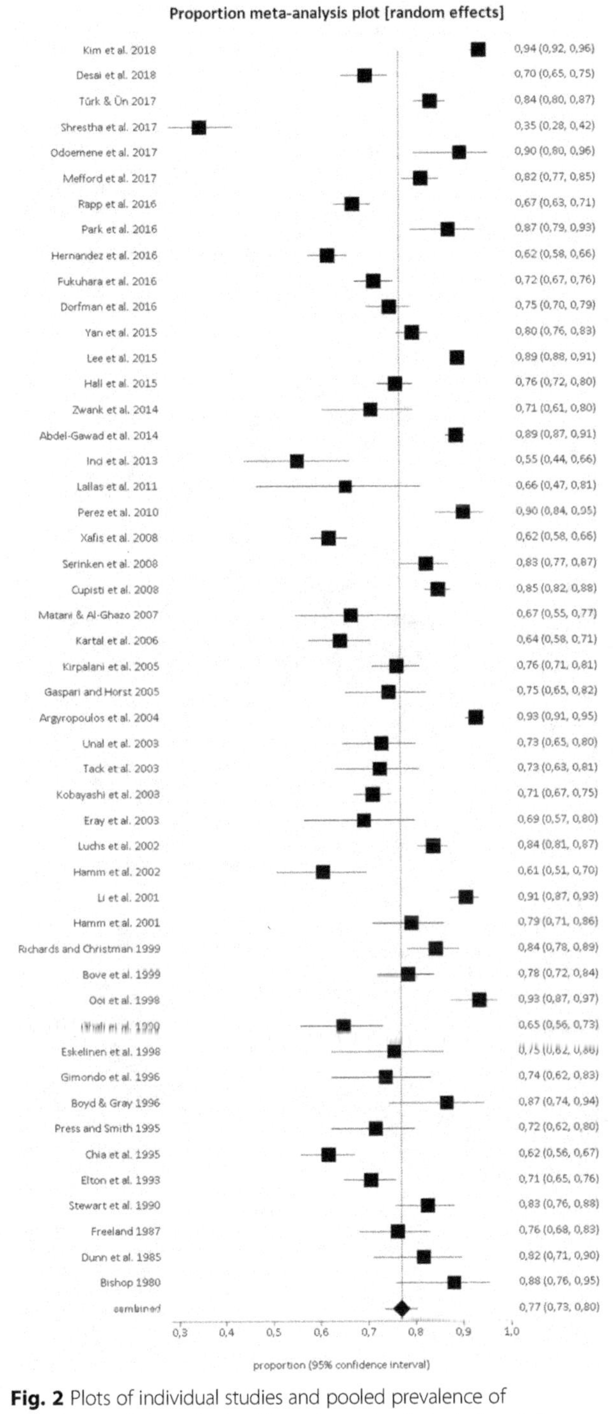

Fig. 2 Plots of individual studies and pooled prevalence of microhematuria in patients with acute renal colic, including 95% confidence intervals (95%CI)

Microhematuria prevalence and confirmed urolithiasis

Secondary outcomes regarding main findings on microhematuria prevalence in patients with acute renal colic and confirmed urolithiasis are summarized in Table 3 and Fig. 3.

Prevalence of microhematuria ranged from 44 to 100%, with a pooled estimate of 84% (95%CI: 80–87%) (Fig. 3). Heterogeneity among the included studies was significant ($I^2 = 93\%$). A publication bias was detected by Egger's test ($p = 0.0008$).

Performing sub-group analyses taking into account different microhematuria tests, the pooled prevalence of microhematuria using urinalysis or urine dipstick was 78% (95%CI: 74–82%) and 90% (95%CI: 83–95%), respectively.

Discussion

Many studies have evaluated the prevalence of microhematuria in patients with suspected acute renal colic (Table 1); this meta-analysis pooled data reported in the published studies to derive a more precise assessment. Overall, this systematic review and meta-analysis revealed a high prevalence of microhematuria in patients with acute renal colic (77%), including those with confirmed urolithiasis (84%). However, intending this prevalence as sensitivity, we reached moderate values, which make microhematuria alone a poor diagnostic test for acute renal colic, respectively for urolithiasis. In our meta-analysis heterogeneity was high; indeed, we found a poor definition regarding urine analysis across studies (see positive microhematuria definition in Table 2), with different cells count on microscopy, but also with various dipstick brands. Argyropoulos et al. [8] carried out a microscopic urinalysis when the dipstick was in doubt or with blood traces; microhematuria was confirmed in all of these cases. Thus, the authors concluded that urinary dipstick test is not inferior to microscopy. Bataille et al. [59] compared the sensitivity of urinary dipstick with microscopy and flow cytometry on in vitro contaminated human urine with human blood of volunteers at different concentrations. Urinary dipstick reached the best sensitivity, probably due to the ability to detect red blood cells after lysis, and was suggested as preferred test for screening of hematuria. Same results were previously reported by Kobayashi et al. [40] and Press et al. [52]. De facto we detected a trend toward a higher pooled prevalence of microhematuria by using urine dipstick compared to microscopic urinalysis. Some studies analyzed the characteristics of patients with renal colic and negative microhematuria, the most without correlation between size, location or composition of the stones, or grade of the obstruction [44, 52, 55, 57]. Kobayashi et al. [40] found a relation between hematuria and pain onset, with the highest incidence of negative hematuria on day 3 and 4. Kim et al. [13] found negative microhematuria in patients with lower stones or elevated serum blood urea nitrogen (BUN). Mefford et al. [18] showed an increased prevalence of hydronephrosis in patients with urolithiasis and negative microhematuria. As hydronephrosis is easy to screen with ultrasonography, Daniel et al. [60] developed the STONE PLUS

Table 3 Data on microhematuria in patients presenting with confirmed urolithiasis at the emergency department

Authors	Microhematuria test	No. patients with microhematuria	Microhematuria prevalence	Diagnostic test for urolithiasis
Kim et al. [13]	Urinalysis	750	750/798 (94%)	Unenhanced MDCT
Desai et al. [14]	Urinalysis	231	231/282 (81.9%)	Non-contrast CT
Türk et al. [15]	Urinalysis	344	344/388 (88.7%)	Non-contrast complete abdominal CT
Shrestha et al. [16]	Urinalysis	27	27/61 (44.3%)	Renal US
Odoemene et al. [17][a]	Urinalysis	62	62/69 (89.9%)	Abdominal US, IVU, CT
Mefford et al. [18]	Urinalysis	321	321/393 (81.7%)	Non-contrast abdominal or pelvic CT
Rapp et al. [19][a]	Urinalysis	177	177/222 (79.7%)	Non-contrast CT
Fukuhara et al. [22][a]	Urinalysis or urine dipstick	323	323/358 (90.2%)	Plain abdominal X-ray, helical contrast enhanced or non-contrast CT
Dorfman et al. [23]	Urinalysis	254	245/339 (74.9%)	Abdominal CT
Hall et al. [26][a]	Urine dipstick	193	193/233 (82.8)	Non-enhanced CT
Zwank et al. [27]	Urinalysis	52	52/62 (83.9)	CT
Abdel-Gawad et al. [28]	Urinalysis	835	835/939 (88.9)	Color doppler or gray-scale US, abdomen X-ray, helical CT
Inci et al. [7]	Urinalysis	46	46/83 (55.4)	Unenhanced MDCT
Lallas et al. [29]	Urinalysis	18	18/32 (56.3)	US, Abdomen X-ray, IVU, CT
	Urine dipstick	21	21/32 (65.6)	
Xafis et al. [31]	Urinalysis	341	341/507 (67.3)	Unenhanced MDCT
Kartal et al. [35]	Urinalysis	121	121/176 (68.8)	IVU, US, spiral CT, stone passage
Gaspari *and* Horst [37]	Urinalysis	54	54/58 (93.1)	US, CT
Argyropoulos et al. [8]	Urine dipstick	539	539/564 (95.6)	Abdomen X-ray, US
Unal et al. [38]	Urinalysis	92	92/114 (80.7)	US, excretory urography, non-enhanced helical CT
Tack et al. [39]	Urinalysis or Urine dipstick	37	37/38 (97.4)	Excretory urography, non-enhanced helical MDCT
Kobayashi et al. [40]	Urine dipstick	346	346/452 (76.5)	Abdomen X-ray, US, CT
	Urinalysis	317	317/452 (70.1)	
Eray et al. [41]	Urinalysis	37	37/54 (68.5)	Abdomen X-ray, spiral CT, stone passage
Luchs et al. 42[]	Urinalysis	492	492/587 (83.8)	CT, stone passage
Hamm et al. [43]	Urinalysis	53	53/80 (66.3)	Unenhanced low dose elical CT
Li et al. [44]	Urinalysis or Urine dipstick	360	360/397 (90.7)	CT, IVP
Hamm et al. [45]	Urinalysis	76	76/91 (83.5)	Helical CT
Richards *and* Christman [46]	Urinalysis	88	88/98 (89.8)	IVU
Bove et al. [47]	Urine dipstick	70	70/87 (80.5)	CT
	Urinalysis	77	77/95 (81.1)	
	Urinalysis or Urine dipstick	82	82/95 (86.3)	
Ooi et al. [9]	Urine dipstick	62	62/65 (95.4)	Abdomen X-ray, IVU
	Urinalysis	46	46/65 (70.8)	
Ghali et al. [48]	Urinalysis	64	64/82 (78)	Abdomen X-ray, IVU, US
Gimondo et al. [50][a]	Urine dipstick	29	29/29 (100)	US
Boyd *and* Gray [51]	Urine dipstick	29	29/29 (100)	Abdomen X-ray, IVU
Press *and* Smith [52]	Urinalysis	78	78/109 (71.6)	IVU
Stewart et al. [55]	Urinalysis	132	132/160 (82.5)	IVP
Freeland [56]	Urine dipstick	72	72/76 (94.7)	IVU or stone passage
Dunn et al. [57]	Urinalysis	62	62/76 (81.6)	IVU or stone passage
Bishop [58]	Urine dipstick	33	33/35 (94.3)	IVU

Abbreviations (alphabetical order): *CT* computed tomography, *HFU* High-power field, *IVU* Intravenous Urography, *MDCT* multidetector CT, *NR* not reported, *RBC* Red Blood Cell, *SD* standard deviation, *US* ultrasound

[a]This study included also patients with gross hematuria

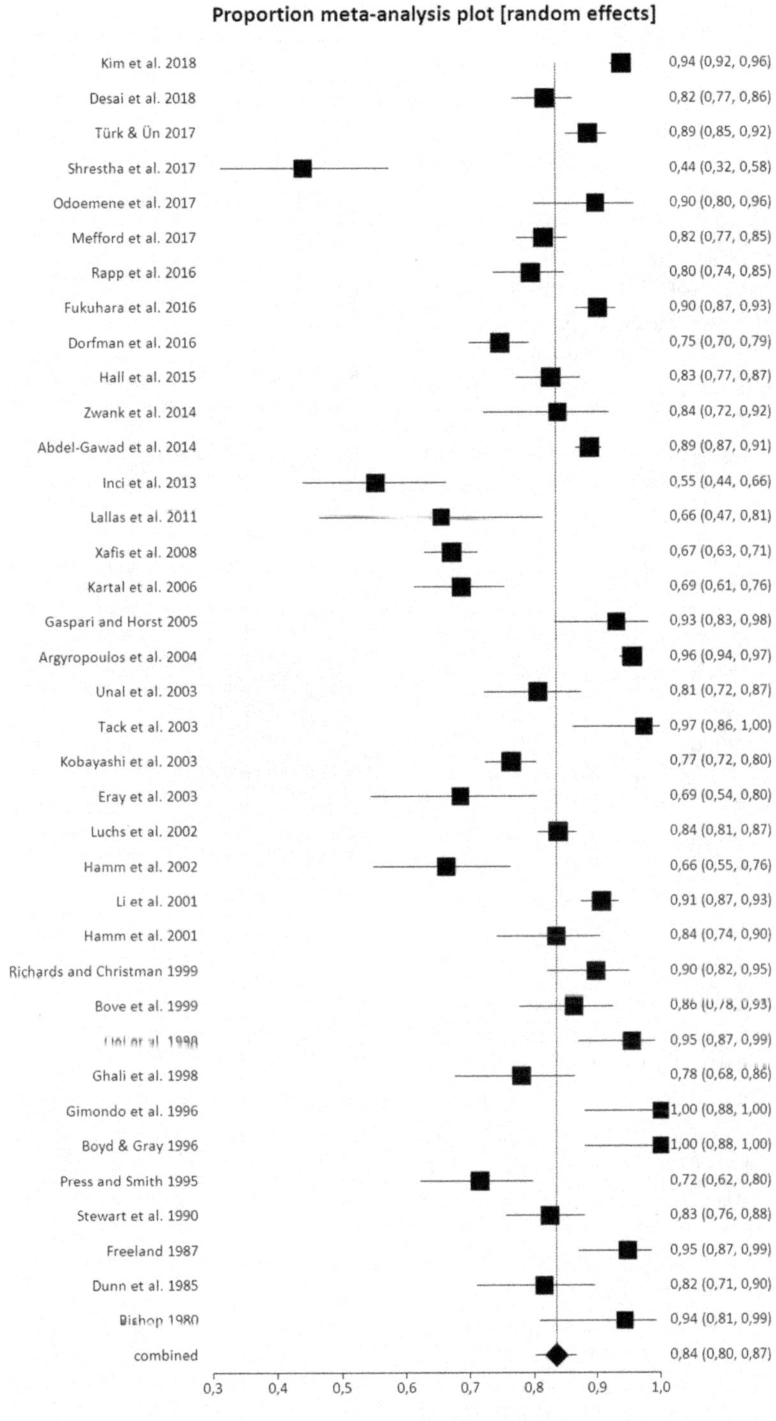

Fig. 3 Plots of individual studies and pooled prevalence of microhematuria in patients with confirmed urolithiasis, including 95% confidence intervals (95%CI)

Score with addition of point-of-care ultrasound of the kidney to the original STONE Score. Presence of hydronephrosis improved the specificity up to 98% and helped to identify patients requiring urological intervention, without remarkably increasing risk stratification.

Considering the moderate sensitivity of microhematuria in patients with renal colic, Xafis et al. [31] suggested to perform a MDCT without urinalysis as a prerequisite. This approach seems to show the best diagnostic accuracy; however, it would increase the number of MDCT with more costs and radiation exposure. Therefore, the focus should be placed in complicated urolithiasis (e.g., obstructive pyelonephritis) or dangerous alternative diagnosis. Rucker et al. [61] reported numerous diseases mimicking urolithiasis. Moore et al. [6] found a lower likelihood of a dangerous alternative diagnosis (< 2%) by using high STONE scores and suggested for this group the possibility to initially avoid compute tomography because till 90% of stones < 7 mm will pass through spontaneously [62]. With the same approach the American College of Emergency Physicians (ACEP) suggests in the Choosing Wisely group to avoid ordering computed tomography of the abdomen and pelvis in young except healthy emergency department patients (age < 50) with known histories of kidney stones, or ureterolithiasis, presenting with symptoms consistent with uncomplicated renal colic [63]. In fact, taking all studies together, the prevalence of patients with renal colic having effectively urolithiasis was 66% (median, IQR 52–76), which means a higher pre-test probability in the studied population and so a good discerning capacity of the treating physicians. Anyway, alternative diagnoses mimicking renal colic have to be taken into account. Commons diagnoses are pyelonephritis, appendicitis, diverticulitis, adnexal cysts/tumor, cholecystitis, and lumbago/sciatica. Rarer pneumonia, lymphoma or aortic dissection/aneurysm. However CT scan negative rate reach till 31% [42] and Zwank et al. [27] could show that CT scan didn't change management when providers did not expect it would. Finally, alternative diagnosis mimicking renal colic could be found by ultrasonography at least in one study with the same accuracy as MDCT [64].

Some limitations and biases of our meta-analysis should be taken into account. We have no registered a protocol of the systematic review on a database such as PROSPERO. We included some retrospective studies because of the good data quality. Heterogeneity among studies may represent a potential source of bias in a meta-analysis. This heterogeneity is likely to arise through baseline differences among patients in the included studies (Table 1), or diversity in methodological aspects between different studies (Table 2). Unfortunately, we detected a significant heterogeneity in our meta-analysis. We believe that, beyond the various microhematuria tests (urinalysis vs dipstick), the most important source of heterogeneity could be the different definitions of microhematuria (Table 2). Finally, we found presence of publication bias.

In conclusion, microhematuria searched with urine dipstick showed higher diagnostic sensitivity and should be used in this setting as a "gold standard"; it is needed to calculate the STONE score, which can help to identify patients with decreased likelihood of a differential diagnosis, reducing costs and radiation exposure of MDCT. Finally, the concomitant use of ultrasound could increase the specificity till 98% by hydronephrosis, identify patients requiring urological intervention and help to find alternative diagnosis in each risk group. Especially for searching differential diagnosis with ultrasound in patients with suspected renal colic, further studies should be undertaken. Larger prospective multicenter validation study of the STONE score could provide more definitive evidence.

Supplementary information

Additional file 1 Supplemental figure 1. Overall quality assessment of the studies included in the systematic review according to QUADAS-2 tool.

Additional file 2 Appendix 1. Search strategy used for PubMed/MEDLINE and Cochrane Central Register of Controlled Trials (CENTRAL).

Abbreviations

MDCT: multi-detector computed tomography; QUADAS: Quality Assessment of Diagnostic Accuracy Studies; CI: Confidence interval; PRISMA: Preferred Reporting Items for Systematic Reviews and Meta-Analyses; BUN: Blood urea nitrogen; ACEP: American College of Emergency Physicians; IQR: Interquartile range; CT: Computed tomography

Acknowledgments

This work was carried out in collaboration with the Clinical Trial Unit of Ente Ospedaliero Cantonale (Ticino, Switzerland).

Authors' contributions

Concept: BM, AS. Literature search: MP, GT. Statistical analysis: MP, GT. Data interpretation: MP, GT, BM, AS. Manuscript writing: MP, GT, BM, AS. Substantial review: SC, LC, LA. Final approval: all authors.

Author details

[1]Emergency Department, Cantonal Hospital of St. Gallen, Rorschacher Strasse 95, CH-9007 St. Gallen, Switzerland. [2]Heath Technology Assessment Unit, Ente Ospedaliero Cantonale, Bellinzona, Switzerland. [3]Clinical Trial Unit, Ente Ospedaliero Cantonale, Bellinzona, Switzerland. [4]Department of Intensive Care Medicine, Clinica Luganese, Lugano, Switzerland. [5]Department of Anesthesia, Ospedale San Giovanni, Bellinzona, Switzerland.

References

1. Bultitude M, Rees J. Management of renal colic. BMJ. 2012;345:e5499.
2. Tasian GE, Ross ME, Song L, Sas DJ, Keren R, Denburg MR, et al. Annual incidence of nephrolithiasis among children and adults in South Carolina from 1997 to 2012. Clin J Am Soc Nephrol. 2016;11:488–96.
3. Scales CD Jr, Smith AC, Hanley JM, Saigal CS. Prevalence of kidney stones in the United States. Eur Urol. 2012;62:160–5.
4. Curhan G. 47 - nephrolithiasis. In: Gilbert SJ, Weiner DE, editors. National Kidney Foundation primer on kidney diseases. 6th ed. Philadelphia: W.B. Saunders; 2014. p. 405–11.
5. Romero V, Akpinar H, Assimos DG. Kidney stones: a global picture of prevalence, incidence, and associated risk factors. Rev Urol. 2010;12:e86–96.
6. Moore CL, Bomann S, Daniels B, Luty S, Molinaro A, Singh D, et al. Derivation and validation of a clinical prediction rule for uncomplicated ureteral stone--the STONE score: retrospective and prospective observational cohort studies. BMJ. 2014;348:g2191.
7. Inci MF, Ozkan F, Bozkurt S, Sucakli MH, Altunoluk B, Okumus M. Correlation of volume, position of stone, and hydronephrosis with microhematuria in patients with solitary urolithiasis. Med Sci Monit. 2013;19:295 9.

8. Argyropoulos A, Farmakis A, Doumas K, Lykourinas M. The presence of microscopic hematuria detected by urine dipstick test in the evaluation of patients with renal colic. Urol Res. 2004;32:294–7.
9. Ooi SB, Kour NW, Mahadev A. Haematuria in the diagnosis of urinary calculi. Ann Acad Med Singap. 1998;27:210–4.
10. Moher D, Liberati A, Tetzlaff J, Altman DG. Preferred reporting items for systematic reviews and meta-analyses: the PRISMA statement. PLoS Med. 2009;6:e1000097.
11. Higgins JP, Thompson SG. Quantifying heterogeneity in a meta-analysis. Stat Med. 2002;21:1539–58.
12. Harbord RM, Egger M, Sterne JA. A modified test for small-study effects in meta-analyses of controlled trials with binary endpoints. Stat Med. 2006;25:3443–57.
13. Kim TH, Oh SH, Park KN, Kim HJ, Youn CS, Kim SH, et al. Factors associated with absent microhematuria in symptomatic urinary stone patients. Am J Emerg Med. 2018;36(12):2187–91.
14. Desai V, Cox M, Deshmukh S, Roth CG. Contrast-enhanced or noncontrast CT for renal colic: utilizing urinalysis and patient history of urolithiasis to decide. Emerg Radiol. 2018;25:455–60.
15. Turk H, Un S. Predictive factors for stone disease in patients with renal colic. Arch Ital Urol Androl. 2017;89:143–5.
16. Shrestha R, Bista Y, Khan A. Current diagnostic approach and initial treatment patterns for renal colic in emergency department. J Nepal Health Res Counc. 2017;15:38–43.
17. Odoemene CA, Okere P, Ugonabo MC. Ureterolithiasis: management in an environment with limited facilities. Niger J Clin Pract. 2017;20:622–8.
18. Mefford JM, Tungate RM, Amini L, Suh D, Anderson CL, Rudkin SE, et al. A comparison of Urolithiasis in the presence and absence of microscopic hematuria in the emergency department. West J Emerg Med. 2017;18:775–9.
19. Rapp DE, Wood NL, Bassignani M, Gergoudis L, Caulkins S, Kramolowsky EV. Clinical variables and stone detection in patients with flank pain. Can J Urol. 2016;23:8441–5.
20. Park YH, Jung RB, Lee YG, Hong CK, Ahn JH, Shin TY, et al. Does the use of bedside ultrasonography reduce emergency department length of stay for patients with renal colic?: a pilot study. Clin Exp Emerg Med. 2016;3:197–203.
21. Hernandez N, Song Y, Noble VE, Eisner BH. Predicting ureteral stones in emergency department patients with flank pain: an external validation of the STONE score. World J Urol. 2016;34:1443–6.
22. Fukuhara H, Ichiyanagi O, Kakizaki H, Naito S, Tsuchiya N. Clinical relevance of seasonal changes in the prevalence of ureterolithiasis in the diagnosis of renal colic. Urolithiasis. 2016;44:529–37.
23. Dorfman M, Chan SB, Hayek K, Hill C. Pyuria and urine cultures in patients with acute renal colic. J Emerg Med. 2016;51:358–64.
24. Yan JW, McLeod SL, Edmonds ML, Sedran RJ, Theakston KD. Risk factors associated with urologic intervention in emergency department patients with suspected renal colic. J Emerg Med. 2015;49:130–5.
25. Lee DH, Chang IH, Kim JW, Chi BH, Park SB. Usefulness of nonenhanced computed tomography for diagnosing Urolithiasis without Pyuria in the emergency department. Biomed Res Int. 2015;2015:810971.
26. Hall TC, Stephenson JA, Rangaraj A, Mulcahy K, Rajesh A. Imaging protocol for suspected ureteric calculi in patients presenting to the emergency department. Clin Radiol. 2015;70:243–7.
27. Zwank MD, Ho BM, Gresback D, Stuck LH, Salzman JG, Woster WR. Does computed tomographic scan affect diagnosis and management of patients with suspected renal colic? Am J Emerg Med. 2014;32:367–70.
28. Abdel-Gawad M, Kadasne R, Anjikar C, Elsobky E. Value of color Doppler ultrasound, kub and urinalysis in diagnosis of renal colic due to ureteral stones. Int Braz j Urol. 2014;40:513–9.
29. Lallas CD, Liu XS, Chiura AN, Das AK, Bagley DH. Urolithiasis location and size and the association with microhematuria and stone-related symptoms. J Endourol. 2011;25:1909–13.
30. Perez JA, Palmes Mde L, Ferrer JF, Urdangarain OO, Nunez AB. Renal colic at emergency departments. Epidemiologic, diagnostic and etiopathogenic study. Arch Esp Urol. 2010;63:173–87.
31. Xafis K, Thalmann G, Benneker LM, Stoupis C, Buggy DJ, Zimmermann H, et al. Forget the blood, not the stone! Microhaematuria in acute urolithiasis and the role of early CT scanning. Emer Med J. 2008;25:640–4.
32. Serinken M, Karcioglu O, Turkcuer I, Ozkan HI, Keysan MK, Bukiran A. Analysis of clinical and demographic characteristics of patients presenting with renal colic in the emergency department. BMC Res Notes. 2008;1:79.
33. Cupisti A, Pasquali E, Lusso S, Carlino F, Orsitto E, Melandri R. Renal colic in Pisa emergency department: epidemiology, diagnostics and treatment patterns. Intern Emerg Med. 2008;3:241–4.
34. Matani YS, Al-Ghazo MA. Role of helical nonenhanced computed tomography in the evaluation of acute flank pain. Asian J Surg. 2007;30:45–51.
35. Kartal M, Eray O, Erdogru T, Yilmaz S. Prospective validation of a current algorithm including bedside US performed by emergency physicians for patients with acute flank pain suspected for renal colic. Emerg Med J. 2006; 23:341–4.
36. Kirpalani A, Khalili K, Lee S, Haider MA. Renal colic: comparison of use and outcomes of unenhanced helical CT for emergency investigation in 1998 and 2002. Radiology. 2005;236:554–8.
37. Gaspari RJ, Horst K. Emergency ultrasound and urinalysis in the evaluation of flank pain. Acad Emerg Med Off J Soc Acad Emerg Med. 2005;12:1180–4.
38. Unal D, Yeni E, Karaoglanoglu M, Verit A, OF K. Can conventional examinations contribute to the diagnostic power of unenhanced helical computed tomography in urolithiasis? Urol Int. 2003;70:31–5.
39. Tack D, Sourtzis S, Delpierre I, de Maertelaer V, Gevenois PA. Low-dose unenhanced multidetector CT of patients with suspected renal colic. AJR Am J Roentgenol. 2003;180:305–11.
40. Kobayashi T, Nishizawa K, Mitsumori K, Ogura K. Impact of date of onset on the absence of hematuria in patients with acute renal colic. J Urol. 2003;170: 1093–6.
41. Eray O, Cubuk MS, Oktay C, Yilmaz S, Cete Y, Ersoy FF. The efficacy of urinalysis, plain films, and spiral CT in ED patients with suspected renal colic. Am J Emerg Med. 2003;21:152–4.
42. Luchs JS, Katz DS, Lane MJ, Mellinger BC, Lumerman JH, Stillman CA, et al. Utility of hematuria testing in patients with suspected renal colic: correlation with unenhanced helical CT results. Urology. 2002;59:839–42.
43. Hamm M, Knopfle E, Wartenberg S, Wawroschek F, Weckermann D, Harzmann R. Low dose unenhanced helical computerized tomography for the evaluation of acute flank pain. J Urol. 2002;167:1687–91.
44. Li J, Kennedy D, Levine M, Kumar A, Mullen J. Absent hematuria and expensive computerized tomography: case characteristics of emergency urolithiasis. J Urol. 2001;165:782–4.
45. Hamm M, Wawroschek F, Weckermann D, Knopfle E, Hackel T, Hauser H, et al. Unenhanced helical computed tomography in the evaluation of acute flank pain. Eur Urol. 2001;39:460–5.
46. Richards JR, Christman CA. Intravenous urography in the emergency department: when do we need it? Eur J Emerg Med. 1999;6:129–33.
47. Bove P, Kaplan D, Dalrymple N, Rosenfield AT, Verga M, Anderson K, et al. Reexamining the value of hematuria testing in patients with acute flank pain. J Urol. 1999;162:685–7.
48. Ghali AM, Elmalik EM, Ibrahim AI, Abdulhameed E, el Tahir MI. Cost-effective emergency diagnosis plan for urinary stone patients presenting with ureteric colic. Eur Urol. 1998;33:529–37.
49. Eskelinen M, Ikonen J, Lipponen P. Usefulness of history-taking, physical examination and diagnostic scoring in acute renal colic. Eur Urol. 1998;34:467–73
50. Gimondo P, Mastropasqua G, Cremona A, Mucciaccio C. Early and systematic use of ultrasonography in emergency patients with renal colic: analysis of the actual diagnostic efficacy. Radiol Med. 1996;92:421–4.
51. Boyd R, Gray AJ. Role of the plain radiograph and urinalysis in acute ureteric colic. J Accid Emerg Med. 1996;13:390–1.
52. Press SM, Smith AD. Incidence of negative hematuria in patients with acute urinary lithiasis presenting to the emergency room with flank pain. Urology. 1995;45:753–7.
53. Chia SJ, Lau W, Tan PK, Consigliere D, Li MK, Low CH. Ureteric colic: value of initial investigations and the outcome. Ann Acad Med Singap. 1995;24:366–9.
54. Elton TJ, Roth CS, Berquist TH, Silverstein MD. A clinical prediction rule for the diagnosis of ureteral calculi in emergency departments. J Gen Intern Med. 1993;8:57–62.
55. Stewart DP, Kowalski R, Wong P, Krome R. Microscopic hematuria and calculus-related ureteral obstruction. J Emer Med. 1990;8:693–5.
56. Freeland P. No haematuria--no IVU. Ir J Med Sci. 1987;156:270–1.
57. Dunn PM, Keller RT, Jones SR. The absence of hematuria in patients with symptomatic urinary tract stones. Western J Med. 1985;142:717–9.
58. Bishop NL. The influence of emergency urography and haematuria on the diagnosis of ureteric colic. Clin Radiol. 1980;31:605–10.
59. Bataille A, Wetzstein M, Hertig A, Vimont S, Rondeau E, Galichon P. Evidence of dipstick superiority over urine microscopy analysis for detection of hematuria. Res Notes. 2016;9:435.
60. Daniels B, Gross CP, Molinaro A, Singh D, Luty S, Jessey R, et al. STONE PLUS: evaluation of emergency department patients with suspected renal colic, using a clinical prediction tool combined with point-of-care limited ultrasonography. Ann Emerg Med. 2016;67:439–48.

61. Rucker CM, Menias CO, Bhalla S. Mimics of renal colic: alternative diagnoses at unenhanced helical CT. Radiographics. 2004;24(Suppl 1):S11–28 discussion S-33.
62. Tao RZ, Qin ZQ, Liu FD, Lv JL. Efficacy and safety of Tamsulosin in the medical expulsion therapy for distal ureteral calculi: a systematic review and meta-analysis of placebo-controlled trials. Urol J. 2019;16:224–31.
63. Ten Things Physicians and Patients Should Question American College of Emergency Physicians 2013–2014.
64. Catalano O, Nunziata A, Sandomenico F, Siani A. Acute flank pain: comparison of unenhanced helical CT and ultrasonography in detecting causes other than ureterolithiasis. Emerg Radiol. 2002;9:146–54.

25

Gender difference analysis of Xp11.2 translocation renal cell carcinomas's attack rate

Wenyuan Zhuang[1], Ning Liu[1], Hongqian Guo[1], Chunni Zhang[2*] and Weidong Gan[1*]

Abstract

Background: Xp11.2 translocation renal cell carcinoma (tRCC) is recently recognized. As Xp11.2 tRCC involved gene translocation and fusion in X chromosome and the number of X chromosomes in female is twice of male, we wondered whether the gender difference of attack rate is consistent with the proportion of the X chromosome. *Methods*: In the present paper, meta-analysis was performed to find out the difference of morbidity between male and female.

Results: Nine studies with 209 cases calculated. Odds ratios (ORs) and ORs with 95% confidence intervals (CIs) were calculated for attack rate of Xp11.2 RCC with different gender. The result showed that the attack rate of female was higher than that of male with pooled OR of 2.84 (95% CI = 1.48–5.45), while the rate rises even further in adult (OR = 3.37, 95% CI =2.19–5.18). In other types of common kidney cancer, the OR value is less than 1, which means that the incidence of female is lower than that of male.

Conclusions: The result showed that the incidence rate of female patients is much higher than that of male patients with Xp11.2 tRCC, it was reasonable to indicate that this particular incidence rate is related to the X chromosome.

Keywords: Xp11.2, tRCC, TFE3, Gender, X chromosome

Background

Xp11.2 translocation renal cell carcinoma (tRCC) was delineated as a distinct entity in the 2004 World Health Organization (WHO) renal tumor classification [1]. Recently, the published WHO classification of tumors classified the Xp11.2 tRCC as one of MiT (microphthalmia transcription factor) family tRCC [2]. A total of 5 Xp11.2 tRCCs have been identified in RCC tumors, *PRCC-TFE3, ASPSCR1-TFE3, SFPQ-TFE3, NONO-TFE3,* and *CLTC-TFE3,* all of which result in TFE3 (transcription factor binding to IGHM enhancer 3) gene fusions [3]. TFE3 gene is located on the short arm of the X chromosome (Xp11.2). The functional domain of the TFE3 gene fused with the promoter of other genes, housekeeping gene usually, resulting to the TFE3 protein is constitutively overexpressed in Xp11.2 tRCC which can be specifically identified by IHC (immunohistochemistry) [4, 5].

Xp11.2 tRCC is predominantly reported in children and young adults less than 45 years of age with a one-third incidence in juveniles [6]. Adult patients are rare reported with an incident rate of 1%. Xp11.2 tRCC shared similar feature to conventional clear cell and papillary renal carcinomas in histology, which creates diagnostic difficulties, and the fact is one possibility to

* Correspondence: zchunni27@hotmail.com; gwd@nju.edu.cn; dr.gwd@yeah.net

[2]Department of Clinical Laboratory, Jinling Hospital, State Key Laboratory of Analytical Chemistry for Life Science, Jiangsu Engineering Research Center for MicroRNA Biology and Biotechnology, Nanjing University School of Medicine, Nanjing University, Nanjing, China

[1]Department of Urology, Nanjing Drum Tower Hospital, Medical School of Nanjing University, Institute of Urology, Nanjing University, 321 Zhongshan Road, Nanjing 210008, China

explain the problem of its frequency [7, 8]. However, Xp11.2 tRCC showed more aggressive behavior, with metastasis common at presentation, and poorer prognosis than other subtypes of RCC. In addition, previous studies revealed that Xp11.2 tRCC was inherently more aggressive in adults than that in children [9]. Complete surgical removal of the tumor mass including the kidney may be the preferred therapy in patients with lower stage tumors. Today, the clinical characteristic and epidemiology of Xp11.2 tRCC are not very clear for the rarity of Xp11.2 tRCC. Controversy about the gender difference of morbidity remained unclear. Several published studies showed the female predominance in incidence of Xp11.2 tRCC while a few studies reported it is seen more often in males than in females [1].

As Xp11.2 tRCC involved gene translocation and fusion in X chromosome and the number of X chromosomes in female is twice of male, we are interested in the relation of female predominance in attack rate of Xp11.2 tRCC and the sex chromosome. We wondered whether the gender difference of attack rate is consistent with the proportion of the X chromosome. Gender factor was significantly associated with the frequency of many diseases and Xp11.2 tRCC might be one of them [10, 11]. However, up to date, studies on large sample for analysis of the clinical characteristic and epidemiology of Xp11.2 tRCC were still lack. Therefore, we analyzed the difference of morbidity between male and female in this systematic review by using meta-analysis and investigated the potential role of X chromosome on

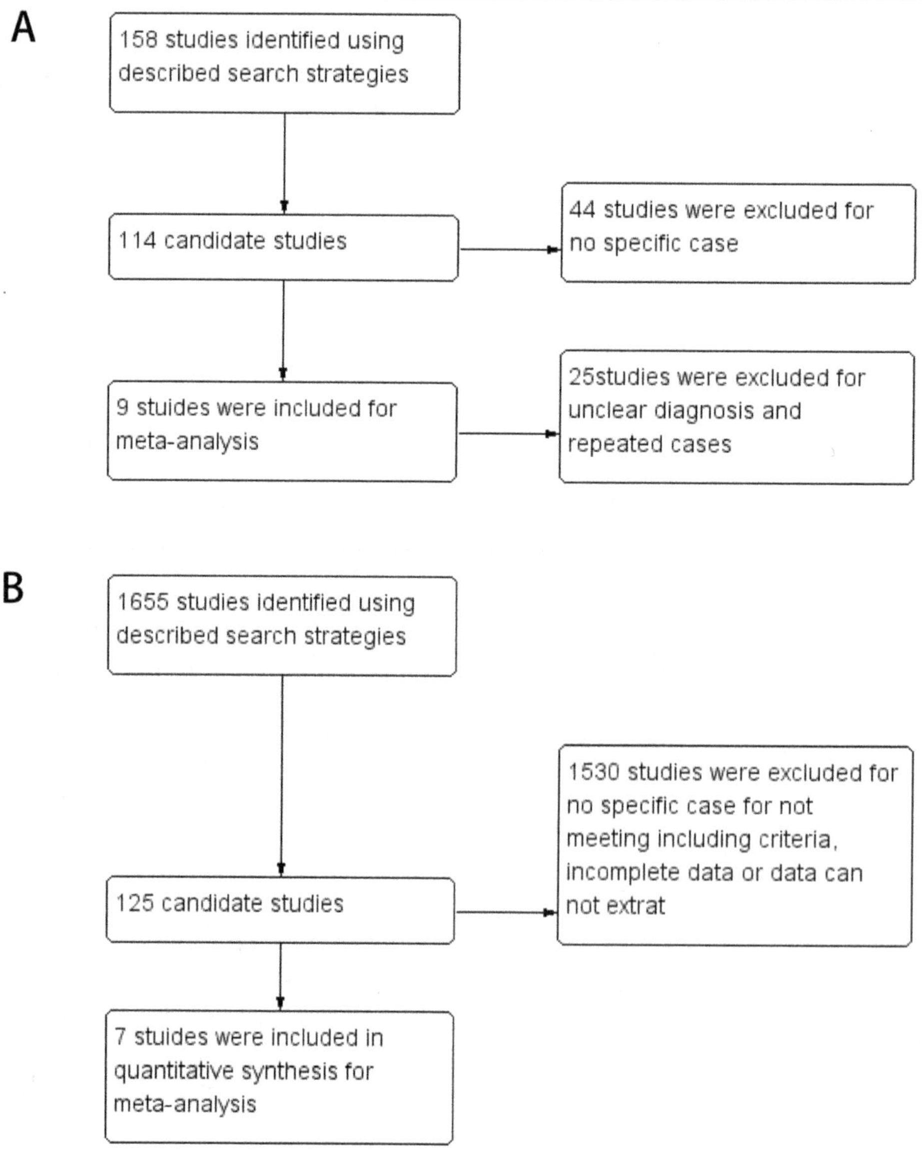

Fig. 1 Flow diagram of study selection. **a** Studies of Xp11.2 tRCC; **b** Studies of ccRCC, pRCC and ChRCC

Table 1 Clinical characteristics of included studies with Xp11.2 tRCC

	Cases				LN metastasis				Distant metastases				Mean age	Main diagnostic method
	male/C	female/C	male/A	female/A	male/C	female/C	male/A	female/A	male/C	female/C	male/A	female/A		
Levevte et al. [12]	1	1	12	14	0/1	0/1	3/12	2/14	0/1	0/1	5/12	6/14	–	FISH
Chenchen et al. [13]	0	0	7	9	–	–	–	–	–	–	–	–	–	IHC + FISH
Ning Liu et al. [14]	2	2	11	19	0/2	0/2	1/11	4/19	0/2	0/2	1/11	2/19	44.5 ± 18.3	FISH
Argani et al. [15]	0	0	6	22	0/0	0/0	2/6	9/22	0/0	0/0	2/6	2/22	37 ± 16.6	IHC + FISH
Green et al. [16]	0	2	10	19	0/0	2/2	0/10	4/19	0/0	1/2	1/10	2/19	30.2 ± 14.1	IHC + FISH
Lim et al. [6]	0	1	8	12	0/0	1/1	3/8	2/12	0/0	1/1	0/8	2/12	43.4 ± 20.0	FISH
Plfueger et al. [17]	3	2	5	12	1/3	0/2	0/5	3/12	1/3	0/2	1/5	0/12	24.6 ± 20.3	IHC + FISH
Song et al. [18]	13	9	0	0	–	–	–	–	–	–	–	–	–	IHC + FISH
Pan et al. [19]	1	0	3	9	0/1	0/0	0/3	4/9	0/1	0/0	0/3	4/9	24.9 ± 9.2	IHC + FISH
total	20	17	72	118	1/7	3/8	9/55	25/97	1/7	2/8	10/55	18/97		

Xp11.2 tRCC. For comparison, we also analyzed clear cell carcinoma (ccRCC), papillary cell carcinoma (pRCC), and chromophobe cell carcinoma (ChRCC).

Methods

Literature search and study selection

A computer-aided literature search was performed with usage of the Cochrane, DARE, MEDLINE, EMBASE, and Science Citation Index. The literature published between July 2004 and May 2019 was searched. An initial search strategy used recognized search terms "TFE3" and "Xp11.2 renal cell carcinoma". Primary studies that meet following criteria were included: (1) All studies that reported cases with definite gender; (2) All cases were confirmed by specific biological technology, such as IHC assay for TFE3, FISH, RT-PCR, and/or other molecular biology methods. (3) The report contained enough cases (≥10). Reviews and mechanism researches were excluded. Studies that performed in the lab with animal or cell models were also excluded. We also collected common types of renal cell carcinoma for comparison, searches included the terms "clear cell renal cell carcinoma" and "papillary renal cell carcinoma" and "chromophobe renal carcinoma". The citations listed in the retrieved articles were reviewed to identify other potentially relevant studies. Primary studies that meet following criteria were included: (1) The patient was diagnosed as renal cell carcinoma. (2) Patients have clear data of treatment and follow-up. (3) There is sufficient data for analysis. All studies were evaluated carefully to eliminate duplicate patient populations. Figure 1 shows a flow diagram.

Data synthesis and analysis

We paid our attention to the difference of morbidity between male and female and all primary studies with gender data were analyzed. The statistical software Review Manager (Version 5.3 for Windows) was applied to carry out all the analysis. Dichotomous data which incidence regarded were expressed as odds ratios (ORs) and ORs with 95% confidence intervals (CIs) were used in the Mantel-Haenszel fixed-effect model when no statistically significant heterogeneity was detected. On the contrary, Mantel-Haenszel random-effect model would be chosen when heterogeneity was significant. Heterogeneity analysis was performed using the Cochran Q-test and I^2 index, the existence of heterogeneity statistically was considered when the p value was less than 0.1. On the other

Table 2 Clinical characteristics of included studies with ccRCC, pRCC and ChRCC

PRCC					
	male	female	LN metastasis	Distant metastases	Mean age
Beck et al. [20]	117	40	–	9/157	62.2 ± 12
Toloken et al. [21]	236	74	7/310	unknown	64
Keengan et al. [22]	1740	538	67/2278	98/2278	–
Sterffens et al. [23]	436	129	50/565	54/565	62.1 ± 11.6
Lee et al. [24]	142	50	unknown	unknown	56.4 ± 13.5
Simone et al. [25]	40	15	13/55	5/55	59.1 ± 14.8
Wagener et al. [26]	1469	474	143/1943	151/1943	–
CCRCC					
	male	female	LN metastasis	Distant metastases	Mean age
Beck et al	487	307	–	95/794	61.5 ± 12
Toloken et al	836	497	23	–	62
Keengan et al	8501	5340	172/13841	1219/12841	–
Sterffens et al	2772	1604	319/4376	618/4376	62.4 ± 11.2
Lee et al	1785	703	–	–	56.1 ± 12.4
Simone et al	599	321	29/920	68/920	59.8 ± 12.6
Wagener et al	3357	2243	210/5600	540/5600	–
Chromophobe					
	male	female	LN metastasis	Distant metastases	Mean age
Beck et al	59	47	–	6/106	57.5 ± 12
Toloken et al	120	100	4	–	59
Keengan et al	568	381	11/949	36/949	–

hand, evaluation of publication bias was performed for each of the pooled study groups using a funnel plot.

Results

Literature and study characteristics

All published cases of Xp11.2 tRCC were enrolled except a few of cases could not meet the inclusion criteria. Nine studies with 209 cases were collected. It was also checked that all cases were unique, no repeated cases were included. For common types of kidney cancer, 7 studies were included in quantitative synthesis for meta-analysis, as shown in Table 1 and Table 2. Publication bias is described as visual assessment of a funnel plot in Fig. 2 and there was no evidence for significant publication bias.

Results of the search

All collected studies

Totally, there were 131 females and 78 males while all the cases according our inclusion criteria were enrolled in. Previous literature has reported significant gender differences in Xp11.2 tRCC between adults and children, so patients of Xp11.2 tRCC was divided into children (≤ 14 years) and adults (> 14 years) for further analysis. The three most common types of renal cell carcinoma, clear cell carcinoma, papillary cell carcinoma, and chromophobe cell carcinoma, were used for comparative analysis.

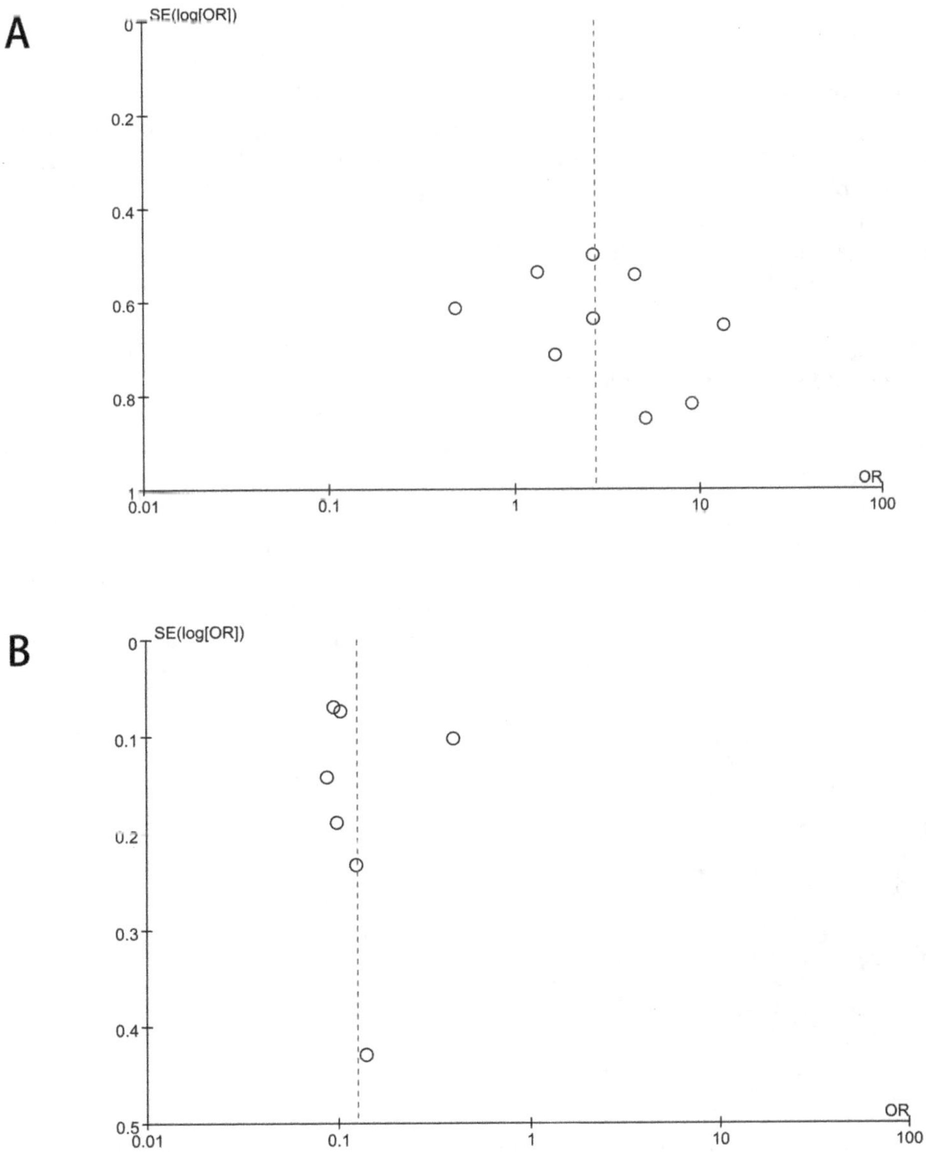

Fig. 2 Publication bias assessment for study. Funnel plots show that there was no evidence for significant publication bias in any of the 2 pooled groups. **a** Studies of Xp11.2 tRCC; **b** Studies of ccRCC, pRCC and ChRCC

Gender-related incidence of all included studies of Xp11.2 tRCC

A total of 209 cases with 131 women and 78 men were included. Tests for heterogeneity showed that $P = 0.002$ and $I^2 = 60\%$. We applied random- effect model while I^2 value> 50%. Pooled OR was 2.84 (95% CI = 1.48–5.45) (Fig. 3a).

Gender-related incidence of included adult studies of Xp11.2 tRCC

A total of 178 cases of Xp11.2 with 116 women and 62 men were included. (I^2 statistic = 31%, $P < 0.00001$), so that Mantel-Haenszel fixed-effect model was still applied. Pooled OR was 3.37 (95% CI =2.19–45.18) (Fig. 3b).

Gender-related incidence of included children studies of Xp11.2 tRCC

For this group, there was no evidence for heterogeneity about incidence of different gender (I^2 statistic = 0%, P = 0.52). Results of meta-analysis demonstrated that The incidence is similar between male and female with pooled OR of 0.76(95% CI = 0.32–1.77) (Fig. 3c).

Gender-related incidence of PRCC, CCRCC and ChRCC

Seven studies were included in quantitative synthesis for meta-analysis. For pRCC, a total of 5500 cases with 1320 women and 4180 men were included. The pooled OR was 0.10(95% CI = 0.09–0.11) (Fig. 4b). For ccRCC, we got similar results. The pooled OR was 0.32 (95% CI = 0.26–0.41) (Fig. 4a). Results of ChRCC showed that the OR of ChRCC was 0.47(95% CI = 0.39–0.56) (Fig. 4c).

Gender-related distant and lymphatic metastases of Xp11.2 tRCC

A total of 209 cases with 131 women and 78 men were included. Tests for heterogeneity showed that no evidence of heterogeneity in the incidence of distant metastasis (I^2 statistic = 32%, $P =$ 0.86) and lymphatic metastasis (I^2 statistic = 0%, $P =$ 0.35) was observed in two pool. The results showed that the rates of lymphatic metastasis (OR = 1.47, 95% CI = 0.66–3.24) (Fig. 5a) and distant metastasis (OR = 1.09, 95% CI = 0.44–1.72) (Fig. 5b) were comparable between male and female patients.

Discussion

Xp11.2 tRCCs, as rare tumors, seen more often in children and young adults, account for less than 5% of all sporadic kidney cancers. It is reported that the prognosis for Xp11 tRCC is similar to that for clear cell RCC in adult while children with Xp11 tRCC may have a more favorable outcome [12, 13, 27, 28]. Since the first described fusion of TFE3 on the short arm of the X chromosome to chromosome 1q21.2 [*PRCC-TFE3* t(X; 1)(p11.2;q21)], several other TFE3 translocation partners have been identified, including at least five different fusion partners of the Xp11.2 chromosome: *ASPL-TFE3, PRCC-TFE3, PSF-TFE3, CLTC-TFE3,* and *NoNo -TFE3* [14–16, 29–31]. Other novel fusion partners in single case, *PARP14, KHSRP,* and *DVL2,* were recently described. Yet despite nearly two decades since the discovery of Xp11.2 tRCCs, the morphology, biological behavior, and molecular biology underlying these cancers remains largely uncharacterized and effective targeted therapies are yet to be identified.

The translocations on chromosome Xp11.2 result in fusions between TFE3 and its respective fusion partners varies and can produce fusions containing differing number of exons in the case of TFE3 and its gene

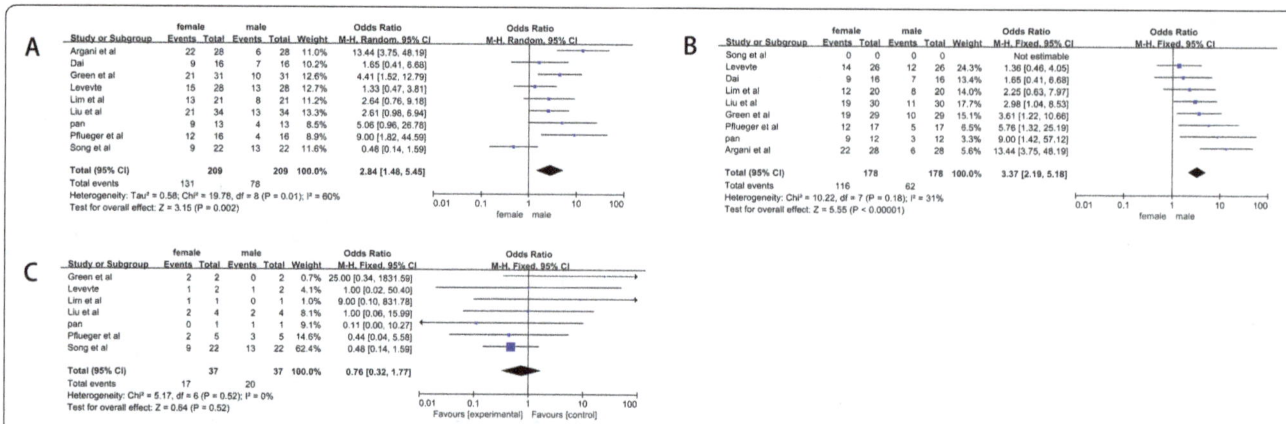

Fig. 3 Forrest plots and meta-analysis of studies with different gender-related incidence showing 95% confidence interval in Xp11.2 tRCC; **a** Different gender-related incidence in included studies; **b** Different gender-related incidence in adults; **c** Different gender-related incidence in children

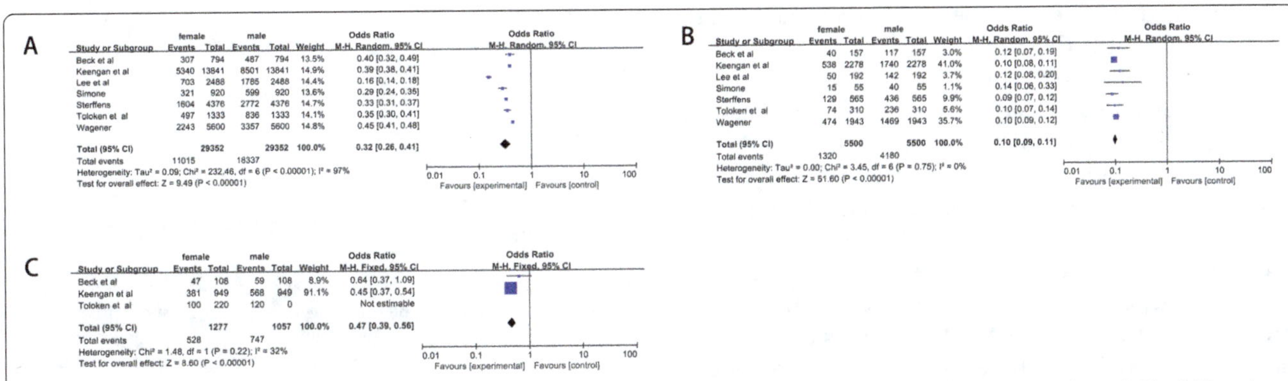

Fig. 4 Forrest plots and meta-analysis of studies with different gender-related incidence showing 95% confidence interval in ccRCC, pRCC and ChRCC. **a** Different gender-related incidence in ccRCC; **b** Different gender-related incidence in pRCC; **c** Different gender-related incidence in ChRCC

partners. All TFE3 fusion partners have constitutively active gene promoters, so TFE3 fusion proteins are expressed at dramatically higher levels than wild-type TFE3. IHC technology is used commonly to diagnose Xp11.2 tRCC and TFE3 protein is the most distinctive immunohistochemical feature of Xp11 tRCC. This immunologic marker of Xp11.2 tRCC has a relatively high sensitivity and specificity [17, 32]. However, TFE3 IHC can show false-positive results, TFE3 IHC combined with other diagnosis tools, such as break-part TFE3 fluorescence in situ hybridization (FISH), Reverse Transcription-Polymerase Chain Reaction (RT-PCR),

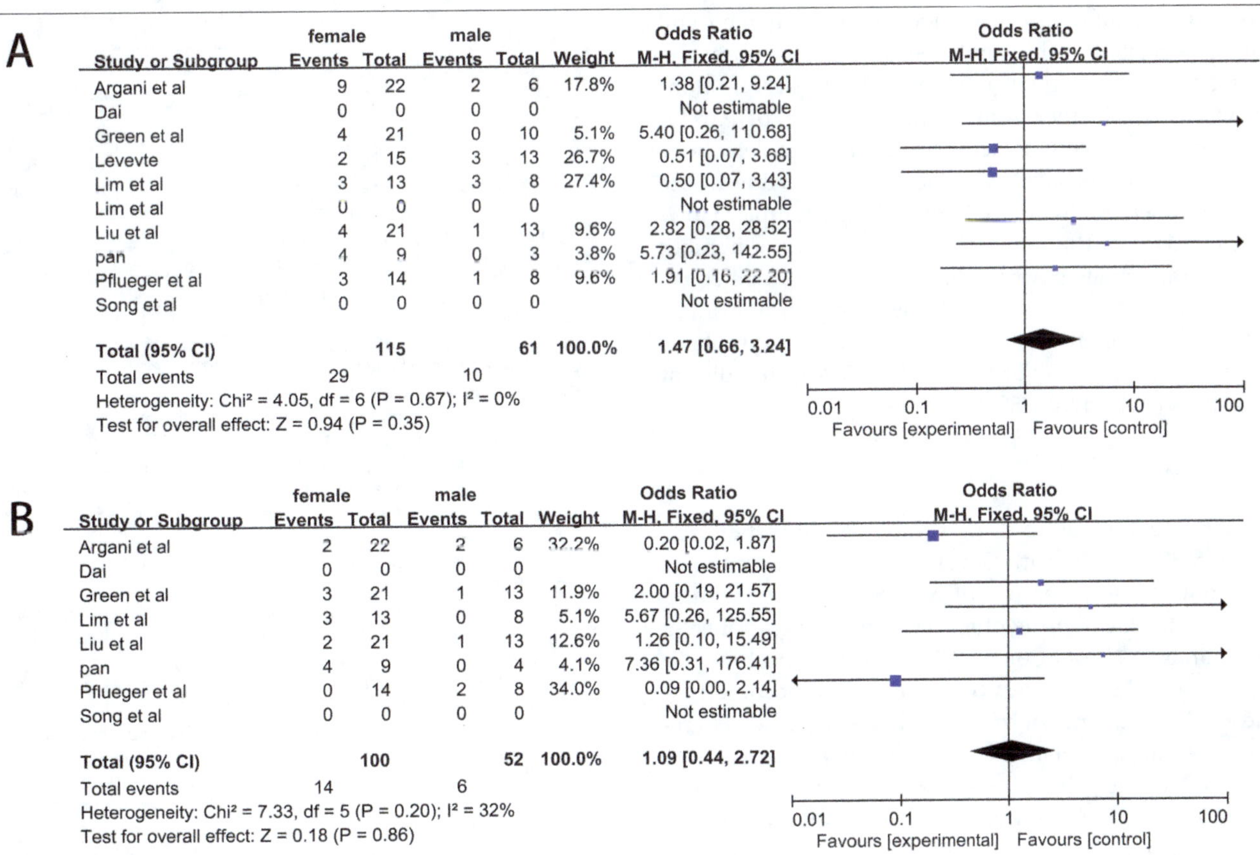

Fig. 5 Forrest plots and meta-analysis of studies showing 95% confidence interval of male Xp11.2 tRCC as compared with female Xp11.2 tRCC. **a** Incidence of lymphatic metastases; **b** Incidence of distant metastases

and cytogenetic analysis can be effective means to diagnose the Xp11.2 tRCC.

Xp11.2 tRCC showed significant differences between men and women compared with the common renal cell carcinoma. According to our results, the incidence of Xp11.2 tRCC is much higher in women than in men (OR = 2.84, 95% CI = 1.48–5.45). In adults, the rate rises even further (OR = 3.37, 95% CI =2.19–5.18). Among the three most common types of kidney cancer, women had a lower incidence than men. We suggest that this significant difference may be due to the particular pathogenesis of Xp11.2 tRCC. In order to balance the difference of X chromosomes between male and female, female have two different X chromosomes, one of them is active (Xa) and the other one is inactive (Xi) while male only have one Xa chromosome. An lncRNA, the X-inactive specific transcript (Xist), is selectively expressed and physically coats one of the X chromosomes in the female, resulting in the one of X chromosomes inactivation [18, 19, 33, 34]. The cause of Xp11.2 tRCC is the fusion of TFE3 on the short arm of the X chromosome. There are differences in the number of X chromosomes between men and women and X chromosome inactivation exists in women. We wonder if there was any effect on the different incidence between men and women. Whether this difference in incidence between men and women is related to the number of X chromosomes, and what role Xa and Xi play respectively, these questions are worthy of further study. The incidence of Xp11.2 tRCC varies between adults and children. Gender differences in child morbidity were not compared due to the small number of children in the included sample. However, in terms of the number of cases alone, the number of male and female cases in children appears to be equal. In other respects, there seems to be no significant difference between men and women in terms of lymphatic metastasis (OR = 1.47, 95% CI = 0.66–3.24) and distant metastasis (OR = 1.09, 95% CI = 0.44–1.72).

Conclusions

Therefore, compared to men, women have a higher incidence for patients with Xp11.2 tRCC. The outcome came out to the difference of X chromosomes between male and female. On the other hand, for the existence of three kinds X chromosomes, Xa of female, Xi of female, and Xa of male, the diversity of the X chromosome may lead to the different source of TFE3 fusion gene. Therefore, it could speculate that the distinction had something to do with the clinical stages, distant metastasis, and prognosis. Further work should be done to confirm this conjecture.

Abbreviations

RCC: Renal cell carcinoma; ccRCC: Clear cell renal cell carcinoma; pRCC: Papillary renal cell carcinoma; ChRCC: Chromophobe renal cell carcinoma; IHC: Immunohistochemistry; FISH: Fluorescence in situ hybridization; TFE3: Transcription factor binding to IGHM enhancer 3; RT-PCR: Transcription-polymerase chain reaction

Acknowledgements

Not applicable.

Authors' contributions

NL, WZ contributed to study conception and design. WZ, NL contributed to data acquisition. WZ contributed to analysis and interpretation of data. WZ, NL contributed to drafting the manuscript. GH, WG, CZ were involved in revising the manuscript. All authors have read and approved the manuscript.

References

1. Wu A, Kunju LP, Cheng L, Shah RB. Renal cell carcinoma in children and young adults: analysis of clinicopathological, immunohistochemical and molecular characteristics with an emphasis on the spectrum of Xp11.2 translocation-associated and unusual clear cell subtypes. Histopathology. 2008;53(5):533–44.
2. Just PA, Letourneur F, Pouliquen C, Dome F, Audebourg A, Biquet P, Vidaud M, Terris B, Sibony M, Pasmant E. Identification by FFPE RNASeq of a new recurrent inversion leading to RBM10-TFE3 fusion in renal cell carcinoma with subtle TFE3 break-apart FISH pattern. Genes Chromosomes Cancer. 2016;55(6):541–8.
3. Argani P, Lui MY, Couturier JM, Bouvier R, Fournet J-C, Ladanyi M. A novel CLTC-TFE3 gene fusion in pediatric renal adenocarcinoma with t(X;17)(p11.2; q23). Oncogene. 2003;22(34):5374.
4. Komai Y, Fujiwara M, Fujii Y, Mukai H, Yonese J, Kawakami S, Yamamoto S, Migita T, Ishikawa Y, Kurata M et al. Adult Xp11 Translocation Renal Cell Carcinoma Diagnosed by Cytogenetics and Immunohistochemistry. Clin Cancer Res. 2009;15(4):1170–6.
5. Magers MJ, Udager AM, Mehra R. MiT Family Translocation-Associated Renal Cell Carcinoma: A Contemporary Update With Emphasis on Morphologic, Immunophenotypic, and Molecular Mimics. Arch Pathol Lab Med. 139(10): 1224–33.
6. Lim B, You D, Jeong IG, Kwon T, Hong S, Song C, Cho YM, Hong B, Hong JH, Ahn H. Clinicopathological features of Xp11.2 translocation renal cell carcinoma. Korean J Urol. 2015;56(3):212–7.
7. Zhong M, Angelo PD, Osborne L, Paniz-Mondolfi AE, Cai D. Translocation renal cell carcinomas in adults. Am J Surg Pathol. 2012;36(5):654–62.
8. Zou H, Kang X, Pang LJ, Hu W, Zhao J, Qi Y, Hu J, Liu C, Li H, Liang W. Xp11 translocation renal cell carcinoma in adults: a clinicopathological and comparative genomic hybridization study. 2014;7(1):236–45.
9. Rao Q, Guan B, Zhou XJ. Xp11.2 translocation renal cell carcinomas have a poorer prognosis than non-Xp11.2 translocation carcinomas in children and young adults: a meta-analysis. Int J Surg Pathol. 2010;18(6):458–64.
10. Sirchia SM, Ramoscelli L, Grati FR, Barbera F, Coradini D, Rossella F, Porta G, Lesma E, Ruggeri A, Radice P et al. Loss of the Inactive X Chromosome and Replication of the Active X in BRCA1-Defective and Wild-type Breast Cancer Cells. Cancer Res. 2005;65(6):2139–46.
11. Chaligné R, Heard E. X-chromosome inactivation in development and cancer. FEBS Lett. 2014;588(15):2514–22.
12. Kuthi L, Somorácz Á, Micsik T, Jenei A, Hajdu A, Sejben I, Imre D, Pósfai B, Kóczián K, Semjén D et al. Clinicopathological Findings on 28 Cases with XP11.2 Renal Cell Carcinoma. Pathology oncology research. POR 2020.
13. Dai C, Ruofan S, Yuqin D, Minglei Y, Jun H, Jianjun Z: Magnetic resonance imaging findings of renal cell carcinoma associated with Xp11.2 translocation/TFE3 gene fusion in adults: a pilot study. Abdominal radiology (New York). 2019;44(1):209–17.
14. Liu N, Wang Z, Gan W, Xiong L, Li D: Renal Cell Carcinoma Associated with Xp11.2 Translocation/TFE3 Gene Fusions: Clinical Features, Treatments and Prognosis. Plos One 2016, 11(11):e0166897.
15. Argani P, Olgac S, Tickoo SK, Goldfischer M, Moch H, Chan DY, Eble JN, Bonsib SM, Jimeno M, Lloreta J, et al. Xp11 Translocation Renal Cell Carcinoma in Adults: Expanded Clinical, Pathologic, and Genetic Spectrum. Am J Surg Pathol. 2007;31(8):1149–60.

16. Green WM, Yonescu R, Morsberger L, Morris K, Netto GJ, Epstein JI, Illei PB, Allaf M, Ladanyi M, Griffin CA. Utilization of a TFE3 break-apart FISH assay in a renal tumor consultation service. Am J Surg Pathol. 2013;37(8):1150–63.
17. Pflueger D, Sboner A, Storz M, Roth J, Moch H. Identification of molecular tumor markers in renal cell carcinomas with TFE3 protein expression by RNA sequencing. Neoplasia. 2013;15(11):1231–40.
18. Hong, Cheng, Song, Ning, Sun, Wei, Ping, Zhang, LeJian, He: Biological characteristics of pediatric renal cell carcinoma associated with Xp11.2 translocations/TFE3 gene fusions. Journal of Pediatric Surgery 2014.
19. Pan CC, Sung MT, Huang HY, Yeh KT. High chromosomal copy number alterations in Xp11 translocation renal cell carcinomas detected by Array comparative genomic hybridization are associated with aggressive behavior. Am J Surg Pathol. 2013;37(7):1116–9.
20. Beck SDW, Patel MI, Snyder ME, Kattan MW, Motzer RJ, Reuter VE, Russo P. Effect of papillary and chromophobe cell type on disease-free survival after nephrectomy for renal cell carcinoma. Ann Surg Oncol. 2004.
21. Teloken, PE, and, Thompson, R H, and, Satish, K.: Prognostic Impact of Histological Subtype on Surgically Treated Localized Renal Cell Carcinoma. *Journal of Urology* 2009.
22. Keegan KA, Schupp CW, Chamie K, Hellenthal NJ, Evans CP, Koppie TM. Histopathology of surgically treated renal cell carcinoma: survival differences by subtype and stage. J Urol. 2012;188(2):391–7.
23. Steffens S, Janssen M, Roos FC, Becker F, Schumacher S, Seidel C, Wegener G, Thüroff JW, Hofmann R, Stöckle M. Incidence and long-term prognosis of papillary compared to clear cell renal cell carcinoma – a multicentre study. Eur J Cancer. 2012;48(15):2347–52.
24. Lee WK, Sang EL, Hong SK, Chang WJ, Byun SS. Characteristics and prognostic value of papillary histologic subtype in non-metastatic renal cell carcinoma in Korea: a multicenter study. Urol J. 2014;11(5):1884–90.
25. Costantini, M., Guaglianone, S., Simone, G., Ferriero, Papalia, Misuraca, R: Papillary type 2 versus clear cell renal cell carcinoma: Survival outcomes. European Journal of Surgical Oncology the Journal of the European Society of Surgical Oncology & the British Association of Surgical Oncology 2016.
26. Wagener N, Edelmann D, Benner A, Zigeuner R, Brookman-May SD. Outcome of papillary versus clear cell renal cell carcinoma varies significantly in non-metastatic disease. PLoS One. 2017;12(9):e0184173.
27. Ellis CL, Eble JN, Subhawong AP, Martignoni G, Zhong M, Ladanyi M, Epstein JI, Netto GJ, Argani P. Clinical heterogeneity of Xp11 translocation renal cell carcinoma: impact of fusion subtype, age, and stage. Mod Pathol. 2014;27(6):875–86.
28. Sukov WR, Hodge JC, Lohse CM, Leibovich BC, Houston TR, Pearce KE, Wiktor AE, Cheville JC, Bedd P. TFE3 rearrangements in adult renal cell carcinoma: clinical and pathologic features with outcome in a large series of consecutively treated patients. Am J Surg Pathol. 2012,36(5):663.
29. Argani P, Aulmann S, Illei PB, Netto GJ, Weiss SW. A distinctive subset of PEComas harbors TFE3 gene fusions. Am J Surg Pathol. 2010;34(10):1395–406.
30. Next-Generation Sequencing of Translocation Renal Cell Carcinoma Reveals Novel RNA Splicing Partners and Frequent Mutations of Chromatin-Remodeling Genes. Clin Cancer Res Official J Am Assoc Cancer Res. 2014; 20(15):4129–40.
31. Argani P, Zhong M, Reuter VE, Fallon JT, Epstein JI, Netto GJ, Antonescu CR. TFE3-fusion variant analysis defines specific Clinicopathologic associations among Xp11 translocation cancers. Am J Surg Pathol. 2016;40(6):723–37.
32. Argani P, Lal P, Hutchinson B, Man YL, Ladanyi M. Aberrant nuclear Immunoreactivity for TFE3 in neoplasms with TFE3 gene fusions a sensitive and specific Immunohistochemical assay. Am J Surg Pathol. 2003;27(6):750–61.
33. Brown CJ, Ballabio A, Rupert JL, Lafreniere RG, Grompe M, Tonlorenzi R, Willard HF. A gene from the region of the human X inactivation Centre is expressed exclusively from the inactive X chromosome. Nature. 1991; 349(6304):38–44.
34. Panning B, Jaenisch R. DNA hypomethylation can activate Xist expression and silence X-linked genes. Genes Dev. 1996;10(16):1991–2002.

26

Comprehensive study of altered proteomic landscape in proximal renal tubular epithelial cells in response to calcium oxalate monohydrate crystals

Zhu Wang[1*†], Ming-xing Li[2†], Chang-zhi Xu[3†], Ying Zhang[1], Qiong Deng[1], Rui Sun[1], Qi-yi Hu[1], Sheng-ping Zhang[1], Jian-wen Zhang[1] and Hui Liang[1*]

Abstract

Background: Calcium oxalate monohydrate (COM), the major crystalline composition of most kidney stones, induces inflammatory infiltration and injures in renal tubular cells. However, the mechanism of COM-induced toxic effects in renal tubular cells remain ambiguous. The present study aimed to investigate the potential changes in proteomic landscape of proximal renal tubular cells in response to the stimulation of COM crystals.

Methods: Clinical kidney stone samples were collected and characterized by a stone component analyzer. Three COM-enriched samples were applied to treat human proximal tubular epithelial cells HK-2. The proteomic landscape of COM-crystal treated HK-2 cells was screened by TMT-labeled quantitative proteomics analysis. The differentially expressed proteins (DEPs) were identified by pair-wise analysis. Gene Ontology (GO) analysis and Kyoto Encyclopedia of Genes and Genomes (KEGG) pathway analysis of DEPs were performed. Protein interaction networks were identified by STRING database.

Results: The data of TMT-labeled quantitative proteomic analysis showed that a total of 1141 proteins were differentially expressed in HK-2 cells, of which 699 were up-regulated and 442 were down-regulated. Functional characterization by KEGG, along with GO enrichments, suggests that the DEPs are mainly involved in cellular components and cellular processes, including regulation of actin cytoskeleton, tight junction and focal adhesion. 3 high-degree hub nodes, CFL1, ACTN and MYH9 were identified by STRING analysis.

Conclusion: These results suggested that calcium oxalate crystal has a significant effect on protein expression profile in human proximal renal tubular epithelial cells.

Keywords: Calcium oxalate crystal, Kidney stone, Protein expression profile, Renal epithelial cells

* Correspondence: wangzhu1223@hotmail.com; dr.1ianghui@aliyun.com
†Zhu Wang, Ming-xing Li and Chang-zhi Xu contributed equally to this work.
[1]Department of Urology, People's Hospital of Longhua, Southern Medical University, Shenzhen 518109, Guangdong, China
Full list of author information is available at the end of the article

Background

Kidney stone is a common disease with prevalence and incidence increasing across the world that seriously affects human health. Generally, it can cause urinary retention, renal pelvis and ureteral hydrops, ureteral dilatation, renal function damage, and infection. The prevalence of kidney stones exhibited a significant increasing trend in the past decades in the mainland of China [1, 2]. The latest research shows that the prevalence of Chinese adult kidney stones is 5.8%, and the life-time prevalence in South China is as high as 26.6% [3]. Kidney stone disease mainly affects people aged 30–50 years old, and half the patients suffered kidney stone recurrence [4]. Kidney stone seriously affects the health and quality of life of patients, and has become a public health problem across the world.

Calcium Oxalate Monohydrate (COM) accounts for over 80% of the incidence of stones [5]. COM caused renal tubular epithelial cells expressing a variety of macromolecules [6], thus affecting adhesion, aggregation and growth of calcium oxalate crystals plays an important role in the formation of kidney stones [6, 7]. Studies reported that the COM crystal-cell interaction stimulates the expression of NADPH oxidase in renal tubular epithelial cells, triggers the massive production of reactive oxygen species, activates the nuclear factor-κB signal transduction pathway, and releases a large number of inflammatory factors and activates the inflammatory cascade, links to local intrarenal inflammation and kidney injury [8–11].

Recently, the mechanism of kidney stone formation has been increasingly concerned. Serval studies demonstrated that kidney stones are initiated by COM crystals deposition due to supersaturation of urinary calcium and oxalate ions [12]. These deposits may act as nidus for stone growth, adhere to apical surface of renal tubular epithelial cells via several crystal-binding molecules or potential crystal receptors [13]. Calcium oxalate stone matrix has been reported to include a large number of protein molecules, which were identified and evidenced to promote the aggregation, nucleation and growth of calcium oxalate crystals in kidney, which ultimately leads to the formation of stones [6, 7, 14–16]. CD44, OPN, MCP-1 and HA are the most widely studied proteins which calcium oxalate crystal attachment depends upon [8, 17]. However, various theories of pathogenesis of human kidney stones suggest that calcium oxalate stone formation is a multistep process which is too complex for simple understanding, a large number of protein molecules involved are still unknown and uninvestigated.

Crystal-cell interaction model is widely used for kidney stone research for better understanding of the pathogenic mechanisms of kidney stone formation [18]. MDCK renal tubular cells (a cell line derived from dog kidney exhibiting distal renal tubule phenotype) and HK-2 cells (an immortalized human kidney proximal tubule epithelial cell line) are the most frequently used cells in crystal-cell interaction model [18]. Although several previous studies have found some new candidate proteins, further studies are necessary, since the COM-crystals prepared by calcium chloride dihydrate and sodium oxalate are different from the clinical COM-stone samples and use of cells from different species of the nephron may result in different findings. We used HK-2 cells for it was derived from adult human kidney proximal tubule which is the major site of renal oxalate handling [19], represents a major potential advantage over currently available animal or human embryonic derived cell lines [20].

In this study, we aim to use TMT (Tandem Mass Tag)–based quantitative proteomics analysis to investigate the effects of calcium oxalate crystal on the differential protein expression profiles of human renal tubular epithelial cell HK-2, screen differentially expressed protein molecules and initially explore their functional roles in calcium oxalate stone formation and its resulting renal damage.

Methods

Cell culture

The immortalized proximal tubule epithelial cell line HK-2 (human kidney-2) was purchased from Bogoo Biotechnology.Co., Ltd. (Cat. BG005, Shanghai, China), and cultured with DMEM medium supplemented with 10% fetal bovine serum, 100 units/ml penicillin sodium, and 100 μg/ml streptomycin as described previously [14]. Cultures were maintained at 37 °C with 5% CO_2 and saturated humidity [21–23].

COM crystal preparation

The calcium oxalate kidney stone specimen used in this study was obtained from the Department of Urology, People's Hospital of Longhua Shenzhen in 2018. After characterization by a stone component analyzer (LIIR-20, Lambda scientific, Tianjin China), the calcium oxalate kidney stone was fully crushed into powder by sterilized mortar and pestle and then prepared into COM suspension. Briefly, the crystals were suspended with serum-free DMEM at a final concentration of 100 μg/mL (per volume of medium) [14, 24], which was demonstrated not to cause severe cytotoxicity to renal tubular cells or increase percentage of cell death [24], but induce alterations in cellular proteome and reflect response of the renal epithelial cells to the COM crystals in vivo [18, 24, 25]. The kidney stone specimen was used in accordance with the hospital ethical review and the patient's informed consent.

Protein extraction and quality analyzation

HK-2 cells were seeded into 6-well plates at a density of 1×10^5 cells per well and divided into two groups ($n = 3$ per group) when the cell density reached 70–80% confluence. The culture medium was replaced by either COM-crystal containing medium (with 100 μg/mL COM crystals) or COM-free medium. The cells were further maintained for 24 h. Cell pictures were taken after incubation by a microscope (GMSP-5, Shanghai Guangmi instrument Co.,ltd). Cell samples were harvested by cell scraping, repeatedly frozen and thawed, and then sonicated on ice for 2 min; After 4 °C, 12000 g centrifugation for 20 min, protein supernatant was collected for BCA quantification and SDS-PAGE electrophoresis.

TMT-based quantitative proteomic analysis

TMT (Tandem Mass Tag) technology is a peptide in vitro labeling technology developed by Thermo Scientific, USA. The technology uses 10 isotopic labels to label the amino group of the peptide. After LC-MS/MS analysis, peak identification was performed to obtain a peak list and a reference database was established to identify peptides and proteins. Samples were analyzed by Shanghai Majorbio bio-pharm Biotechnology Co. Ltd. (Shanghai, China). The differential expressed proteins were screened based on the significance of p values, and the differentially expressed proteins were subjected to bioinformatics.

GO and KEGG enrichment analysis

GO (Gene Ontology, http://www.geneontology.ory/) is a comprehensive database of gene-related research results from all over the world. The significant functional enrichment analysis of the differential proteins can explain the functional enrichment of the differential proteins and clarify the differences in the sample components at the functional level. This study used Goatools for enrichment analysis using Fisher's exact test. KEGG (Kyoto Encyclopedia of Genes and Genomes) is a database resource for understanding high-level functions and utilities of the biological system, so we used KOBAS software to test the statistical enrichment of differential expression proteins in KEGG pathways.

Differential protein interaction network analysis

The Search Tool for the Retrieval of Interacting Genes (STRING) database (http://string-db.org/), a database that provides experimental and predicted proteins interaction information [26], was used to build protein-protein interaction networks. In addition to mining data including experimental data and various databases, comprehensive scoring (0.4–1) is performed from the aspects of chromosome proximity, gene fusion, phylogenetics and gene-based co-expression based on chip data, thereby predicting the inter-protein interactions. Each node in the network represents a protein molecule, and the line represents the interaction between proteins. The wider the line, the higher the score, and the narrower the line, the lower the score. In this study, the cutoff confidence score of protein-interactions was ≥0.4.

Statistics

Statistical analysis was performed using SPSS17.0 software. Quantitative data were analyzed by one-way ANOVA. Those with irregular variance were analyzed by rank sum test. Differences between samples were analyzed by LSD method, and the results were expressed as mean ± standard deviation. The difference was statistically significant at $p < 0.05$.

Results

Preparation of kidney stone treated HK-2 cells and quality control of TMT mass spectrometry samples

The human proximal tubular epithelial cell HK-2 cells were suspended into single cells, seeded onto 6-well plates overnight. Crystal suspension of calcium oxalate stone with a final concentration of 100 μg/ml was added and incubated for 24 h. The calcium oxalate crystals adhered to the surface of HK-2 cells was clearly observed by phase-contrast microscopy (Fig. 1a). These COM crystals adhere tightly to the surface of the cells, which even cannot be removed by several washes with PBS. After incubation, cells were harvested by scraping, and prepared for quality control prior to TMT analysis. Quality control results showed that 24,224 proteins were identified in 122,920 identified spectrum (Fig. 1b). Protein coverage distribution analysis showed that 4137 proteins were covered over 10% (Fig. 1c), suggesting that the sample preparation was successful and could be proceeded for TMT analyzation.

Proteome alterations of HK-2 cells after adhered by calcium oxalate crystals

The screening criteria for significant differentially expressed proteins (DEPs) were $p < 0.05$ and $FC < 0.83$ or $FC > 1.20$. The scatter plot of the DEPs is shown in Fig. 2a. Results showed that among the total number of 6407 target proteins, 1141 (17.8%) proteins changed significantly, of which 699 (61.3%) proteins were upregulated (Fig. 2b), 442 (38.7%) proteins were downregulated expression. The proteins with $p > 0.05$ and $FC > 2$ (Table 1) or $FC < 0.6$ (Table 2) were selected for further bioinformatics analyzation.

Cluster analysis of differentially expressed proteins

Two-dimensional hierarchical clustering feature of the 40 selected DEPs was presented in a heatmap (Fig. 3). Columns in the heat map represents COM-treated

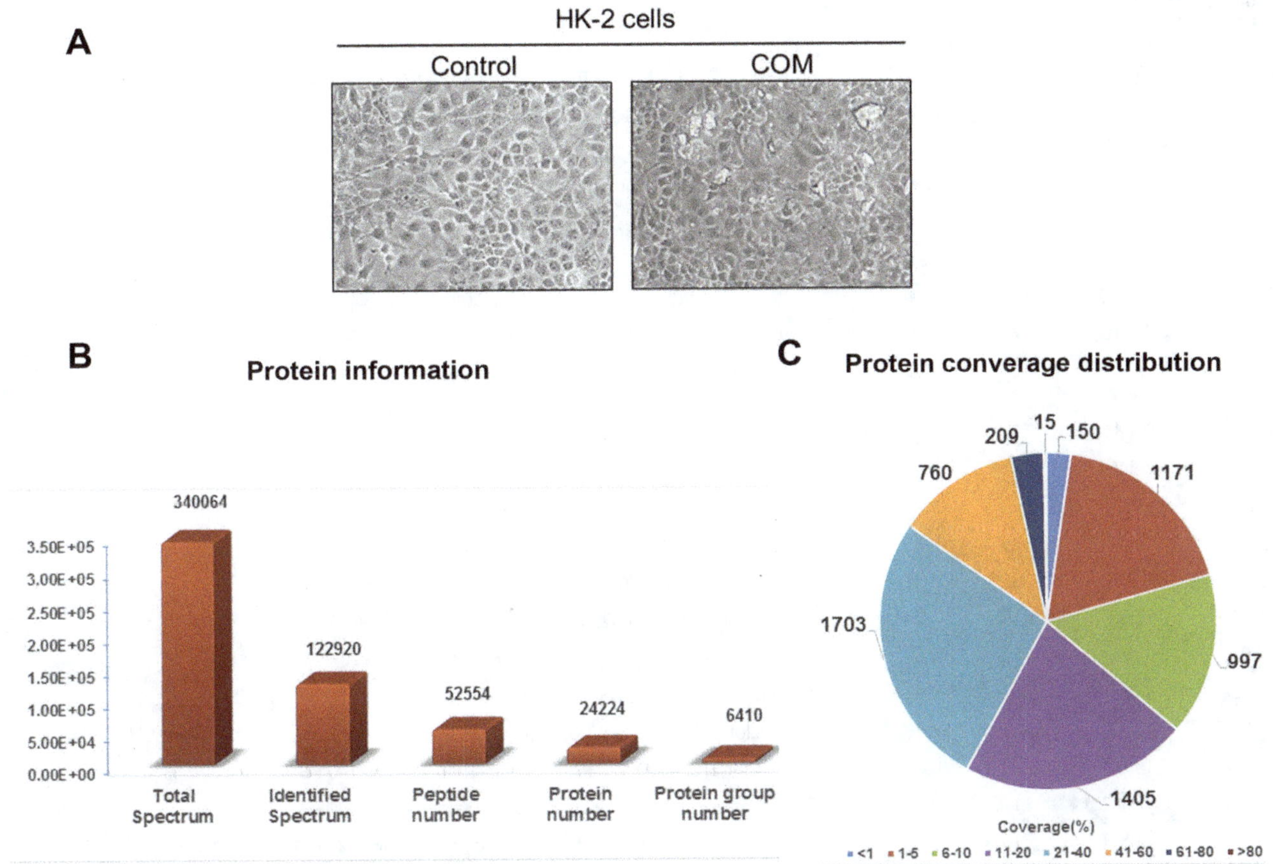

Fig. 1 COM-HK-2 cell preparation and protein sample quality control. **a**. Representative pictures of calcium oxalate monohydrate crystals treated HK-2 cells and its' parental control. COM crystal adhesion and cell-crystal interactions. Images were taken using phase-contrast microscopy. **b**. Protein information of quality control. **c**. Protein coverage distribution of quality control

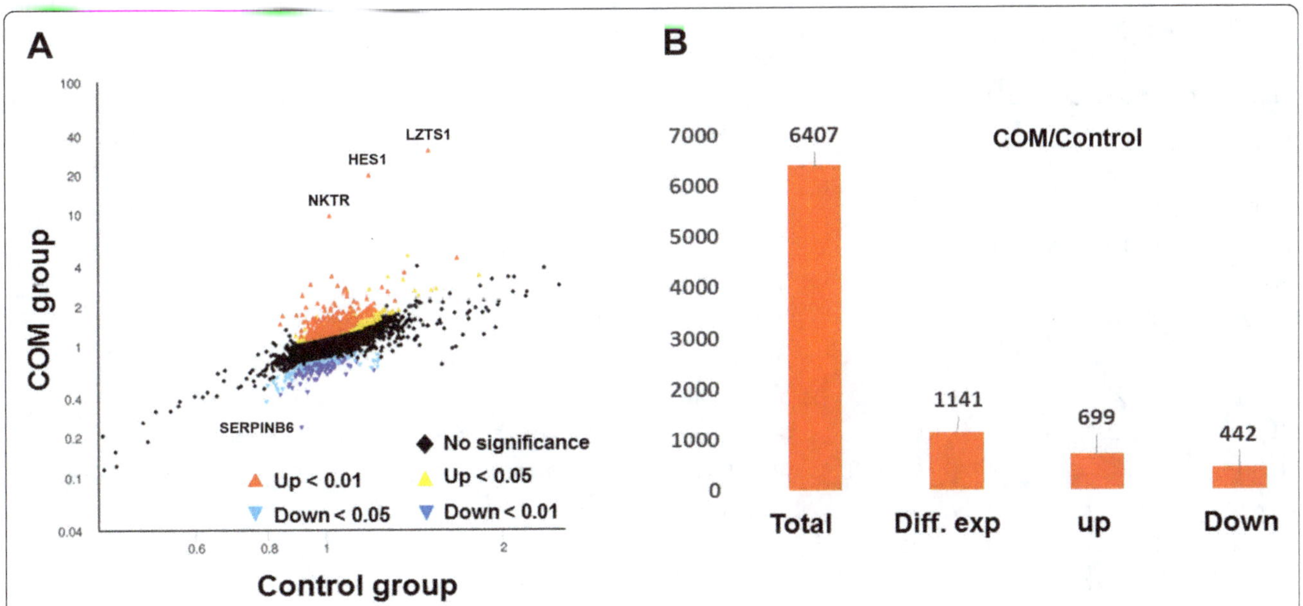

Fig. 2 Proteome alterations of HK-2 cells after treated with calcium oxalate crystals. **a**. Scatter plot of differential expressed proteins statistics. **b**. Histogram of differential expressed proteins

Table 1 Upregulated proteins in COM-stimulated HK-2 cells ($P < 0.05$, $FC > 2$)

Gene name	Accession	FC (C/H)	**P** value (C/H)	Description
LZTS1	Q9Y250	20.20	0.001	Leucine zipper putative tumor suppressor 1 OS=Homo sapiens GN = LZTS1 PE = 1 SV = 3
HES1	Q14469	16.53	0.001	Transcription factor HES-1 OS=Homo sapiens GN=HES1 PE = 1 SV = 1
NKTR	P30414	9.53	0.001	NK-tumor recognition protein OS=Homo sapiens GN=NKTR PE = 1 SV = 2
KLK15	M0R2F7	3.51	0.033	Kallikrein-15 (Fragment) OS=Homo sapiens GN=KLK15 PE = 4 SV = 1
CLPS	P04118	3.30	0.002	Colipase OS=Homo sapiens GN=CLPS PE = 1 SV = 2
DPP8	Q6V1X1	3.09	0.004	Dipeptidyl peptidase 8 OS=Homo sapiens GN = DPP8 PE = 1 SV = 1
CEP128	Q6ZU80	2.77	0.004	Centrosomal protein of 128 kDa OS=Homo sapiens GN=CEP128 PE = 1 SV = 2
PHRF1	Q9P1Y6	2.74	0.003	PHD and RING finger domain-containing protein 1 OS=Homo sapiens GN=PHRF1 PE = 1 SV = 3
HNRNPD	D6RBQ9	2.64	0.007	Heterogeneous nuclear ribonucleoprotein D0 (Fragment) OS=Homo sapiens GN=HNRNPD PE = 1 SV = 1
ANXA2	H0YL33	2.63	0.015	Annexin (Fragment) OS=Homo sapiens GN = ANXA2 PE = 1 SV = 1
TMEM141	Q96I45	2.61	0.000	Transmembrane protein 141 OS=Homo sapiens GN = TMEM141 PE = 1 SV = 1
FAU	E9PM49	2.53	0.001	40S ribosomal protein S30 (Fragment) OS=Homo sapiens GN=FAU PE = 1 SV = 8
TMSB10	P63313	2.49	0.009	Thymosin beta-10 OS=Homo sapiens GN = TMSB10 PE = 1 SV = 2
CFL1	E9PP50	2.38	0.013	Cofilin-1 (Fragment) OS=Homo sapiens GN=CFL1 PE = 1 SV = 8
RPS29	P62273	2.35	0.024	40S ribosomal protein S29 OS=Homo sapiens GN = RPS29 PE = 1 SV = 2
ACTB	C9JTX5	2.34	0.000	Actin, cytoplasmic 1 (Fragment) OS=Homo sapiens GN = ACTB PE = 1 SV = 1
ZNF12	P17014	2.32	0.001	Zinc finger protein 12 OS=Homo sapiens GN = ZNF12 PE = 1 SV = 3
GCHFR	P30047	2.27	0.013	GTP cyclohydrolase 1 feedback regulatory protein OS=Homo sapiens GN = GCHFR PE = 1 SV = 3
ZNF146	Q15072	2.23	0.000	Zinc finger protein OZF OS=Homo sapiens GN = ZNF146 PE = 1 SV = 2
TMEM222	Q9H0R3	2.17	0.002	Transmembrane protein 222 OS=Homo sapiens GN = TMEM222 PE = 1 SV = 2
ZNF574	A0A0C4DFM2	2.16	0.000	HCG1643764, isoform CRA_b OS=Homo sapiens GN = ZNF574 PE = 1 SV = 1
TSHZ1	Q6ZSZ6	2.11	0.006	Teashirt homolog 1 OS=Homo sapiens GN = TSHZ1 PE = 1 SV = 2
ITGA5	P08648	2.04	0.007	Integrin alpha-5 OS=Homo sapiens GN=ITGA5 PE = 1 SV = 2
BTF3	D6RDG3	2.02	0.004	Transcription factor BTF3 (Fragment) OS=Homo sapiens GN=BTF3 PE = 1 SV = 3

Table 2 Down-regulated proteins in COM-stimulated HK-2 cells ($P < 0.05$, $FC < 0.6$)

Gene name	Accession	FC (C/H)	**P** value (C/H)	Description
PRDX1	Q06830	0.57	0.001	Peroxiredoxin-1 OS=Homo sapiens GN=PRDX1 PE = 1 SV = 1
NME2P1	O60361	0.57	0.029	Putative nucleoside diphosphate kinase OS=Homo sapiens GN=NME2P1 PE = 5 SV = 1
SLC39A10	Q9ULF5	0.57	0.001	Zinc transporter ZIP10 OS=Homo sapiens GN=SLC39A10 PE = 1 SV = 2
SERPINB1	P30740	0.56	0.006	Leukocyte elastase inhibitor OS=Homo sapiens GN=SERPINB1 PE = 1 SV = 1
FAM133B	Q5BKY9	0.56	0.014	Protein FAM133B OS=Homo sapiens GN=FAM133B PE = 1 SV = 1
PRDX2	P32119	0.56	0.003	Peroxiredoxin-2 OS=Homo sapiens GN=PRDX2 PE = 1 SV = 5
MYL12A	J3QRS3	0.56	0.012	Myosin regulatory light chain 12A OS=Homo sapiens GN = MYL12A PE = 1 SV = 1
MYH14	Q7Z406	0.55	0.002	Myosin-14 OS=Homo sapiens GN = MYH14 PE = 1 SV = 2
MAP10	Q9P2G4	0.55	0.017	Microtubule-associated protein 10 OS=Homo sapiens GN = MAP10 PE = 1 SV = 2
PADI2	Q9Y2J8	0.54	0.012	Protein-arginine deiminase type-2 OS=Homo sapiens GN=PADI2 PE = 1 SV = 2
C14orf1	Q9UKR5	0.54	0.003	Probable ergosterol biosynthetic protein 28 OS=Homo sapiens GN=C14orf1 PE = 1 SV = 1
MYH9	P35579	0.53	0.010	Myosin-9 OS=Homo sapiens GN = MYH9 PE = 1 SV = 4
MT-ND2	P03891	0.50	0.010	NADH-ubiquinone oxidoreductase chain 2 OS=Homo sapiens GN = MT-ND2 PE = 1 SV = 2
APITD1-CORT	A0A087WT10	0.47	0.001	APITD1-CORT readthrough OS=Homo sapiens GN = APITD1-CORT PE = 1 SV = 1
TUFT1	Q9NNX1	0.47	0.015	Tuftelin OS=Homo sapiens GN = TUFT1 PE = 1 SV = 1
SERPINB6	A0A087X1N8	0.26	0.000	Serpin B6 OS=Homo sapiens GN=SERPINB6 PE = 1 SV = 1

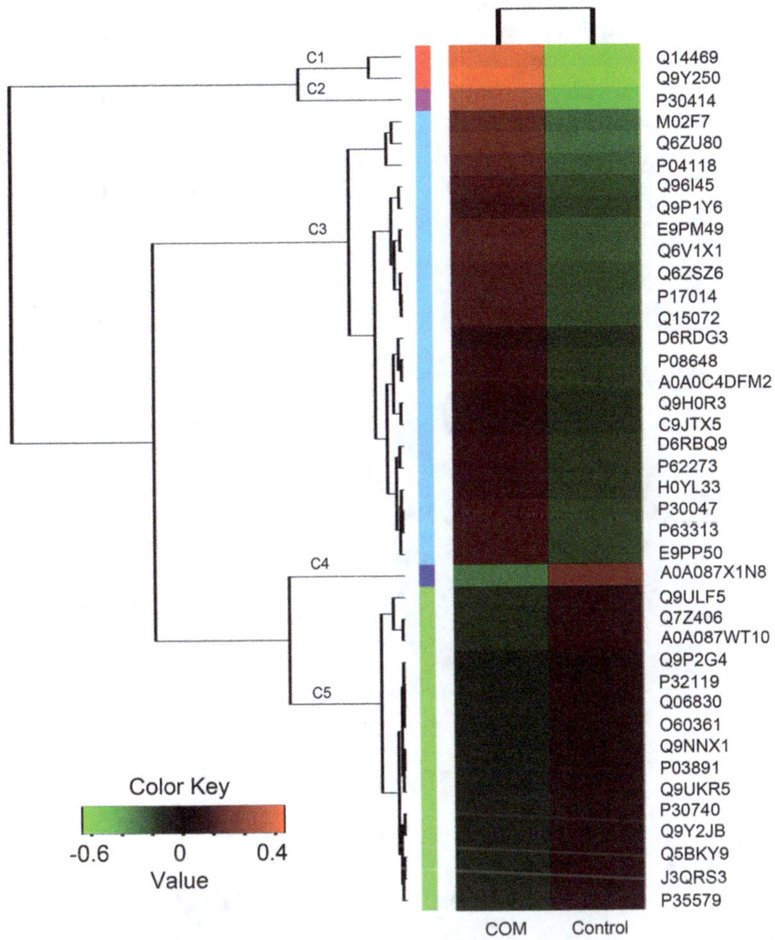

Fig. 3 Heatmap and cluster analysis of differential expressed proteins. Proteins fold change (FC) > 2 or < 0.6 and $p < 0.05$ were enriched

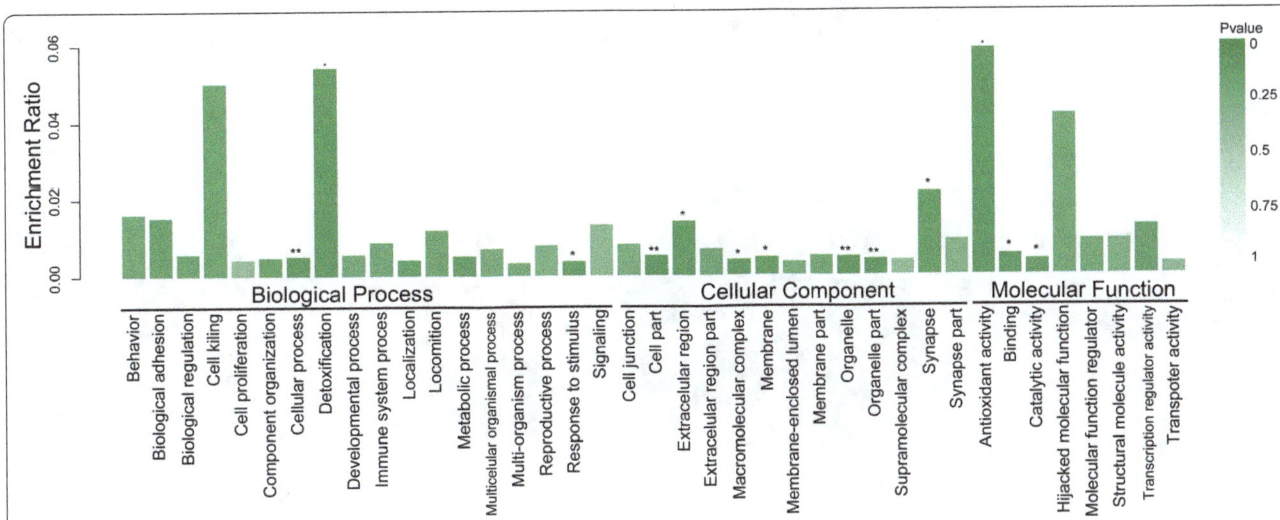

Fig. 4 GO analysis. Each column is a GO term, the abscissa indicates the GO name and the classification, the height of the column indicates the enrichment rate, and the p value is represented by the color. The darker the color, the more significant. ***, $p < 0.001$; **, $p < 0.01$; *, $p < 0.05$

group ($n = 3$) and Control group ($n = 3$) respectively. The color in the figure indicates the relative expression of the protein in the sample, the red color indicates that the protein is expressed higher in the sample, and the green color represents the lower expression level. The trend of the amount of expression is shown in the color code. On the left is a dendrogram of protein clustering. Cluster analysis showed that the selected DEPs can be divided into 5 clusters (C1 to C5) based on the heat map signal intensity. The cluster 1 (C1) included two proteins (LZTS1, HES1) which showed the highest expression level in the COM treated group compare to that in control group. The cluster 3 (C3) included 21 proteins which were higher expressed in COM treated group. By contrast, the cluster 5 (C5) consisted 15 proteins which were decreased in COM treated group.

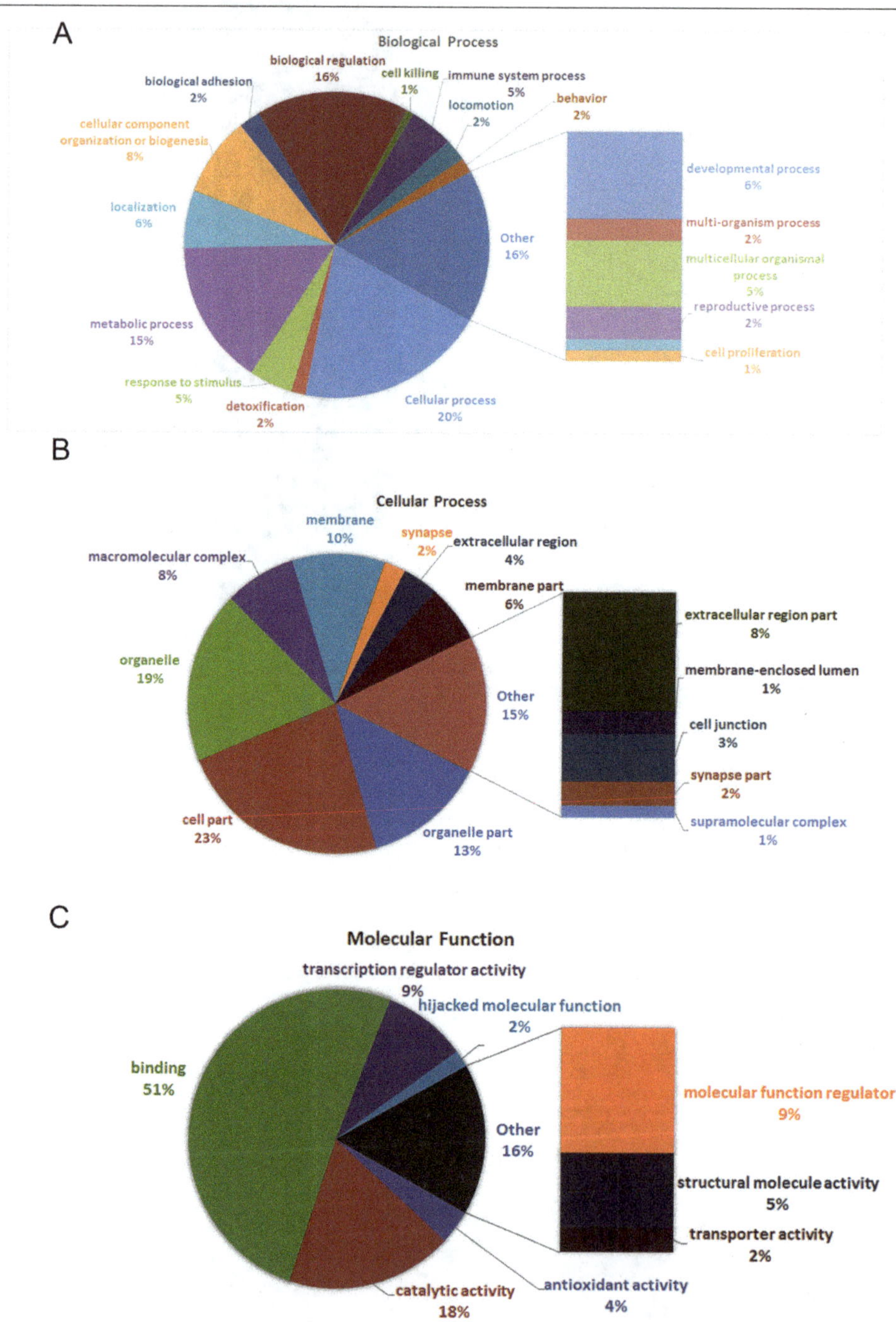

Fig. 5 GO level-2 distribution of differential expression proteins. **a**. Biological process. **b**. Cellular process. **c**. Molecular function. Results showed that most of the differential expressed proteins are related to cellular process, cell part and binding

Table 3 GO terms of the differentially expressed proteins involved in COM-stimulated HK-2 cells

Name	Namespace	Count	*P* value
Cell part	Cellular component	30	0.002
Organelle	Cellular component	24	0.003
Membrane	Cellular component	13	0.038
Organelle part	Cellular component	17	0.001
Macromolecular complex	Cellular component	10	0.021
Extracellular region	Cellular component	5	0.046
Synapse	Cellular component	3	0.044
Cellular process	Biological process	26	0.009
Response to stimulus	Biological process	6	0.046
Detoxification	Biological process	2	0.020
Antioxidant activity	Molecular function	2	0.017
Binding	Molecular function	28	0.019
Catalytic activity	Molecular function	10	0.018

GO and KEEG enrichment analyses

The significant functional enrichment analysis of GO proteins on differential proteins can explain the functional enrichment of differential proteins and clarify the differences exhibited in the samples at the functional level. To investigate the biological roles of the DEPs altered by COM crystals in HK-2 cells, a categorized GO enrichment analysis was performed. According to the gene function classification of GO, the selected DEPs were mainly related to cellular process, cell part, organelles, binding and catalytic activity (Figs. 4 and 5). For the response to the COM crystals, cell part ($p = 0.002$) and cellular process ($p = 0.009$) were the most significantly enriched functional terms for cellular component (CC) and biological processes (BP), respectively. Most of the candidate proteins are involved in cellular component (CC) as showed in Table 3.

There were 11 significant pathways identified in HK-2 cells in response to COM crystals (Fig. 6 and Table 4), among which the regulation of actin cytoskeleton pathway was the most significant ($p = 0.0001$), suggested that the regulation of the actin cytoskeleton was a critical part of cellular activities in response to COM crystals adhesion.

Biological interaction of differentially expressed proteins

According to the information of STRING database, the protein-interaction networks of the selected DEPs contained 8 main nodes and 21 connects (Fig. 7). The top 3 high-score hub nodes included β-Actin (ACTN), Cofilin-1 (CFL1) and Myosin-9 (MYH9). Among these proteins, the interaction between CFL1 and ACTN, which were both up-regulated in COM-treated HK-2 cells, exhibited the highest combined score of 0.999. These proteins and interactions may play vital roles in HK-2 cells in response to the COM crystals adhesion.

Discussion

Kidney stone is a common urological disease with high incidence, which remains a common health problem worldwide. At present, the mechanism of kidney stone formation is not fully understood. One of the favored

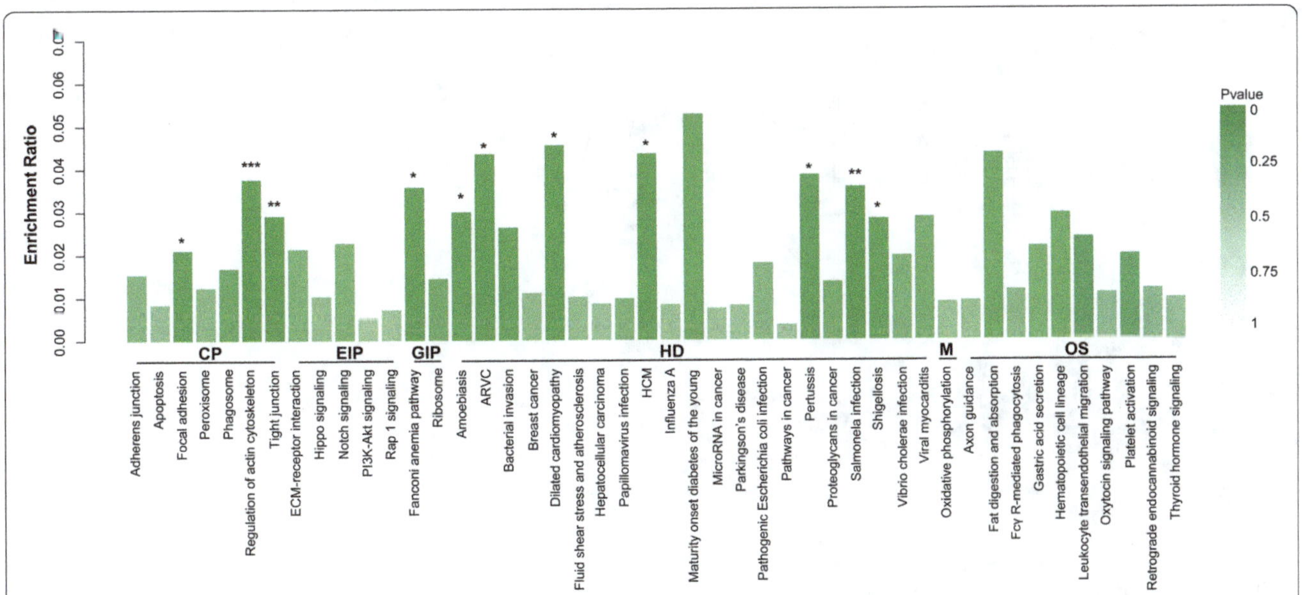

Fig. 6 KEEG analysis. Each column is a pathway, the abscissa indicates the name and the classification, the height of the column indicates the enrichment rate, and the *p* value is represented by the color. The darker the color, the more significant. Results showed that 11 pathways were significant changed in the COM treated HK-2 cells as compared to its untreated control. ***, $p < 0.001$; **, $p < 0.01$; *, $p < 0.05$

Table 4 KEGG pathway analysis of the differentially expressed proteins involved in COM-stimulated HK-2 cells

Pathway	Class	Count	***p*** value
Regulation of actin cytoskeleton	Cellular Processes	6	0.0001
Tight junction	Cellular Processes	4	0.004
Focal adhesion	Cellular Processes	3	0.0294
Salmonella infection	Human Diseases	3	0.0076
Dilated cardiomyopathy (DCM)	Human Diseases	2	0.0195
Arrhythmogenic right ventricular cardiomyopathy (ARVC)	Human Diseases	2	0.0211
Hypertrophic cardiomyopathy (HCM)	Human Diseases	2	0.0211
Pertussis	Human Diseases	2	0.0264
Amoebiasis	Human Diseases	2	0.041
Shigellosis	Human Diseases	2	0.0453
Fanconi anemia pathway	Genetic Information Processing	2	0.0301

theories suggests that the calcium oxalate-induced injury to renal tubular epithelial cells promotes the adherence and acumination of calcium oxalate crystals results in stone formation [27]. Given proteins are the major component of kidney stone organic matrix and considered to play a regulatory function in cell-crystal interactions and lithogenesis inside the kidney [28–31], we selected immortalized human proximal tubular epithelial cells HK-2 exposure to COM crystals to generate the cell-crystal interaction model and analyzed the altered proteomic landscape in HK-2 cells in response to COM adhesion.

In this study, we first systematically screened the DEPs profiles in COM-HK-2 model by TMT-labeled quantitative proteomics analysis. Of the 1141 identified DEPs, 699 (61.3%) proteins were up-regulated, 442 (38.7%) proteins were down-regulated. By contrast, a similar previous study performed by Chen et al. in 2010 [32] demonstrated that only 12 DEPs were identified in HK-2 cells after COM crystals stimulation. This different observation may due to the limits of methodology used by Chen et al. in their study. Here, gel-free TMT-based quantitative proteomic approach uses isobaric labels and allows for genome-wide quantitation of differences in protein expression levels [33], proved to be a more reliable and reproducible technology to analyze complex samples.

Several of proteins have been characterized to play critical roles in kidney stone formation, however, the

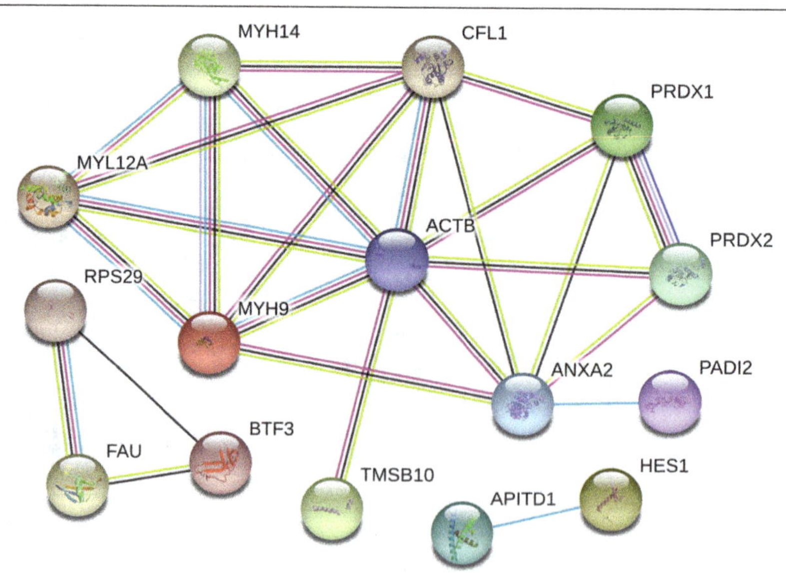

Fig. 7 Protein interaction networks of differential expressed proteins. According to the STRING database, the protein interaction networks of the DEPs contained 8 main nodes and 21 connections. Each node in the network represents a protein molecule, and the line represents the interaction between proteins. The wider the line, the higher the score, and the narrower the line, the lower the score. The top 3 high-score hub nodes included CFL1, ACTN and MYH9. The interaction between CFL1 and ACTN exhibited the highest combined score of 0.999, suggested that may play vital roles in the adhesion of COM to the HK-2 cells

mechanisms involved are far from clear. Tamm-Horsfall protein (THP) was identified as a kidney-specific protein, serve as a key regulator in promoting the aggregation of calcium-salt crystals and stone formation [34, 35], which is a potent immunomodulatory molecule and a disease biomarker in the urinary system [35]. Osteopontin (OPN) is another important component of calcium oxalate stone matrix [29], plays an important role in preventing the formation of calcium oxalate monohydrate (COM) kidney stones, which controls switching of calcium oxalate monohydrate morphologies in urine [36] to promote the formation of stones by promoting crystal adhesion and mediating oxidative stress and apoptosis [17, 37].

In this study, we identified that the LZTS1 (leucine zipper hypothetical tumor suppressor gene 1) protein, a full-length 596 amino acid protein with a molecular weight of 67 kD, was significantly upregulated in COM adhered HK-2 cells. Though the role and mechanism involved of LZTS1 protein was well studied in various types of malignant tumors such as stomach, lung, bladder, ovary, and kidney [38], the functional role of LZTS1 in kidney stone disease is unreported. The HES1 (hairy enhancer of split 1) protein, the core effector of NOTCH signaling pathway and considered to be a good indicator of the activation of the NOTCH signaling pathway [39, 40], exhibited significant reduce expression in COM adhered HK-2 cells. Present study is the first report to demonstrate the relation between the HES1 protein and kidney stone formation and its associated kidney injury, however, further study of the mechanism involved is in need.

Our bioinformatics analysis indicated that the GO terms of cellular process, cell part, organelles, binding and catalytic activity are significant changed in COM adhered HK-2 cells, suggested that these processes or cell structures and its related proteins are widely involved in kidney stone formation. The enriched signaling pathway identified by KEEG analysis were regulation of the actin cytoskeleton, tight junction and focal adhesion. Of these, the regulation of actin cytoskeleton showed the most significance, which plays vital roles in response to extracellular signals, spatially and temporally regulates adhesions, protrusion, contraction, and retraction [41]. Meanwhile, we analyzed the protein interaction networks of the selected DEPs and found that the CFL1, ACTN and MYH9 were the 3 high-degree hub nodes and may be involved in the pathological processes of HK-2 cells in response to the COM crystals adhesion. These findings suggested that the cell structure- and cell actin cytoskeleton dynamics had been significantly changed by COM crystals.

Conclusion

We screened and identified key protein molecules that may be involved in the formation of calcium oxalate kidney stones, and revealed the possible signaling pathways and related disease processes, providing important potential targets and interactions for further elucidation of the pathogenesis of kidney stones. However, despite these comprehensive bioinformatics analyses, the current study has several limitations. HK-2 cells are not normal proximal tubular cells, which is a big limitation of the present study. Furthermore, the in vitro COM concentration could not perfectly mimic the status of crystals in kidney, the dose-dependent and time-dependent effects of COM stimulation were not involved. In our future investigations, we hope to perform additional proteomics analyses on normal proximal tubular cells/animal models of different time points and experimental validation to enrich this study.

Abbreviations

COM: Calcium Oxalate Monohydrate; DEP: Differential expression protein; TMT: Tandem Mass Tag; KEEG: Kyoto Encyclopedia of Genes and Genomes; GO: Gene Ontology; CC: Cellular Component; BP: Biological Processes; MF: Molecular Function; OS: Organismal Systems; HD: Human Diseases; CP: Cellular Processes; EIP: Environmental Information Processing; GIP: Genetic Information Processing; M: Metabolism

Acknowledgments

Not applicable.

Authors' contributions

ZW and ML examined and scripted the manuscript. ZW obtained funding for the study, drafted and revised the manuscript. CX, QD and RS performed the experiments and statistical analysis; YZ, JZ and SZ helped to analyze the data and draft the manuscript. QH and HL supported for the critical revision of the manuscript for intellectual content. All authors read and approved the final manuscript.

Author details

[1]Department of Urology, People's Hospital of Longhua, Southern Medical University, Shenzhen 518109, Guangdong, China. [2]Laboratory of Molecular Pharmacology, Department of Pharmacology, School of Pharmacy, Southwest Medical University, Luzhou 646000, Sichuan, China. [3]Department of Laboratory Medicine, Third Affiliated Hospital of Sun Yat-sen University, Guangzhou, Guangdong 510630, People's Republic of China.

References

1. Trinchieri A, Coppi F, Montanari E, Del Nero A, Zanetti G, Pisani E. Increase in the prevalence of symptomatic upper urinary tract stones during the last ten years. Eur Urol. 2000;37(1):23–5. https://doi.org/10.1159/000020094.
2. Wang W, Fan J, Huang G, Li J, Zhu X, Tian Y, Su L. Prevalence of kidney stones in mainland China: a systematic review. Sci Rep. 2017;7:41630. https://doi.org/10.1038/srep41630.
3. Zeng G, Mai Z, Xia S, Wang Z, Zhang K, Wang L, Long Y, Ma J, Li Y, Wan SP, Wu W, Liu Y, Cui Z, Zhao Z, Qin J, Zeng T, Liu Y, Duan X, Mai X, Yang Z, Kong Z, Zhang T, Cai C, Shao Y, Yue Z, Li S, Ding J, Tang S, Ye Z. Prevalence of kidney stones in China: an ultrasonography based cross-sectional study. BJU Int. 2017;120(1):109–16. https://doi.org/10.1111/bju.13828.
4. Leveridge M, D'Arcy FT, O'Kane D, Ischia JJ, Webb DR, Bolton DM, Lawrentschuk N. Renal colic: current protocols for emergency presentations. Eur J Emerg Med. 2016;23(1):2–7. https://doi.org/10.1097/MEJ.0000000000000324.

5. Worcester EM, Coe FL. Clinical practice. Calcium kidney stones. N Engl J Med. 2010;363(10):954–63. https://doi.org/10.1056/NEJMcp1001011.
6. Wang B, Wu B, Liu J, Yao W, Xia D, Li L, Chen Z, Ye Z, Yu X. Analysis of altered microRNA expression profiles in proximal renal tubular cells in response to calcium oxalate monohydrate crystal adhesion: implications for kidney stone disease. PLoS One. 2014;9(7):e101306. https://doi.org/10.1371/journal.pone.0101306.
7. Khan SR. Role of renal epithelial cells in the initiation of calcium oxalate stones. Nephron Exp Nephrol. 2004;98(2):e55–60. https://doi.org/10.1159/000080257.
8. Qin B, Wang Q, Lu Y, Li C, Hu H, Zhang J, Wang Y, Zhu J, Zhu Y, Xun Y, Wang S. Losartan ameliorates calcium oxalate-induced elevation of stone-related proteins in renal tubular cells by inhibiting NADPH oxidase and oxidative stress. Oxidative Med Cell Longev. 2018;2018:1271864. https://doi.org/10.1155/2018/1271864.
9. Joshi S, Peck AB, Khan SR. NADPH oxidase as a therapeutic target for oxalate induced injury in kidneys. Oxidative Med Cell Longev. 2013;2013: 462361. https://doi.org/10.1155/2013/462361.
10. Zuo J, Khan A, Glenton PA, Khan SR. Effect of NADPH oxidase inhibition on the expression of kidney injury molecule and calcium oxalate crystal deposition in hydroxy-L-proline-induced hyperoxaluria in the male Sprague-Dawley rats. Nephrol Dial Transplant. 2011;26(6):1785–96. https://doi.org/10.1093/ndt/gfr035.
11. Narula S, Tandon S, Singh SK, Tandon C. Kidney stone matrix proteins ameliorate calcium oxalate monohydrate induced apoptotic injury to renal epithelial cells. Life Sci. 2016;164:23–30. https://doi.org/10.1016/j.lfs.2016.08.026
12. Evan AP, Worcester EM, Coe FL, Williams J Jr, Lingeman JE. Mechanisms of human kidney stone formation. Urolithiasis. 2015;43(Suppl 1):19–32. https://doi.org/10.1007/s00240-014-0701-0.
13. Vinaiphat A, Aluksanasuwan S, Manissorn J, Sutthimethakorn S, Thongboonkerd V. Response of renal tubular cells to differential types and doses of calcium oxalate crystals: integrative proteome network analysis and functional investigations. Proteomics. 2017;17(15–16). https://doi.org/10.1002/pmic.201700192.
14. Wang Z, Zhang JW, Zhang Y, Zhang SP, Hu QY, Liang H. Analyses of long non-coding RNA and mRNA profiling using RNA sequencing in calcium oxalate monohydrate-stimulated renal tubular epithelial cells. Urolithiasis. 2019;47(3):225–34. https://doi.org/10.1007/s00240-018-1065-7.
15. Martelli C, Marzano V, Iavarone F, Huang L, Vincenzoni F, Desiderio C, Messana I, Beltrami P, Zattoni F, Ferraro PM, Buchholz N, Locci G, Faa G, Castagnola M, Gambaro G. Characterization of the protein components of matrix stones sheds light on S100-A8 and S100-A9 relevance in the inflammatory pathogenesis of these rare renal calculi. J Urol. 2016;196(3): 911–8. https://doi.org/10.1016/j.juro.2016.04.064.
16. Kolbach-Mandel AM, Mandel NS, Cohen SR, Kleinman JG, Ahmed F, Mandel IC, Wesson JA. Guaifenesin stone matrix proteomics: a protocol for identifying proteins critical to stone formation. Urolithiasis. 2017;45(2):139–49. https://doi.org/10.1007/s00240-016-0907-4.
17. Asselman M, Verhulst A, De Broe ME, Verkoelen CF. Calcium oxalate crystal adherence to hyaluronan-, osteopontin-, and CD44-expressing injured/regenerating tubular epithelial cells in rat kidneys. J Am Soc Nephrol. 2003; 14(12):3155–66. https://doi.org/10.1097/01.asn.0000099380.18995.f7.
18. Thongboonkerd V. Proteomics of crystal-cell interactions: a model for kidney stone research. Cells. 2019;8(9). https://doi.org/10.3390/cells8091076.
19. Shum DK, Liong E. Calcium oxalate crystallizing properties of polyanions elaborated by cultured renal proximal tubular cells. Urol Res. 1995;23(2):103–10. https://doi.org/10.1007/bf00307940.
20. Ryan MJ, Johnson G, Kirk J, Fuerstenberg SM, Zager RA, Torok-Storb B. HK-2: an immortalized proximal tubule epithelial cell line from normal adult human kidney. Kidney Int. 1994;45(1):48–57. https://doi.org/10.1038/ki.1994.6.
21. Wang Z, Wang Y, Zhang J, Hu Q, Zhi F, Zhang S, Mao D, Zhang Y, Liang H. Significance of the TMPRSS2:ERG gene fusion in prostate cancer. Mol Med Rep. 2017;16(4):5450–8. https://doi.org/10.3892/mmr.2017.7281.
22. Wang Z, Yin J, Li M, Shen J, Xiao Z, Zhao Y, Huang C, Zhang H, Zhang Z, Cho CH, Wu X. Combination of shikonin with paclitaxel overcomes multidrug resistance in human ovarian carcinoma cells in a P-gp-independent manner through enhanced ROS generation. Chin Med. 2019; 14:7. https://doi.org/10.1186/s13020-019-0231-3.
23. Wu D, Wang Z, Lin M, Shang Y, Wang F, Zhou J, Wang F, Zhang X, Luo X, Huang W. In vitro and in vivo antitumor activity of Cucurbitacin C, a novel natural product from cucumber. Front Pharmacol. 2019;10:1287. https://doi.org/10.3389/fphar.2019.01287
24. Thongboonkerd V, Semangoen T, Sinchaikul S, Chen ST. Proteomic analysis of calcium oxalate monohydrate crystal-induced cytotoxicity in distal renal tubular cells. J Proteome Res. 2008;7(11):4689–700. https://doi.org/10.1021/pr8002408.
25. Semangoen T, Sinchaikul S, Chen ST, Thongboonkerd V. Proteomic analysis of altered proteins in distal renal tubular cells in response to calcium oxalate monohydrate crystal adhesion: implications for kidney stone disease. Proteomics Clin Appl. 2008;2(7–8):1099–109. https://doi.org/10.1002/prca.200780136.
26. Franceschini A, Szklarczyk D, Frankild S, Kuhn M, Simonovic M, Roth A, Lin J, Minguez P, Bork P, von Mering C, Jensen LJ. STRING v9.1: protein-protein interaction networks, with increased coverage and integration. Nucleic Acids Res. 2013;41(Database issue):D808–15. https://doi.org/10.1093/nar/gks1094.
27. Aggarwal KP, Narula S, Kakkar M, Tandon C. Nephrolithiasis: molecular mechanism of renal stone formation and the critical role played by modulators. Biomed Res Int. 2013;2013:292953. https://doi.org/10.1155/2013/292953.
28. Wesson JA, Kolbach-Mandel AM, Hoffmann BR, Davis C, Mandel NS. Selective protein enrichment in calcium oxalate stone matrix: a window to pathogenesis? Urolithiasis. 2019. https://doi.org/10.1007/s00240-019-01131-3.
29. Narula S, Tandon S, Baligar P, Singh SK, Tandon C. Human kidney stone matrix: latent potential to restrain COM induced cytotoxicity and inflammatory response. Chem Biol Interact. 2017;278:114–22. https://doi.org/10.1016/j.cbi.2017.10.018.
30. Taguchi K, Hamamoto S, Okada A, Unno R, Kamisawa H, Naiki T, Ando R, Mizuno K, Kawai N, Tozawa K, Kohri K, Yasui T. Genome-wide gene expression profiling of Randall's plaques in calcium oxalate stone formers. J Am Soc Nephrol. 2017;28(1):333–47. https://doi.org/10.1681/ASN.2015111271.
31. Okumura N, Tsujihata M, Momohara C, Yoshioka I, Suto K, Nonomura N, Okuyama A, Takao T. Diversity in protein profiles of individual calcium oxalate kidney stones. PLoS One. 2013;8(7):e68624. https://doi.org/10.1371/journal.pone.0068624.
32. Chen S, Gao X, Sun Y, Xu C, Wang L, Zhou T. Analysis of HK-2 cells exposed to oxalate and calcium oxalate crystals: proteomic insights into the molecular mechanisms of renal injury and stone formation. Urol Res. 2010; 38(1):7–15. https://doi.org/10.1007/s00240-009-0226-0.
33. van Ulsen P, Kuhn K, Prinz T, Legner H, Schmid P, Baumann C, Tommassen J. Identification of proteins of Neisseria meningitidis induced under iron-limiting conditions using the isobaric tandem mass tag (TMT) labeling approach. Proteomics. 2009;9(7):1771–81. https://doi.org/10.1002/pmic.200800642.
34. Rhodes DCJ. Human Tamm-Horsfall protein, a renal specific protein, serves as a cofactor in complement 3b degradation. PLoS One. 2017;12(7): e0181857. https://doi.org/10.1371/journal.pone.0181857.
35. Wu TH, Li KJ, Yu CL, Tsai CY. Tamm-Horsfall protein is a potent Immunomodulatory molecule and a disease biomarker in the urinary system. Molecules. 2018;23(1). https://doi.org/10.3390/molecules23010200.
36. Langdon A, Grohe B. The osteopontin-controlled switching of calcium oxalate monohydrate morphologies in artificial urine provides insights into the formation of papillary kidney stones. Colloids Surf B: Biointerfaces. 2016; 146:296–306. https://doi.org/10.1016/j.colsurfb.2016.06.030.
37. Xi Q, Ouyang J, Pu J, Hou J, Wang S. High concentration of calcium stimulates calcium oxalate crystal attachment to rat tubular epithelial NRK cells through Osteopontin. Urology. 2015;86(4):844 e841–5. https://doi.org/10.1016/j.urology.2015.07.018.
38. Ishii H, Baffa R, Numata SI, Murakumo Y, Rattan S, Inoue H, Mori M, Fidanza V, Alder H, Croce CM. The FEZ1 gene at chromosome 8p22 encodes a leucine-zipper protein, and its expression is altered in multiple human tumors. Proc Natl Acad Sci U S A. 1999;96(7):3928–33. https://doi.org/10.1073/pnas.96.7.3928.
39. Gao F, Huang W, Zhang Y, Tang S, Zheng L, Ma F, Wang Y, Tang H, Li X. Hes1 promotes cell proliferation and migration by activating Bmi-1 and PTEN/Akt/GSK3beta pathway in human colon cancer. Oncotarget. 2015; 6(36):38667–80. https://doi.org/10.18632/oncotarget.5484.
40. Kay SK, Harrington HA, Shepherd S, Brennan K, Dale T, Osborne JM, Gavaghan DJ, Byrne HM. The role of the Hes1 crosstalk hub in Notch-Wnt interactions of the intestinal crypt. PLoS Comput Biol. 2017;13(2):e1005400. https://doi.org/10.1371/journal.pcbi.1005400.
41. Tang DD, Gerlach BD. The roles and regulation of the actin cytoskeleton, intermediate filaments and microtubules in smooth muscle cell migration. Respir Res. 2017;18(1):54. https://doi.org/10.1186/s12931-017-0544-7

27

Can serum procalcitonin levels be useful in predicting spontaneous ureteral stone passage?

Nusret Can Cilesiz[1*], Arif Ozkan[1], Arif Kalkanli[1], Ali Eroglu[2], Cem Tuğrul Gezmis[3], Berkan Simsek[4] and Burak Arslan[1]

Abstract

Background: Medical expulsive therapy (MET) is recommended for ureteral stones when there is no indication for interventional treatment. Spontaneous passage (SP) may not always be perceived in patients undergoing MET. We aimed to demonstrate the effects of inflammatory factors on spontaneous ureteral stone passage in patients undergoing MET.

Methods: Our study was conducted between August and November, 2016, in healthy volunteers and patients with a single distal ureteral stone between 5 and 10 mm in diameter and no indications for interventional therapy. Blood and urine samples from all patients and healthy volunteers were tested. The patients were followed up every 2 weeks for 1 month unless emergency situations appeared. Patients with stone-free status at follow-up were concluded to have achieved complete stone passage [SP(+)], and failure [SP(−)] was concluded if the patient had not passed the stone by the end of the study. Blood samples of the patients and the control group were analyzed, recording WBC (white blood cell), CRP (c-reactive protein), SED (sedimentation), MPV (mean platelet volume), NLR (neutrophil-to-lymphocyte ratio), and serum procalcitonin levels. Abnormalities in urine samples were recorded. All patients received diclofenac sodium 75 mg/day, tamsulosin 0.4 mg/day, and at least 3 l/day fluid intake. Patients were followed for a month with kidney, ureter, bladder (KUB) plain films, ultrasonography (USG), and unenhanced abdominal CT scans while undergoing MET. Comparative statistical analyses were performed between the SP(+) and SP(−) groups.

Results: The procalcitonin levels of the SP(−) group were significantly higher (207 ± 145.1 pg/ml) than in the SP(+) group (132.7 ± 28.1 pg/ml) ($p = 0.000$). The leucocyturia rate of the SP(−) group was significantly higher than in the SP(+) group ($p = 0.004$). Based on the ROC curve analysis, 160 pg/ml (86.7% sensitivity, 70.8% specificity, $p < 0.001$; AUC: 0.788 95% CI (0.658–0.917) was identified as the optimal cut-off value for procalcitonin. In logistic regression analysis, a significant efficacy of procalcitonin and leucocyturia was observed in the univariate analysis on spontaneous passage. In the multivariate analysis, significant independent activity was observed with procalcitonin. ($p < 0.05$).

Conclusion: Our findings suggest that high procalcitonin levels and the presence of leucocyturia have a strong negative effect on SP of ureteral stones between 5 and 10 mm in diameter. This relationship can be explained by stone impaction, possibly caused by increased mucosal inflammation.

Keywords: Ureteral stone, Spontaneous stone passage, Medical expulsive therapy, Serum procalcitonin, Leucocyturia

* Correspondence: nusretcancilesiz@gmail.com
Department of Urology, GOP Taksim Education Training and Research Hospital, Karayolları Str. No:621 Gaziosmanpasa, İstanbul, Turkey
Full list of author information is available at the end of the article

Background

Urinary tract stones' localization is usually on the kidney, while ureteral stones make up 20% of all urinary system stones [1]. Patients with a ureteral stone usually present with complaints such as flank pain, nausea-vomiting, and lower urinary tract symptoms [1, 2]. The most important parameter in determining the treatment to be applied is the size of the ureteral stones. Ureteral stones classified as non-complicated and smaller than 10 mm in diameter may be followed up for a month due to the possibility of spontaneous passage (SP).

Medical expulsive therapy (MET) is a non-invasive treatment modality that is especially recommended for ureteral stones > 5 mm. MET consists of high fluid intake and medical agents such as anti-inflammatory drugs, alpha-blockers, calcium channel blockers, corticosteroids or phosphodiesterase inhibitors. It has been proven elsewhere that the likelihood and speed of spontaneous passage are increased with MET [1, 3]. Furthermore, MET decreases hospital visits, costs, and the requirement of interventional treatment [4–7].

Ureteral stones can cause inflammation in the ureteral wall, and this mucosal inflammation was found to be related to the impaction of the stone. In studies using serum inflammation markers to predict the impaction of ureteral stones, serum white blood cell (WBC), neutrophil count, c-reactive protein (CRP), and neutrophil-lymphocyte ratio (NLR) values were found to be related to the spontaneous passage of ureteral stones [8–11].

Procalcitonin is a polypeptide consisting of 116 amino acids, with a molecular weight of approximately 13 kilodaltons. Ghillani et al., 1989, first described this hormone as the precursor of calcitonin, which is made up of 32 amino acids [12]. In sepsis and inflammation, serum procalcitonin levels have been shown to increase following release of endotoxins and immunomodulators [13]. Furthermore, it has been reported that the elevation of procalcitonin may be used to indicate a relapse of chronic prostatitis, the rate of infection in obstructed ureteral stones, and the severity of inflammation in cholecystitis [14–16].

Despite MET, the spontaneous passage of ureteral stones smaller than 10 mm may not be observed in clinical practice. In recent years, many studies have investigated the reasons behind this circumstance [10, 11]. In light of these studies, we aimed to investigate the effect of serum procalcitonin and other inflammation markers at the time of diagnosis, for patients with ureteral stones sized 5-10 mm.

Methods

This prospective observational study was conducted between August and November of 2016, after receiving institutional review board approval. The patients gave informed consent for participation at the beginning of the study.

Patients aged 20 to 60 years with renal colic and having a single distal ureteral stone 5-10 mm in diameter, detected by an unenhanced CT scan, were included in this study. Exclusion criteria from the study were the patients with severe hydronephrosis, symptomatic urinary system infection, findings of acute renal failure, congenital ureteral anomaly, a history of ureteral stenosis or reconstructive ureteral surgery, and those who had received anti-inflammatory or anti-microbial drugs for the ureteral stone. Patients with active infective disease, chronic inflammatory disease (e.g., ulcerative colitis, rheumatoid arthritis, ankylosing spondylitis), active neoplasia, thyroid disease with or without thyroid surgery, immunosuppression or immunosuppressive treatment were also excluded from the study. The control group included 33 healthy volunteers of the same age range and socio-demographic characteristics, no history of stone disease and no active or chronic disease.

The patients' characteristics including age, gender, BMI (body mass index), smoking history, chronic illnesses, drug allergies, previous stone interventions (nephropyelolithotomy, percutaneous surgery, URS-L or ESWL) were all recorded. Unenhanced abdominal CT scans were used to determine the stone size (dimension at its greatest diameter), area (width x length × 0.8), laterality (left/right), and the degree of hydronephrosis.

Complete blood cell count, C-reactive protein (CRP), sedimentation, serum procalcitonin, urinalysis and urine culture were performed for both groups. In the complete blood cell count, values for white blood cells (WBC), neutrophil/lymphocyte ratio (NLR), mean platelet volume (MPV), and red cell distribution width (RDW) were noted. In the urinalysis, the presence or absence of leucocyturia and bacteriuria were noted. The BioVendor® (Czechia) Human Procalcitonin ELISA (RD191006200R) kit was used to measure the procalcitonin level. Serums were analyzed using the Biotek Elx-800 microplate reader and Biotek Gen5 software.

All patients received diclofenac sodium 75 mg/day, tamsulosin 0.4 mg/day and at least 3 l/day fluid intake. The patients were followed up with kidney, ureter, bladder (KUB) plain films, ultrasonography (USG) and unenhanced abdominal CT scan every 2 weeks for 1 month unless emergency situations appeared. Patients with stone-free status at follow-up were concluded to have achieved complete stone passage [SP(+)], and failure [SP(−)] was concluded if the patient had not passed the stone by the end of the study.

Statistical analyses

Mean, standard deviation, median, lowest and highest scores, frequency and ratio values were used for the descriptive statistics of the data. Distribution of variables was obtained using the Kolmogorov Smirnov test. The Mann-Whitney U test was utilized for analyses of the independent quantitative data. For the analyses of independent categorical data, the chi square test was preferred, and when it was not applicable, Fischer's exact test was substituted. Impact level and cut-off values were determined using the ROC curve. The effect level was investigated by univariate and multivariate logistic regression. All analyses were conducted with SPSS 22.0; the accepted level of statistical significance was $p < 0.05$.

Results

According to the exclusion criteria, 11 patients were excluded from the study, and the data of the case ($n = 54$) and control ($n = 33$) groups were analyzed. None of the patients showed symptoms requiring intervention treatment, such as high fever, renal colic attacks that cannot be controlled with analgesics, progressive hydronephrosis or renal failure, during the follow-up period.

There were no significant differences between the case and the control groups in terms of bacteriuria ratio, WBC or CRP values. However, the leucocyturia ratio, RDW, NLR, sedimentation and procalcitonin values were significantly higher in the case group ($p < 0.05$) (Table 1).

Based on the follow-up controls, 30 patients (55.5%) passed the stone [SP(+)], whereas passage did not occur in 24 patients (44.5%) [SP(−)]. Age, gender, BMI, smoking history, and previous stone-related intervention rates were similar in both groups except stone distributions ($p < 0.05$) (Table 2).

Table 1 Comparison of case and control groups's sosyodemographic characteristics and biochemichal inflammation markers

	Case Group	Control Group	P
Age (years)	37,1 ± 10,2	33,9 ± 8,3	0,159
Gender	Male 38 (70,4%)	Male 27 (81,8%)	0,233
BMI (kg/m^2)	26,5 ± 4,1	24,8 ± 5,1	0,245
WBC (10^3/μL)	8,8 ± 2,3	8,0 ± 1,9	0,553
RDW (%)	15,5 ± 1,9	12,8 ± 0,9	**0,000**
NLR (%)	2,8 ± 1,7	2,0 ± 0,3	**0,009**
MPV (fL)	8,6 ± 1,0	8,5 ± 0,7	0,451
CRP (mg/L)	10,4 ± 12,6	4,0 ± 1,1	0,088
Sedimentation (mm/h)	13,4 ± 9,9	4,2 ± 1,3	**0,000**
Procalcitonin (pg/ml)	165,7 ± 104,7	128,2 ± 36,6	**0,004**
Bacteriuria (+)	3,7%	0%	0,524
Leucocyturia (+)	37%	0%	**0,000**

BMI Body mass index; *WBC* White blood cell; *NLR* Neutrophil-lymphocite ratio; *MPV* Mean platelet volume; *CRP* C-reactive protein

Table 2 Sosyodemographic characteristics and stone history of SP(−) and SP(+) groups

	SP(−)	SP(+)	p
Age (years)	35,8 ± 9,3	38,0 ± 10,9	0,381
Gender (F/M) %	41,7/58,3	20/80	0,083
BMI (kg/m^2)	26,4 ± 4,7	26,5 ± 3,6	0,781
Smoking history	%50	%53,3	0,808
Previous ESWL	%12,5	%16,7	0,668
Previous Stone surgery	%8,3	%6,7	0,816
Stone burden (mm^2)	30 ± 8.2	29.1 ± 10.3	0,310
Stone distrubition (R/L)	16/14	13/11	0,745

BMI Body mass index; *ESWL* Extracorporeal shock wave lithotripsy

Between the SP(−) and SP(+) groups, bacteriuria ratios, WBC, RDW, NLR, MPV, CRP, and sedimentation values were not significantly different ($p > 0.05$).

Compared to the SP (+) group, mean serum procalcitonin levels (207 ± 145.1 vs 132.7 ± 28.1 pg/ml, $p = 0.000$) and the leucocyturia ratio (58.3 vs. 20%, $p = 0.004$) were significantly higher in the SP (−) group (Table 3). Based on the ROC curve analysis, 160 pg/ml (86.7% sensitivity, 70.8% specificity, $p < 0.001$; AUC: 0.788 95% CI (0.658–0.917) was identified as the optimal cut-off value for procalcitonin (Fig. 1). In logistic regression analysis, a significant efficacy of procalcitonin and leucocyturia was observed in the univariate analysis of spontaneous passage. In the multivariate analysis, significant independent activity was observed with procalcitonin. (Table 4) ($p < 0.05$).

Discussion

Observation with MET protocol, ESWL and URS-L are the treatment options for the ureteral stones and could be preferred based on the patient's clinical condition and size of the stone. Treatment success for ESWL and URS-L depends on localization and size of the stone and is reported to be 68–90% and 80–97% respectively [1]. Even though high success rates occur from these treatment modalities, high costs and complication risks must

Table 3 Effect of biochemichal inflammation markers for spontaneous ureteral stone passage

	SP(−)	SP(+)	p
WBC (10^3/μL)	8,4 + 2,3	9,1 + 2,4	0,261
RDW (%)	15,5 + 2,4	15,4 + 1,5	0,657
NLR (%)	2,8 + 1,7	2,9 + 1,7	0,821
MPV (fL)	8,7 + 0,6	8,5 + 1,3	0,721
CRP (mg/L)	9,0 + 8,2	11,5 + 15,4	0,875
Sedimentation (mm/h)	11,8 + 7	14,7 + 11,7	0,558
Procalcitonin (pg/ml)	207 + 145,1	132,7 + 28,1	**0,000**
Leucocyturia (+)(%)	58,3%	20%	**0,004**

WBC White blood cell; *NLR* Neutrophil-lymphocite ratio; *MPV* Mean platelet volume; *CRP* C-reactive protein

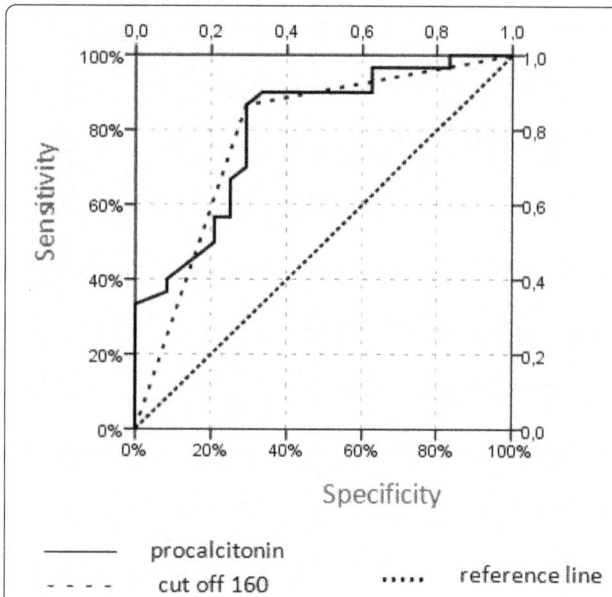

Fig. 1 ROC curve for cutoff value of 160 pg/ml of procalcitonin on prediction of spontaneous ureteral stone passage

be weighed as to their primary disadvantages [17, 18]. Moreover, the financial burden of having additional laboratory tests is another controversy about whether a ureteral stone can be spontaneously evacuated or not [18]. Similarly, complications such as recurrent renal colic attacks, urosepsis, and urinary tract infections may occur; observation or MET is therefore to be preferred for those patients. During the observation, ureteral stone impaction may also be observed due to ureteral mucosal inflammation, resulting in a more difficult and complicated treatment process of the ureteral stone [11]. For these reasons, accurate prediction of spontaneous passage has taken on greater importance in recent years, and several studies have been conducted in this area.

Recent studies have determined the likelihood of spontaneous passage in ureteral stones < 5 mm to be 71–100%, and 25–46% in stones measuring 5-10 mm. Also, for ureteral stones < 4 mm, the possibility of spontaneous passage within 40 days was reported to be 95% [1, 19]. One study classified stones into three groups based on size and reported spontaneous passage rates of 89.9, 63.4 and 9.1% for < 5 mm, 5-10 mm and > 10 mm ureteral stones, respectively [20]. In another study, which compared observation and MET for 5-10 mm ureteral stones, SP ratios were reported to be 50 and 81.8% respectively [21]. In our study, when medical expulsive therapy was conducted for the 5-10 mm ureteral stones, the SP rate was calculated to be 55.5%.

Another important factor affecting the possibility of SP in ureteral stones is localization. Studies indicate that as the stone approaches to distal, both the SP ratio and the greatest benefit from MET increase [22–24]. Although

Table 4 Logistic regression analysis for spontaneous passage in 5-10 mm distal ureteral stones

	Univariate analysis			Multivariate analysis		
	OR	95% Confidence Interval	p	OR	95% Confidence Interval	p
Age (years)	1,02	0,97-1,08	0,447			
Gender	2,86	0,85-9,56	0,088			
BMI	1,00	0,88–1,15	0,962			
Primary/secondary	1,27	0,43-3,82	0,665			
History of SWL	0,96	0,32-2,93	0,950			
History of stone passage	1,40	0,30-6,56	0,669			
History of stone surgery	0,79	0,10-6,03	0,817			
Smoking history	1,14	0,39-3,35	0,808			
Hydronephrosis	0,58	0,19-1,72	0,326			
Stone burden	0,99	0,95-1,04	0,732			
WBC	1,14	0,89-1,46	0,287			
RDW	0,97	0,73-1,28	0,807			
NLR	1,03	0,74-1,43	0,855			
MPV	0,84	0,47-1,48	0,547			
CRP	1,02	0,97-1,07	0,470			
Sedimentation	1,03	0,97-1,10	0,307			
Procalcitonin	0,96	0,94-0,99	***0,002***	0,94	0,89- 0,98	***0,005***
Leucocyturia	0,18	0,05-0,60	***0,005***			

BMI Body mass index; *ESWL* Extracorporeal shock wave lithotripsy; *WBC* White blood cell; *NLR* Neutrophil-lymphocite ratio; *MPV* Mean platelet volume; *CRP* C-reactive protein

MET was employed in our study, the SP rate was lower than in other studies. AUA panels showed superior SFR for patients treated with MET (77.3%) compared with placebo (54.4%) on distal ureteral stones < 10 mm [22]. We believe that the lower rate of SFR (55.5%) in our study was due to the 5-10 mm stone size in the patients in our research.

Lifestyle factors, such as smoking habits and sexual intercourse, have also been investigated in recent years as potential factors of spontaneous passage. Fazlıoğlu et al. reported similar SP ratios in < 4 mm distal ureter stones for smokers and non-smokers, but for ≥ 4 mm distal ureter stones, the SP ratio was reported to be lower in smokers [25]. In another study, Bayraktar et al. investigated three groups of patients with 5-10 mm distal ureteral stones receiving different treatments. Group 1 received tamsulosin 0.4 mg/day, Group 2 was asked to have intercourse three times per week, and Group 3 received medical treatment. The authors reported that, based on their results, having sexual intercourse three times a week could be as beneficial as tamsulosin treatment [26]. We also compared SP levels in terms of BMI and smoking habits, but the differences were not significant ($p > 0.05$).

In recent years, the effect of some biochemical factors on the SP ratio has been reported. Ahmed et al. reported that patients with small stones, distal localization, high serum WBC level, low perinephric fat thickness, and lack of tissue-rim sign had increased SP ratios [27]. Similarly, another study reported significant correlations between the increase of WBC and neutrophil levels and the SP ratio, in < 10 mm ureteral stones ($p < 0.001$) [11]. According to the authors, this correlation was associated with increased ureteral peristalsis, caused by inflammation in the ureteral wall. By contrast, Aldaqodossi et al. reported that an increase in ureteral inflammation could decrease the SP ratio [8]. In this study, the authors reported that the SP(−) group was significantly higher than the SP(+) group for initial CRP values ($p = 0.001$). Furthermore, based on ROC curve analysis, it was found that sensitivity and specificity of the 21.9 mg/dl cut-off value for CRP, were 78.6 and 89.3% respectively [8]. In our study, the mean serum WBC value was higher in the SP(+) group, when compared to the SP(−) group (9.1 ± 2.4 vs. 8.4 ± 2.3), although this difference is not statistically significant. Similarly, mean CRP values were higher in the SP(+) group (11.5 ± 15.4) than in the SP(−) group (9.0 ± 8.2), and again, there is no statistically significant difference.

To our knowledge, the available literature does not include a study investigating the effect of serum procalcitonin on SP. However, procalcitonin has been reported to be valuable in showing a correlation between urinary tract infection and impacted ureteral stones. Papagiannopoulos et al. reported that procalcitonin > 100 pg/ml was detected in 18% of patients treated with MET, 45% of whom had undergone URS-L or ureteral stenting [16]. In our study, the mean serum procalcitonin level of the SP(−) group (207.0 ± 145.1 pg/ml) was significantly higher than in the SP(+) group (132.7 ± 28.1 pg/ml) ($p = 0.000$). Furthermore, leucocyturia rates of the SP(−) group were significantly higher than in the SP(+) group (58.3% vs. 20%) ($p = 0.004$). This finding could better explain the relationship between high serum procalcitonin and mucosal inflammation. It has been reported in previous studies that leucocyturia did not effect on spontaneous passage; this finding should be re-evaluated through studies with larger sample sizes [9, 27].

The fact that procalcitonin is significant even in multivariant analysis increases the possibility of using this marker in daily practice in the future. Of course, the accuracy of this information should be supported by a larger series.

Based on these results, it could be argued that procalcitonin plays a role in predicting SP, but this hypothesis needs to be supported with studies having higher sample sizes. Also, measuring the procalcitonin level again at the end of the study could increase the strength of the study. Our sample size was not large enough for subgroup analysis, a limitation of our study. Particularly, evaluating the serum procalcitonin and leucocyturia through subgroup analysis may provide a more objective argument for our hypothesis.

Conclusion

This study reports that distal ureteral stones sized 5-10 mm presenting with high procalcitonin levels and leucocyturia may have a negative effect on spontaneous passage. This relationship can be explained by stone impaction, possibly caused by increased mucosal inflammation.

Abbreviations

MET: Medical expulsive therapy; SP: Spontaneous passage; KUB: Kidney, ureter, bladder plain films; USG: Ultrasonography; CT: Computerized tomography; URS-L: Ureterorenoscopic lithotripsy; ESWL: Extracorporeal shock wave lithotripsy; VAS: Visual Analogue Scale; BMI: Body mass index; AUA: American Urological Association

Acknowledgements

Not applicable.

Authors' contributions

NCC conceived the idea for the study, made the protocol and wrote the manuscript with NCC. NCC,CTG,AE performed the data collection, conducted the analyses and wrote the manuscript with BA. AK, AO and BS made the protocol and assisted with the data collection. AO, NCC, BS and AK had access to all of the research data. BA revised necessary pathology. NCC, AK, AO and BA assisted with protocol development. NCC, AO, AK, CTG, AE, BS and BA contributed to the interpretation of the data and critically revised earlier draft versions. All authors read and approved the final manuscript.

Author details

[1]Department of Urology, GOP Taksim Education Training and Research Hospital, Karayolları Str. No:621 Gaziosmanpasa, İstanbul, Turkey. [2]Department of Urology, Yeniyüzyıl University Medicine Faculty, Gaziosmanpaşa Hospital, İstanbul, Turkey. [3]Bitlis State Hospital, Bitlis, Turkey 4 10 Sancaktepe State Hospital, İstanbul, Turkey. [4]Department of Urology, Sancaktepe State Hospital, İstanbul, Turkey.

References

1. Türk C, Petřík A, Sarica K, Seitz C, Skolarikos A, Straub M, et al. EAU guidelines on diagnosis and conservative Management of Urolithiasis. Eur Urol. 2016;69(3):468–74.
2. Pak CY. Kidney stones. Lancet. 1998;351(9118):1797–1801. Review.
3. Ordon M, Andonian S, Blew B, Schuler T, Chew B. Pace KT CUA, guideline: management of ureteral calculi. Can Urol Assoc J. 2015;9(11–12):E837–51.
4. Singh A, Alter HJ, Littlepage A. A systematic review of medical therapy to facilitate passage of ureteral calculi. Ann Emerg Med. 2017;50:552–63.
5. Loftus C, Nyame Y, Hinck B, Greene D, Chaparala H, Alazem K, et al. Medical expulsive therapy is underused for the management of renal colic in the emergency setting. J Urol. 2016;195(4 Pt 1):987–91.
6. Brede C, Hollingsworth JM, Faerber GJ, Taylor JS, Wolf JS Jr. Medical expulsive therapy for ureteral calculi in the real world: targeted education increases use and improves patient outcome. J Urol. 2010;183:585–9.
7. Furyk JS, Chu K, Banks C, Greenslade J, Keijzers G, Thom O et al Distal Ureteric Stones and Tamsulosin: A Double-Blind, Placebo-Controlled, Randomized, Multicenter Trial. Ann Emerg Med. 2016;67(1):86–95.e2.
8. Aldaqadossi HA. Stone expulsion rate of small distal ureteric calculi could be predicted with plasma C-reactive protein. Urolithiasis. 2013;41(3):235–9.
9. Lee KS, Ha JS, Koo KC. Significance of neutrophil-to-lymphocyte ratio as a novel Indicator of spontaneous ureter stone passage. Yonsei Med J. 2017; 58(5):988–93.
10. Özcan C, Aydoğdu O, Senocak C, Damar E, Eraslan A, Oztuna D, et al. Predictive factors for spontaneous stone passage and the potential role of serum C-reactive protein in patients with 4 to 10 mm distal ureteral stones: a prospective clinical study. J Urol. 2015;194(4):1009–13.
11. Sfoungaristos S, Kavouras A, Katafigiotis I, Perimenis P. Role of white blood cell and neutrophil counts in predicting spontaneous stone passage in patients with renal colic. BJU Int. 2012;110(8 Pt B):E339–45.
12. Aouifi A, Piriou V, Blanc P, et al. Effect of cardiopulmonary bypass on serum procalcitonin and C-reactive protein concentrations. Br J Anaesth. 1999;83: 602–7.
13. Meisner M. Procalcitonin: a new innovative infection parameter. In: Meisner M, ed. Biochemistry. Stuttgart: Brahms Diagnostica; 2000: 15.
14. Çakıroğlu B, Eyyüpoğlu E, Balcı MBC, Hazar Aİ, Uyanık BS, Doğan AN. The evaluation of the procalcitonin levels in chronic prostatitis patients. Nobel Med. 2016;12(2):60–5.
15. Yuzbasioglu Y, Duymaz H, Tanrikulu CS, Halhalli HC, Koc MO, Tandoğan M, et al. Role of Procalcitonin in evaluation of the severity of acute Cholecystitis. Eurasian J Med. 2016;48(3):162–6.
16. Papagiannopoulos D, Whelan P, Ahmad W, Rybak J, Hota B, Deane L, et al. Procalcitonin is a strong predictor of urine culture results in patients with obstructing ureteral stones: a prospective, pilot study. Urol Ann. 2016;8(3): 277–80.
17. Skolarikos A, Alivizatos G, de la Rosette J. Extracorporeal shock wave lithotripsy 25 years later: complications and their prevention. Eur Urol. 2006; 50(5):981–90 discussion 990.
18. Perez Castro E, Osther PJ, Jinga V, Razvi H, Stravodimos KG, Parikh K, et al. CROES Ureteroscopy global study group. Differences in ureteroscopic stone treatment and outcomes for distal, mid-, proximal, or multiple ureteral locations: the clinical research Office of the Endourological Society ureteroscopy global study. Eur Urol. 2014;66(1):102–9.
19. Skolarikos A, Laguna MP, Alivizatos G, Kural AR, de la Rosette JJ. The role for active monitoring in urinary stones: a systematic review. J Endourol. 2010; 24(6):923–30.
20. Demehri S, Steigner ML, Sodickson AD, Houseman EA, Rybicki FJ, Silverman SG. CT-based determination of maximum ureteral stone area: a predictor of spontaneous passage. AJR Am J Roentgenol. 2012;198(3):603–8.
21. Chau LH, Tai DC, Fung BT, Li JC, Fan CW, Li MK. Medical expulsive therapy using alfuzosin for patient presenting with ureteral stone less than 10mm: a prospective randomized controlled trial. Int J Urol. 2011;18(7):510–4.
22. Türk C, Knoll T, Seitz C, Skolarikos A, Chapple C, McClinton S;European Association of Urology. Medical expulsive therapy for Ureterolithiasis: the EAU recommendations in 2016. Eur Urol 2017;71(4):504–507. doi:https://doi.org/10.1016/j.eururo.2016.07.024. Epub 2016 Aug 6. PubMed PMID: 27506951.
23. Brubaker WD, Dallas KB, Elliott CS, Pao AC, Chertow GM, Leppert JT, Conti SL. Payer type, race/ethnicity, and the timing of surgical Management of Urinary Stone Disease. J Endourol. 2019;33(2):152–8.
24. Matlaga BR, Jansen JP, Meckley LM, Byrne TW, Lingeman JE. Treatment of ureteral and renal stones: a systematic review and meta-analysis of randomized, controlled trials. J Urol. 2012;188(1):130–7.
25. Fazlioglu A, Salman Y, Tandogdu Z, Kurtulus FO, Bas S, Cek M. The effect of smoking on spontaneous passage of distal ureteral stones. BMC Urol. 2014; 14:27.
26. Bayraktar Z, Albayrak S. Sexual intercourse as a new option in the medical expulsive therapy of distal ureteral stones in males: a prospective, randomized, controlled study. Int Urol Nephrol. 2017;49(11):1941–6.
27. Ahmed AF, Gabr AH, Emara AA, Ali M, Abdel-Aziz AS, Alshahrani S. Factors predicting the spontaneous passage of a ureteric calculus of ⩽10 mm. Arab J Urol. 2015;13(2):84–90.

28

A comparison among PCNL, Miniperc and Ultraminiperc for lower calyceal stones between 1 and 2 cm: A prospective, comparative, multicenter and randomised study

Giorgio Bozzini[1], Tahsin Batuhan Aydogan[2*], Alexander Müller[3], Maria Chiara Sighinolfi[2], Umberto Besana[1], Alberto Calori[1], Berti Lorenzo[1], Alexander Govorov[4], Dmitry Y. Pushkar[4], Giovannalberto Pini[5], Antonio Luigi Pastore[6], Javier Romero-Otero[7], Bernardo Rocco[2] and Carlo Buizza[1]

Abstract

Background: Conventional Percutaneous Lithotripsy (PCNL) has been an effective, successful and easy approach for especially > 1 cm sized calyceal stones however risks of complications and nephron loss are inevitable. Our aim is to compare the efficacy and safety of PCNL, MiniPerc (MP) and UltraMiniPerc (UMP) for lower calyceal stones between 1 and 2 cm with a multicenter prospective randomized study.

Methods: Between January 2015 and June 2018, 132 consecutive patients with single lower calyceal stone were enrolled. Patients were randomized in three groups; A: PCNL; B: MP; C: UMP. 44 patients for the Group A, 47 for Group B and 41 for Group C. Exclusion criterias were the presence of coagulation impairments, age of < 18 or > 75, presence of infection or serious comorbidities. Patients were controlled with computerized tomography scan after 3 months. A negative CT or an asymptomatic patient with stone fragments < 3 mm size were the criteria to assess the stone-free status. Patient characteristics, stone free rates (SFR) s, complications and re-treatment rates were analyzed.

Results: The mean stone size were 16.38, 16.82 and 15.23 mm respectively in Group A, B and C($p = 0.34$). The overall SFR was significantly higher in Group A (86.3%) and B (82.9%) as compared to Group C (78%)($p < 0.05$). The re-treatment rate was significantly higher in Group C (12.1%) and complication rates was higher in Group A (13.6%) as compared to others($p < 0.05$). The hospitalization was significantly shorter in Group C compared to Group A ($p = 0.04$).

Conclusions: PCNL and MP showed higher efficacy than UMP to obtain a better SFR. Auxiliary and re-treatment rates were higher in UMP. On the other hand for such this kind of stones PCNL had more complications. Overall evaluation favors MP as a better indication in stones 1–2 cm size.

Keywords: PCNL, Percutaneous, Miniperc, Ultraminiperc, Lower calyces stones , Stone-free rate

* Correspondence: drbatu@hotmail.com
[2]Department of Urology, University of Modena and Reggio Emilia, Modena, Italy
Full list of author information is available at the end of the article

Background

Lower calyceal (LC) stones approximately account for 35% of all renal stones [1]. Natural history of non-obstructing asymptomatic LC stone is not well defined, and the risk of progression is unclear. Although the question of whether calyceal stones should be treated is still unanswered and patients electing expectant management should be counseled regarding the potential for stone-related symptom progression and need for future intervention [2]. Stone growth, de novo obstruction, associated infection, stone composition, and acute and/or chronic pain are general indications for treatment decision. According to the European Association of Urology (EAU) guidelines as considered for LC stones, in case of unfavorable conditions for extracorporeal shockvawe lithotripsy (ESWL), endourological interventions such as Percutaneous Nephrolithotomy (PCNL) or Retrograde Intrarenal Surgery (RIRS) are recommended at first step [3].

LC stones have been a problem for both patients and urologists. Due to the anatomical variations of LC, especially considering for stone clearance, ESWL has been usually failed in here. Flexible ureterorenoscopic interventions have also gained popularity by time for especially endoscopic treatment of < 2 cm sized LC stones [3, 4]. But again because of some anatomical difficulties and durability of instrument it may not always be easy to perform RIRS for all LC stones [5]. Conventional PCNL has been an effective, successful and easy approach for LC stones however risks of complications and nephron loss are inevitable [2]. But regarded to the invasiveness and morbidities of PCNL, the optimal management of LC stones continue to be a dilemma that has recently received heightened attention among urologists. Moreover with time the miniaturization of PCNL also developed in order to diminish access related complications, bleeding and morbidities [6]. Conventionally the miniaturization of PCNL has defined by diameter less than 20 Fr [7]. The Minipercutaneous (MP)(16–18 Fr), Ultraminiperc (UMP)(11–14 Fr) and Micropercutaneous (MicroPNL) (< 10Fr) are currently feasible and modern alternatives with minimal invasiveness [2]. The MP is accepted as suitable for renal stones < 2 cm in size while UMP is for renal stones < 1.5 cm [7, 8]. A prospective multicenter randomized comparison among PCNL, MP and UMP for LC stones between 1 and 2 cm according to CT scan was performed to evaluate the efficacy and the safety of these procedures.

Methods

Between January 2015 and June 2018, 132 consecutive patients presented with a singular 1–2 cm LC stone were enrolled in this prospective, comparative, multicenter and randomised study. The ethical committee approval was taken in 2014 thus gave the possibility to start at the same time in January 2015 for each participating center. Randomized number table was used for simple randomization. Patients were randomized into three groups; Group A: patients treated with PCNL; Group B: patients treated with MP; Group C: patients treated with UMP. The Hounsfield Unit (HU) of each group was 1234 ± 256, 1113 ± 341 and 1254 ± 289 for Group A, B and C respectively. The main inclusion criteria was related on stone's maximum diameter in coronal images on CT scans. Exclusion criteria were the presence of coagulation impairments, age less than 18 or more than 75 (with increased risks of elongated procedure under general anesthesia leading with incomplete completion of interventions), presence of acute infection, presence of cardiovascular or pulmonary comorbidities. 8 patients for Group A, 9 for Group B and 7 for Group C were excluded. Patients were controlled with CT scan after 3 months. A negative CT or an asymptomatic patient with < 3 mm residual stone fragments and a negative urinary culture were the criteria to obtain the stone-free status (SFR). We accepted stone-free status as inferior to 3 mm and at least if the fragments we more than 2 in number with a residual area less than 9 mm^2. A numerical pain scale from 0 to 10 was used for evaluation and comparison of pain levels. A statistical analysis was carried out to assess patients data, success and complications rates, re-treatment rate and need for auxiliary treatment. The informed written consent has been obtained from each participant, that study has been performed according to the Declaration of Helsinki, and the procedures have been approved by local ethics committee.

PCNL, MP and UMP procedures

All PCNL procedures were started with the ureteral catheterization of stone side via cystoscopy. Under the semi-flex supine positioning access to kidney was performed by combined guidance of intraoperative ultrasonography (US) and fluoroscopy. After a successfully co-axial dilatation on guidewire up to a 30 CH Amplatz sheath, 800 μm Laser fiber with Litho 35 W (Quanta System, Samarate, Lombardia VA) was used for stone fragmentation (0.6–0.8 J 12 Hz) through a 24 Fr nephroscope (Karl-Storz) whereas retrieval grasper for stone extraction. A standart re-entry nephrostomy catheter was placed at the end and left for two days postoperatively.

The initial procedures before access, as cystoscopy and ureteral catheterization were similarly helded also in MP and UMP as during in PCNL. During MP, a 16 Fr nephroscope (Karl-Storz) was used with a smaller sheath size of 16.5/19.5 Fr (Karl-Storz) as compared to conventional PCNL. 550 μm Laser fiber with Cyber Ho was used by the help of a delicate forceps and nitinol basket for clearance of fragments. So at the end a small 10 Fr diameter nephrostomy catheter was placed.

Different than the two techniques, during UMP a gentle single step dilatation was needed for UMP sheath 11–13 Fr and Holmium laser energy was used through a 6 Fr nephroscope (Karl-Storz) for stone fragmentation. Again similar to MP, 550 μm Laser fiber with Cyber Ho was used. Neither graspers nor basket were used. Saline irrigation was mainly used to remove the stone fragments. Differently than other procedures, nephrostomy tube was not used.

For the all groups papilla access technique was used. The conventional PCNL could be used with balistic and ultrasonic lithotriptors as well but we used the laser fragmentation modality in order not to have bias regarding in between all three interventions. The energy settings did not differ in between procedures. Fragmentation method was used during PCNL whereas dusting method was used during MP and UMP. All the surgeons who had performed the procedures were all completed their learning curve on three techniques prior to this study with a minimum case record of 250 procedures for each technique. All the three procedures were done in two centers with six experienced surgeons.

Statistical analyses

The Shapiro-Wilk normality test was used to evaluate the behavior of the continuous variables. The collected data were analysed by an online regression tool (Student's t-test and chi-square test). The calculation of the sample size was done using "Creative Research System Software" indicating 95% as confidence level and a confidence interval (margin of error) of 15%. A post-hoc regression analysis was also performed on 3rd months SFR. For all statistical comparisons, significance was considered at $p < 0.05$.

Results

Group A was consisted of 44 patients while Group B and Group C were consisted of 47 and 41 patients respectively. The mean stone size was 16.38 mm in Group A, 16.82 mm in Group B and 15.23 mm in Group C (p = 0.34). Our patient and stone related characteristics were all statistically similar in between the groups ($p > 0.05$) (Table 1). The overall SFR was 86.3% for Group A, 82.9% for Group B and 78.0% for Group C. The complication rates were 13.6, 4.2 and 2.4% respectively for group A, B and C. The re-treatment rates were significantly higher in group C compared to the other two groups ($p = 0.007$). Our analyze was by intention to treat so further on considering the re-treatment, RIRS was performed to get a stone free situation. The operating time did not show a significant difference in between the groups. The hospitalization was significantly shorter in Group C compared to Group A ($p = 0.04$) (Table 2). The post-hoc regression analysis on 3rd month SFR for groups was shown in Table 3. The complications of all groups were assessed and summarized as based up on clinical evidences (Table 4). The clinically evident complications were significantly higher in Group A as compared to the other groups ($p < 0.05$) (Table 4). The distribution of post-operative complications according to Clavien-Dindo was summarized in Table 5. The Clavien-Dindo scale of scores were higher in Group A as compared to the other groups ($p < 0.05$).

Table 1 The demographic and stone related characteristics of groups

	Group A	Group B	Group C	*p* value
Total patient (*n* = 132)	44	47	41	0.44
Age yrs (mean ± SD)	53.3 ± 14.8	55.8 ± 16.1	54.8 ± 17.2	0.33
Sex (M/F)	23/21	20/27	22/19	0.23
Height cm (mean ± SD)	171.1 ± 2.5	175.8 ± 4.1	173.2 ± 2.3	0.40
Weight Kg (mean ± SD)	73.1 ± 4.6	77.9 ± 4.7	75.5 ± 7.1	0.66
Stone side (Right/Left)	25/19	22/25	21/20	0.52
Stone size (mm) (mean ± SD)	16.38 ± 2.9	16.82 ± 2.7	15.23 ± 3.3	0.34

Group A: PCNL, Group B: MP, Group C: UMP

Discussion

The LC stones have always been problematic in order to obtain a total stone clearance. It is very well discussed in literature as a systematic review and meta-analysis showed PCNL and RIRS were superior to ESWL in stone clearance and even PCNL is more effective then RIRS [9]. In 2017 Bozzini et al. performed a prospective randomized comparison among ESWL, PCNL and RIRS on < 2 cm sized LC stones [10]. ESWL was failed against PCNL and RIRS considering SFR and re-treatment rates($p < 0.05$). The SFRs were significantly higher in PCNL (87.3%) and RIRS (82.1%) as compared to ESWL (61.8%). The duration of procedure and hospital stay, radiation exposure favored RIRS against PCNL [10]. RIRS looks a feasible and better option against PCNL when complication rates were also taken in consideration. But still RIRS may not be performed on all LC stones successfully due to anatomic variations as narrow ureter or calyceal infindibulum. So among with the miniaturized PCNL modalities as MP, UMP and MicroPNL there need of a decision to choice the priority for most effective and safe intervention against < 2 cm LC stones even in case of narrow calyx existence [2].

The MP was first described and experienced with a single step dilatation with usage of 11 Fr sheath on 11 cases at preschool age [11]. At the same year an initial results from an adult study appeared [12]. Nine patients with < 2 cm stones were treated with 13 Fr MP. 89% stone-free rate was achieved while with better outcomes

Table 2 The comparison of re-treatment needs, complications and SFRs percentages of groups

	Group A	Group B	Group C	*p* value A-B	*p* value A-C	*p* value B-C
Need for re-treatment (%)	6.8	4.2	12.1	0.17	0.41	**0.007**
Operating time min ± SD	45.9 ± 7.7	55.8 ± 11.4	59.3 ± 13.8	0.07	0.05	0.17
Hospitalization days ± SD	3.7 ± 1.5	2.7 ± 2.1	2.2 ± 2.1	0.06	**0.04**	0.18
Complication rate (%)	13.6	4.2	2.4	**0.001**	**0.002**	0.25
SFR at 3rd month (%)	86.3	82.9	78	0.33	**0.022**	**0.02**

Group A: PCNL, Group B: MP, Group C: UMP, SFR: Stone-free rate. Re-treatment (Secondary Interventions): Retrograde Intrarenal Surgery (RIRS)

in selected patients favoring MP for blood loss, hospital stay and postoperative pain [12]. Despite this, Giusti et al. declared that MP had no obvious advantage against PCNL and concluded as tubeless PCNL could be a better option [13]. But Knoll et al. defended that not all tubeless PCNL procedures has ended with delighted results. Some cases need auxiliary interventions. Even being a limitation in their study that stone sizes were smaller in MP patients; the results were comparable in means of safety and effectiveness. More, the short hospital stay, less pain and more possibility for tubeless completion of operations has favored MP [14]. The MP studies have showed comparable and equal SFR and reduced comorbidities compared to conventional PCNL [8, 14, 15]. ElSheemy et al. compared MP and standard PCNL through 18 and 30 Fr tracts respectively [16]. According to their results there was significant difference on SFR in between patients who had larger stone burden (>2cm^2). But for those with singular stones or stone burden ≤2 cm^2; there was no significant difference in SFR and also MP showed lower complications compared to standard PCNL [16]. Similar to the current literature, in our study there was no significant difference in between SFR of PCNL and MP($p = 0.33$) while a significant difference in between complication rates ($p = 0.001$) (Table 2).

In 2013, the UMP technique was published with initial experiences in literature [17]. Desai et al. used a 6 Fr mini nephroscope through a 11/13 Fr metal sheath on 36 consecutive patients with stone size of < 2 cm [17]. Similar to our access method, ultrasonographic guidance was also used in addition to fluoroscopy. Not all stones were located in LC. The LC stone ratio and LC access ratio were 27.8 and 38.9% respectively while 8.3% of their patients had multiple calyceal stones. Their immediate (postoperative 1st day) and total (postoperative 1st month) SFR's were 88.9 and 97.2% respectively [17]. More, their significant complication (urosepsis, extravasation and fever) ratio was 16.7% and need for a second intervention was 2.8% whereas ours were 2.4 and 12.1% respectively. This inverse ratio may be explained with the differences between operative time, stone analysis, surgeon experience or other patient characteristics in between the studies.

Table 3 Post-hoc logistic regression analysis on 3rd month SFR

	SFR at 3rd month		
Group	**Log-odds**	**Odds**	**Probability**
A	1.91	7.02	0.87
B	1.81	5.42	0.83
C	0.72	1.88	0.77

Group A: PCNL, Group B: MP, Group C: UMP, SFR: Stone-free rate

In a cohort study of 98 consecutive UMP patients, the mean stone size was 15.85 ± 4.53 mm which was comparable of ours (15.23 ± 3.3 mm) but their postoperative SFR on 1st month control was 83% [18]. Jones et al. published a systematic review study investigating the role of MicroPNL and UMP. Across seven studies a total of 262 patients were undergone UMP with a mean of stone size 18.6 mm, SFR of 88.3% and complication rate of 6.2% [19]. In our study, we calculated the SFR on 3rd month control. The SFR of our UMP was calculated as 78% which was also significantly lower than our PCNL and MP groups.

Ganpula et al. discussed well the differences between PCNL, MP and UMP [7]. The cross-sectional area and length differences of access sheats and more the smaller fragments obtained during MP all create a superior fragment vacuum clearance during MP compared to PCNL. Also sheath sizes of MP may give a chance to use flexible nephroscope for stone fragments in smaller different calyces [7]. So these all may participate to the similar SFR in between PCNL and MP. Again in another study, during the interventions on 15–30 mm renal stones, 16.5 Fr MP showed comparable SFR but lower complications as compared with 24 Fr PCNL [20]. According to a recent review study the terminology seems to be confusing in between the modalities but all miniaturized tract size interventions result with better outcomes in terms of pain and complication rates whereas comparable SFR with standart PCNL [21]. Depending on our comparison in between MP and UMP complication ratios were comparable but our SFR results in between MP and UMP

Table 4 The complications (Clinical evidences)

	Group A (44)	Group B (47)	Group C (41)	*p* value A-B	*p* value A-C	*p* value B-C	Total
UTI n (%)	4 (9.2)	2 (4.2)	1 (2.4)	**0,0320**	**0,0230**	0,2300	7 (5.3)
Gross haematuria n (%)	2 (4.5)	0 (0)	0 (0)	**0,0020**	**0,0030**	10,000	2 (1.5)
Severe pain n (%)	2 (4.5)	1 (2.1)	1 (2.4)	0,0500	0,0510	0,3475	4 (3.0)
Total n (%)	8 (18.2)	3 (6.3)	2 (4.8)	**0,0410**	**0,0320**	0,1300	13 (9.8)

Group A: PCNL, Group B: MP, Group C: UMP, UTI: Urinary tract infection

were statistically significant($p = 0.02$). According to our results mean stone size were similar as 16.38 mm, 16.82 mm and 15.23 mm respectively. The UMP looks like an alternative to MP but may not be satisfactory especially for interventions on stones with > 1.5 cm sized. The UMP may also be a good alternative to RIRS especially for medium sized (< 1.5 cm) LC stones. This mismatch between the ideal indication for UMP and the stone size treated with UMP in this study may have meaningful bias on the results and downgraded the potential efficacy of UMP. However, currently due to the lack of literature there are no clear guideline on MP and UMP.

The PCNL was at highest risk of complication coexistence. The clinically evident complications in Table 4 were all higher in PCNL compared to MP and UMP. Only among those, between PCNL and MP the severe pain seems to be questionable($p = 0.05$). According to Mishra et al. the need of postoperative analgesics were similar between PCNL and MP [8]. More in contrast to PCNL, none of the patients who were undergone MP and UMP procedures needed a further surgical or endoscopic interventions according to Clavien-Dindo classification [22] score of >III (Table 5). Also there was no difference among clinically evident complications between MP and UMP. Careful selection of patients, experience of surgeon and special equipment for each intervention is essential.

The number of the patients in each groups may be a statistical limitation. So we can assume that surely the tendency (obtained by univariate analysis) would be better confirmed by randomized control trial with higher numbers on which we are already working.

Here in our study a limitation may be lack of evaluation according to the stone analysis or Hounsfield unit (HU). We did not include pediatric age group (< 18) in order not to increase the heterogeneity with extra choice of MP and UMP. Moreover, exclusion of patients more than 75 years old seems to be a potential selection bias but but increased risks with older age under general anesthesia may require incomplete termination of procedure which may also be a cause of bias on postoperative outcomes.

Tubeless or non-tubeless comparison may be also considered in future studies. MP may seem to be supported as first choice of PCNL subtype considering the 1–2 cm sized LC stones. UMP may be recommended for certain selected patients. Further studies with giant patient groups may show comparable SFR in between MP and UMP. As last, the use of the same Holmium laser energy during the interventions might give the possibility to focus only on the technique chosen and not a different kind of energy to break the stone.

Conclusion

PCNL and MP showed higher efficacy than UMP in order to obtain a better SFR. Auxiliary and re-treatment rates were similar between PCNL and MP but differed in between MP and UMP. On the other hand for such this kind of stones PCNL had more complications among all. The MP and UMP find a better indication whereas MP seems to be the preferential alternative for 1–2 cm LC stone intervention among the others. Further randomized comparison between RIRS and MP in this setting is needed.

Table 5 The postoperative complications (Clavien-Dindo classification)

	Group A (44)	Group B (47)	Group C (41)	*p* value A-B	*p* value A-C	*p* value B-C	Total
Overall complication n (%)	8 (18.2)	3 (6.3)	2 (4.8)	**0,0410**	**0,0320**	0,1300	13 (9.8)
Clavien score 1–2 n (%)	6 (13.6) 4 UTI 2 Severe Pain	3 (6.3) 2 UTI 1 Severe Pain	2 (4.8) 1 UTI 1 Severe Pain	**0,0280**	**0,0190**	0,0961	11 (8.3)
3a-5 n (%)	2 (4.5) Gross Hematuria	0 (0)	0 (0)	**0,0020**	**0,0030**	10,000	2 (1.5)

Group A: PCNL, Group B: MP, Group C: UMP, UTI: Urinary tract infection

Abbreviations

PCNL: Percutaneous Lithotripsy; MP: Minipercutaneous lithotripsy; UMP: Ultraminiperc lithotripsy; ESWL: Extraschock vawe lithotripsy; RIRS: Retrograde intrarenal surgery; SFR: Stone-free rate; LC: Lower calyceal; EAU: European Association of Urology

Acknowledgements

Not applicable.

Authors' contributions

GB, UB, AC, BL, CB, MCS and BR performed the research, data collection and conception. AG, DYP, GP, ALP and JRO contributed interpretation of the data. GB, TBA and AM wrote the paper and performed the revisions. All authors have read, took active role and approved the submitted version of manuscript.

Author details

[1]Department of Urology, ASST Valle Olona Busto Arsizio, Varese, Italy. [2]Department of Urology, University of Modena and Reggio Emilia, Modena, Italy. [3]Department of Urology, Spital Limmattal, Schlieren, Switzerland. [4]Department of Urology, A.I. Evdokimov Moscow State University of Medicine and Dentistry, Moscow, Russia. [5]Department of Urology, San Raffaele Turro Hospital, Milan, Italy. [6]Department of Urology, ICOT Latina, Latina, Italy. [7]Department of Urology, Hospital Universitario 12 de Octobre, Madrid, Spain.

References

1. Cass AS, Grine WB, Jenkins JM, Jordan WR, Mobley TB, Myers DA. The incidence of lower-pole nephrolithiasis--increasing or not? Br J Urol. 1998; 82(1):12–5.
2. Moore SL, Bres-Niewada E, Cook P, Wells H, Somani BK. Optimal management of lower pole stones: the direction of future travel. Cent European J Urol. 2016;69(3):274–9.
3. Turk C, Petrik A, Sarica K, Seitz C, Skolarikos A, Straub M, et al. EAU guidelines on diagnosis and conservative Management of Urolithiasis. Eur Urol. 2016;69(3):468–74.
4. Mi Y, Ren K, Pan H, Zhu L, Wu S, You X, et al. Flexible ureterorenoscopy (F-URS) with holmium laser versus extracorporeal shock wave lithotripsy (ESWL) for treatment of renal stone <2 cm: a meta-analysis. Urolithiasis. 2016;44(4):353–65.
5. Monga M, Best S, Venkatesh R, Ames C, Lee C, Kuskowski M, et al. Durability of flexible ureteroscopes: a randomized, prospective study. J Urol. 2006; 176(1):137–41.
6. Ghani KR, Andonian S, Bultitude M, Desai M, Giusti G, Okhunov Z, et al. Percutaneous Nephrolithotomy: update, trends, and future directions. Eur Urol. 2016;70(2):382–96.
7. Ganpule AP, Bhattu AS, Desai M. PCNL in the twenty-first century: role of Microperc, Miniperc, and Ultraminiperc. World J Urol. 2015;33(2):235–40.
8. Mishra S, Sharma R, Garg C, Kurien A, Sabnis R, Desai M. Prospective comparative study of miniperc and standard PNL for treatment of 1 to 2 cm size renal stone. BJU Int. 2011;108(6):896–9 discussion 9-900.
9. Donaldson JF, Lardas M, Scrimgeour D, Stewart F, MacLennan S, Lam TB, et al. Systematic review and meta-analysis of the clinical effectiveness of shock wave lithotripsy, retrograde intrarenal surgery, and percutaneous nephrolithotomy for lower-pole renal stones. Eur Urol. 2015;67(4):612–6.
10. Bozzini G, Verze P, Arcaniolo D, Dal Piaz O, Buffi NM, Guazzoni G, et al. A prospective randomized comparison among SWL, PCNL and RIRS for lower calyceal stones less than 2 cm: a multicenter experience : a better understanding on the treatment options for lower pole stones. World J Urol. 2017;35(12):1967–75.
11. Jackman SV, Hedican SP, Peters CA, Docimo SG. Percutaneous nephrolithotomy in infants and preschool age children: experience with a new technique. Urology. 1998;52(4):697 701.
12. Jackman SV, Docimo SG, Cadeddu JA, Bishoff JT, Kavoussi LR, Jarrett TW. The "mini-perc" technique: a less invasive alternative to percutaneous nephrolithotomy. World J Urol. 1998;16(6):371–4.
13. Giusti G, Piccinelli A, Taverna G, Benetti A, Pasini L, Corinti M, et al. Miniperc? No, thank you! Eur Urol. 2007;51(3):810–4 discussion 5.
14. Knoll T, Wezel F, Michel MS, Honeck P, Wendt-Nordahl G. Do patients benefit from miniaturized tubeless percutaneous nephrolithotomy? A comparative prospective study. J Endourol. 2010;24(7):1075–9.
15. Yamaguchi A, Skolarikos A, Buchholz NP, Chomon GB, Grasso M, Saba P, et al. Operating times and bleeding complications in percutaneous nephrolithotomy: a comparison of tract dilation methods in 5,537 patients in the clinical research Office of the Endourological Society Percutaneous Nephrolithotomy Global Study. J Endourol. 2011;25(6):933–9.
16. ElSheemy MS, Elmarakbi AA, Hytham M, Ibrahim H, Khadgi S, Al-Kandari AM. Mini vs standard percutaneous nephrolithotomy for renal stones: a comparative study. Urolithiasis. 2019;47(2):207–14.
17. Desai J, Zeng G, Zhao Z, Zhong W, Chen W, Wu W. A novel technique of ultra-mini-percutaneous nephrolithotomy: introduction and an initial experience for treatment of upper urinary calculi less than 2 cm. Biomed Res Int. 2013;2013:490793.
18. Desai JD. Prospective outcomes of 11-13Ch. Ultra-mini percutaneous nephrolithotomy (UMP): a consecutive cohort study. Arch Esp Urol. 2017; 70(1):202–10.
19. Jones P, Elmussareh M, Aboumarzouk OM, Mucksavage P, Somani BK. Role of minimally invasive (micro and ultra-mini) PCNL for adult urinary stone disease in the modern era: evidence from a systematic review. Curr Urol Rep. 2018;19(4):27.
20. Kukreja RA. Should mini percutaneous nephrolithotomy (MiniPNL/Miniperc) be the ideal tract for medium-sized renal calculi (15-30 mm)? World J Urol. 2018;36(2):285–91.
21. Heinze A, Gozen AS, Rassweiler J. Tract sizes in percutaneous nephrolithotomy: does miniaturization improve outcome? Curr Opin Urol. 2019;29(2):118–23.
22. Dindo D, Demartines N, Clavien PA. Classification of surgical complications: a new proposal with evaluation in a cohort of 6336 patients and results of a survey. Ann Surg. 2004;240(2):205–13.

Machine learning prediction of stone-free success in patients with urinary stone after treatment of shock wave lithotripsy

Seung Woo Yang[1†], Yun Kyong Hyon[2†], Hyun Seok Na[1], Long Jin[1], Jae Geun Lee[1], Jong Mok Park[1], Ji Yong Lee[1], Ju Hyun Shin[1], Jae Sung Lim[1], Yong Gil Na[1], Kiwan Jeon[2], Taeyoung Ha[2], Jinbum Kim[3] and Ki Hak Song[1*]

Abstract

Background: The aims of this study were to determine the predictive value of decision support analysis for the shock wave lithotripsy (SWL) success rate and to analyze the data obtained from patients who underwent SWL to assess the factors influencing the outcome by using machine learning methods.

Methods: We retrospectively reviewed the medical records of 358 patients who underwent SWL for urinary stone (kidney and upper-ureter stone) between 2015 and 2018 and evaluated the possible prognostic features, including patient population characteristics, urinary stone characteristics on a non-contrast, computed tomographic image. We performed 80% training set and 20% test set for the predictions of success and mainly used decision tree-based machine learning algorithms, such as random forest (RF), extreme gradient boosting trees (XGBoost), and light gradient boosting method (LightGBM).

Results: In machine learning analysis, the prediction accuracies for stone-free were 86.0, 87.5, and 87.9%, and those for one-session success were 78.0, 77.4, and 77.0% using RF, XGBoost, and LightGBM, respectively. In predictions for stone-free, LightGBM yielded the best accuracy and RF yielded the best one in those for one-session success among those methods. The sensitivity and specificity values for machine learning analytics are (0.74 to 0.78 and 0.92 to 0.93) for stone-free and (0.79 to 0.81 and 0.74 to 0.75) for one-session success, respectively. The area under curve (AUC) values for machine learning analytics are (0.84 to 0.85) for stone-free and (0.77 to 0.78) for one-session success and their 95% confidence intervals (CIs) are (0.730 to 0.933) and (0.673 to 0.866) in average of methods, respectively.

Conclusions: We applied a selected machine learning analysis to predict the result after treatment of SWL for urinary stone. About 88% accurate machine learning based predictive model was evaluated. The importance of machine learning algorithm can give matched insights to domain knowledge on effective and influential factors for SWL success outcomes.

Keywords: Lithotripsy, Machine learning, Artificial intelligence

* Correspondence: urosong@cnu.ac.kr
†Seung Woo Yang and Yun Kyong Hyon contributed equally to this work.
[1]Department of Urology, Chungnam National University College of Medicine, Chungnam National University Hospital, 282 Monwha-ro, Jung-gu, Daejeon, Republic of Korea 35015
Full list of author information is available at the end of the article

Background

Shock wave lithotripsy (SWL), which was first introduced by Chaussy in 1980 [1], has been recognized as convenient, noninvasive management for urinary stones, and now it is widely used as primary treatment for urinary stones smaller than 2 cm sized due to high stone-free rate [2–4]. However, the stone-free rate of SWL in the treatment of urinary stone is affected by the size, location, composition, and radiological density of the stone. Especially in cases of large stones, the success rate is relatively low, and the rate of retreatment is high, thus requiring more time and resulting in low cost-effectiveness [5].

Ineffective procedures can be avoided, and unnecessary resource waste can be prevented by choosing better treatment methods for stone management by evaluating whether patients with urinary stones can respond well to SWL or not. The popular use of non-contrast computed tomography (NCCT) in the diagnosis of urinary stone has allowed accurate measurement of stone characteristics such as size, shape, location, and consistency, using Hounsfield units (HU). Therefore, considering the factors that may affect the stone-free rate, it is possible to reduce such retreatment and economic costs by selectively applying SWL. Many researchers have tried to determine these factors by using statistical methods, and various studies have been reported to predict the stone-free rate after SWL [6–8].

Recently, the importance of machine learning and artificial intelligence technology has increased, and get more attention in medical areas with the advent of big data. In the medical field, researchers applied machine learning methodology to various disease diagnoses and predictions [9, 10]. The purposes of this study are to investigate retrospective information on patients with a diagnosis of urinary stone who underwent SWL and to establish a machine learning model in binary classification for predicting the stone-free, or not and one-session success, or not after SWL. Furthermore, the resulting machine learning prediction models can be implemented as an actual diagnostic support system for urinary stone treatment and provide more capability or new functionality for it.

Methods

We retrospectively identified patients with kidney and upper-ureter stones who underwent the first start session of SWL at our institution between January 2015 and December 2018. All data analysis was carried out in accordance with applicable laws and regulations described in the Declaration of Helsinki and approved by Chungnam national university hospital institutional review board approval (CNUH 2018–07-047). Three hundred fifty-eight patients with previously untreated stones and a solitary stone diameter of 5 to 20 mm were included. Patients were excluded if they were younger than 18 years old; had a congenital genitourinary tract anomaly, history of previous open urinary-tract surgery, or multiple stones, or who had not undergone imaging for 4 weeks after SWL. We retrospectively reviewed the medical records and picture archiving and communication system (PACS) data of these patients and evaluated the possible prognostic features, including age and sex; presence of diabetes mellitus (DM) or hypertension (HTN); stone characteristics such as stone laterality, location, maximal length, stone volume, skin to stone distance (SSD), mean stone density (MSD), and stone heterogeneity index (SHI); double-J stenting and percutaneous nephrostomy (PCN) procedure before SWL; simple psoas muscle cross-sectional area measurement for sarcopenia; complete blood cell count; liver function test; renal function test; electrolyte test; and urinalysis.

Stone characteristics on NCCT

The stone characteristics were interpreted by NCCT, and each maximal length was measured on axial, coronal, and sagittal NCCT scan. The volume of the stone was computed by the ellipsoid method (X-axis length x Y-axis length x Z-axis length x $\pi/6$). The SSD was calculated using radiographic calipers from the point of the largest stone diameter at 90° from the horizontal plane because of vertical shockwave delivery through the patient's back. HU was carefully calculated on the magnified, axial NCCT image from a circle with a diameter of about 2–3 mm in the center of the middle cross-section without including the adjacent tissue. MSD was identified as the mean value of HU, and SHI was identified as the standard deviation of HU.

SWL protocol

SWL was performed on an outpatient basis, without anesthesia. The same lithotripter was used to treat all patients, with fluoroscopic guidance. The lithotripter was an electromagnetic lithotripter made by the DirexGroup (Integra SL, Initia Ltd., Israel). The intensity of the shock wave started from 10.0 kV and gradually increased less than 18.0 kV to improve stone fragmentation and reduce the risk of adjacent tissue trauma. The number of shock waves per SWL session varied from 2300 to 2500 at a rate of 60 shock waves per minute.

Additional SWL was performed at intervals of 1 week if evidence of stones remained. The stone-free was defined as the absence of observed stone with X-ray studies or asymptomatic condition and clinically insignificant residual fragments ≤3 mm in maximal length 4 weeks after the first SWL treatment as measured by simple abdominal radiography or NCCT. One-session success was defined as patients who were stone-free after a single

SWL treatment. Enough water intake and appropriate exercise were recommended for all patients.

Data analytics

The SWL data has 42 features including the two target variables, stone-free and one- session success, and a total of 358 cases. The SWL data were analyzed using well-known machine learning methods such as random forest (RF), which is a statistical machine learning method [11] and extreme gradient boosting trees (XGBoost), which is a decision tree–based gradient boosting regression method [12] and light gradient boosting method (LightGBM) [13]. The machine learning models were trained in binary classifications for predicting the targets, stone-free and one-session success. Experiments were performed with 80% of the data for training the prediction model (training set) and 20% for testing the trained model (test set). For the experiment, we randomly sampled 10 times, and then take average of its results, which is similar to n-fold validation method, and performed the prediction for stone-free and one-session success. The sampling strategy shows a certain capability of predictive models obtained from the given SWL data set. For calculating sensitivity, specificity, PPV, we computed the confusion matrix and do computed their values in average over sample data sets for prediction tests, and AUCs, we adopted sklearn.metric module in Python. For 95% CIs, we used bootstrapping methods with 1000 bootstraps for each sampled data sets, and then took the average over samples.

Results

The number of cases with stone-free and one-session success were 253 (70.7%) and 154 (43.0%). Table 1 shows the patient and stone characteristics of the patient data, which we used for predictions. We present the prediction accuracies in Table 2. The prediction accuracies for the stone-free were 86.0, 87.5%, and 87.9 and those for one-session success were 78.0, 77.4, and 77.0% using RF, XGBoost, and LightGBM, respectively. In predictions for the stone-free, LightGBM offers better accuracy than XGBoost and RF; and for one-session success, RF algorithms showed better accuracy than XGBoost and LightGBM.

The sensitivity, specificity, positive predictive value, confidence interval and area under the roc curve (AUC) for machine learning analytics are presented in Table 3. As the result in Table 3, the specificity of stone-free was better than the sensitivity. The result implied that the predictive models were more accurate in prediction stone-free. On the contrary, the models were good in the prediction of one-session fail. In AUC for the stone-free, RF and LightGBM offered higher value than XGBoost; and for one-session success, RF offered higher value than XGBoost and LightGBM. Here, we also have shown the feature importance, which had certain interpretability of prediction results related to domain insights. In Fig. 1, we present the feature importance of LightGBM for stone-free predictions. It shows that MSD was the main factor that had decided the stone-free and stone volume (mm^3) and SSD 90° (mm) played an important role in supporting the stone-free decision. It

Table 1 General characteristics of all urinary stone patients

	Kidney stone	Ureter stone	*P*-value
Patient characteristics			
Numbers of patients	167	191	
Age, mean ± SD	56.4 ± 13.9	60.4 ± 13.7	0.007
Sex, numbers of men, %	90, 53.9	108, 56.5	0.615
Diabetes mellitus, %	48, 28.7	57, 29.8	0.820
Hypertension, %	65, 38.9	86, 45.0	0.243
Psoas muscle cross-sectional area (mm^2), mean ± SD	1105.9 ± 373.1	1067.4 ± 368.7	0.326
Stone characteristics			
Stone laterality, numbers on left side, %	87, 52.1	93, 48.7	0.520
Stone length (mm, X-axis), mean ± SD	9.2 ± 3.5	6.6 ± 1.5	< 0.001
Stone length (mm, Y-axis), mean ± SD	9.3 ± 3.2	7.4 ± 1.7	< 0.001
Stone length (mm, Z-axis), mean ± SD	9.7 ± 3.1	9.4 ± 2.8	0.345
Stone volume (mm^3), mean ± SD	516.8 ± 479.6	268.2 ± 182.2	< 0.001
Skin to stone distance 90° (mm), mean ± SD	87.9 ± 14.8	108.9 ± 16.3	< 0.001
Mean stone density, mean ± SD	834.3 ± 296.9	766.6 ± 274.7	0.025
Stone heterogeneity index, mean ± SD	178.0 ± 83.9	174.2 ± 84.9	0.669

SD standard deviation

Table 2 Comparison of prediction accuracies for stone-free and one-session success according to three machine learning methods

	Stone-free	One-session success
Random forest (RF)		
Training Accuracy (%)	86.47	76.83
Test Accuracy (%)	85.98	78.02
Extreme gradient boosting trees (XGBoost)		
Training Accuracy (%)	87.50	75.60
Test Accuracy (%)	87.46	77.39
Light Gradient Boosting Method (LightGBM)		
Training Accuracy (%)	88.09	74.92
Test Accuracy (%)	87.95	77.04

might match a typical intuition of stone-free; however, with the machine learning method, LightGBM caught the intuition for that. In addition, in the prediction of one-session success, stone volume (mm^3) was the main factor (Fig. 2).

Discussion

To be able to predict the result of treatment and the patient's condition with easy measurement would be beneficial for all concerned. The prediction could provide the ability to choose an effective treatment for urinary tract stones and reduce unnecessary resource waste. One promising approach to obtain an appropriate prediction is to adopt machine learning based artificial intelligence methods.

Table 3 Comparison of Receiver Operating Characteristic (ROC) values for stone-free and one-session success according to three machine learning methods

	Stone-free	One-session success
Random forest (RF)		
Sensitivity	0.74	0.81
Specificity	0.92	0.75
AUC	0.85	0.78
CI (95%)	(0.75–0.94)	(0.67–0.86)
PPV	0.82	0.79
Extreme gradient boosting trees (XGBoost)		
Sensitivity	0.75	0.80
Specificity	0.93	0.75
AUC	0.84	0.77
CI (95%)	(0.74–0.93)	(0.68–0.87)
PPV	0.78	0.79
Light Gradient Boosting Method (LightGBM)		
Sensitivity	0.78	0.79
Specificity	0.92	0.74
AUC	0.85	0.77
CI (95%)	(0.73–0.93)	(0.67–0.87)
PPV	0.81	0.78

AUC area under ROC curve, *CI* confidence interval, *PPV* positive predictive value

The machine learning methods can show the potential to make decisions that are best suited to the situation without the involvement of emotions, based solely on thorough statistics and calculations. There are some advantages to analyzing data by using machine learning methods. First, machine learning can provide interpretability for analysis and prediction results. Second, insufficient number of data set to apply deep learning algorithms can be handled by certain types of machine learning algorithms, such as tree-based ones; statistical machine learning especially is more effective in predicting with small data, even though more data usually yield more accuracy. Third, machine learning treats heterogeneous data, which is statistically and structurally quite different, simultaneously; for instance, data about kidney stone and ureter stone properties differ distinctly [14, 15]. Machine learning could find new values from data and derives important factors for predicted target variables from the analytical/predicting perspective of machine learning. These factors can be used to validate known domain insights and sometimes reveal factors that were not previously recognized. The main factors of them derived from machine learning are expected to play a major role in developing an auxiliary system for diagnosing diseases and a supporting system.

In this study, data on SWL is accumulated in the treatment of urinary stone, and valid data is available, and we applied three well-known tree-based machine learning methods and compared their results. The decision tree-based methods, such as RF, XGBoost, and LightGBM increased the interpretability of the predicted results by providing the importance of the properties used in the prediction, suggesting new functionality of the machine learning methodology. The reason, why we applied the above decision tree-based machine learning algorithms rather than well-known deep learning ones, is that the tree-based predictive models give better performance in prediction accuracy in case of the relatively small number of data for deep learning ones, in general. Moreover, the algorithms give certain interpretation of their results in feature importance. Another strategy to overcome the relatively small number of data, we collected SWL treatment data for both the upper ureter and kidney stones without their positional information. Then the trained machine learning model with the collected data can show the capability of prediction for stone-free and one-session success. Even though the positional information for urinary stones is neglected, the predictive model can

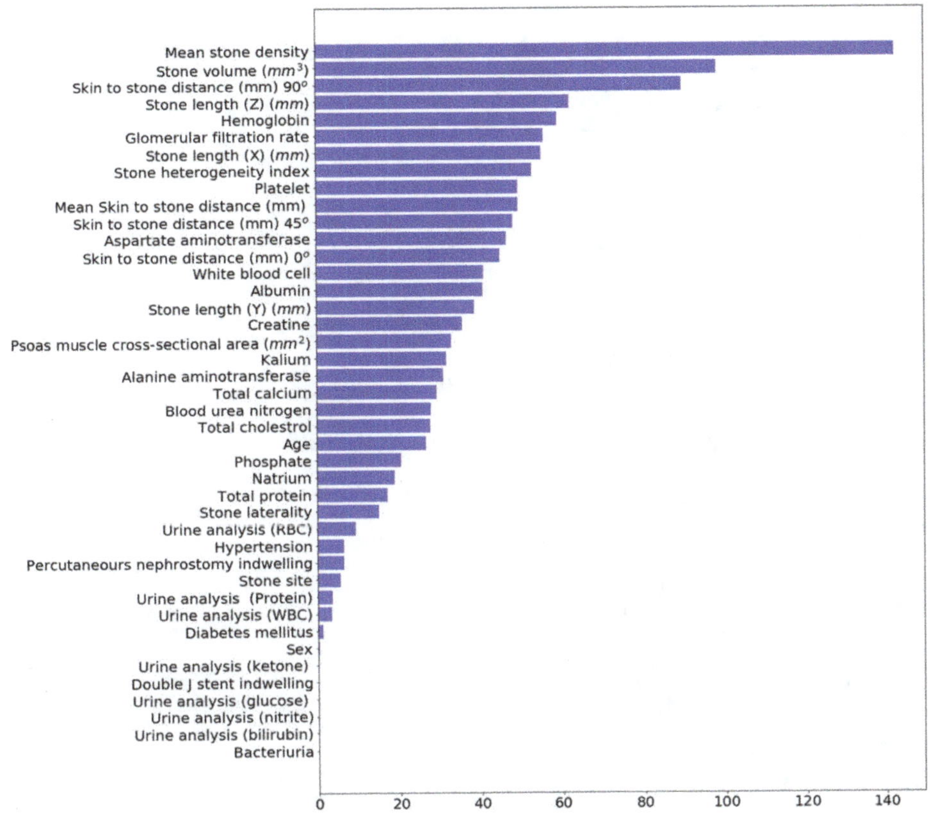

Fig. 1 Feature importance of LightGBM for stone-free prediction. Stone-free was affected with mean stone density, stone volume, and skin to stone distance

catch the effective accuracy in predictions. After filtering the missing data, carefully, three hundred and fifty-eight cases were obtained for applying machine learning algorithms. The experiment results obtained by taking an average of ten samplings of the given data set. In these prediction experiments, the parameter tuning was not performed for comparison purpose, because parameter tuning shows different results for different sampling of given data.

The major contribution of this study was to enable urologists to choose patients who would realize the most optimal results from SWL. After prediction analysis, patients who have a high risk of stone-free failure can select another method, such as percutaneous nephrolithotomy or retrograde intrarenal surgery, using flexible ureteroscopy to manage urinary stone. The first objective of this study was achieved because each outcome in the predictive analysis exceeded 85% for stone-free and 77% for one-session success, especially, LightGBM and XGBoost showed good prediction outcomes of more than 87% in stone-free prediction.

In most cases of the SWL, the stone analysis could not be done without analyzing the stone fragments that had been discharged from the body directly. Therefore, patients and stone characteristics should have an important role in the pretreatment prediction of treatment outcomes. Even though stone volume, MSD, and SSD are known as important factors that can affect the stone-free rate after SWL, controversy about SSD still exists [16, 17]. In our feature importance analysis, as with the results from various other studies that have been analyzed using general statistical methods, MSD and stone volume were the most influential factors, and SSD was less affected than MSD and stone volume.

MSD is the mean value of the HU of each pixel in a specific stone area and is known as a potential predictor of successful treatment of urinary stone with SWL [18–20]. Eisner et al. found that by measuring the mean HU of defined regions just smaller than the stone in magnified images on each slice of the transverse planes with a standard bone window was the most accurate method of determining MSD [21]. In addition, PACS may provide pixel statistics such as minimum, maximum, and standard deviation of HU values. Lee et al. [22] defined SHI as the standard deviation of stone density on NCCT and assessment that SHI was independently associated with SWL success in patients with ureter stone. In our study, we easily determined MSD by measuring the mean HU from NCCT by using a PACS in the same way. It was significant that MSD was a more important feature than SHI in the prediction of stone-free. All things are taken

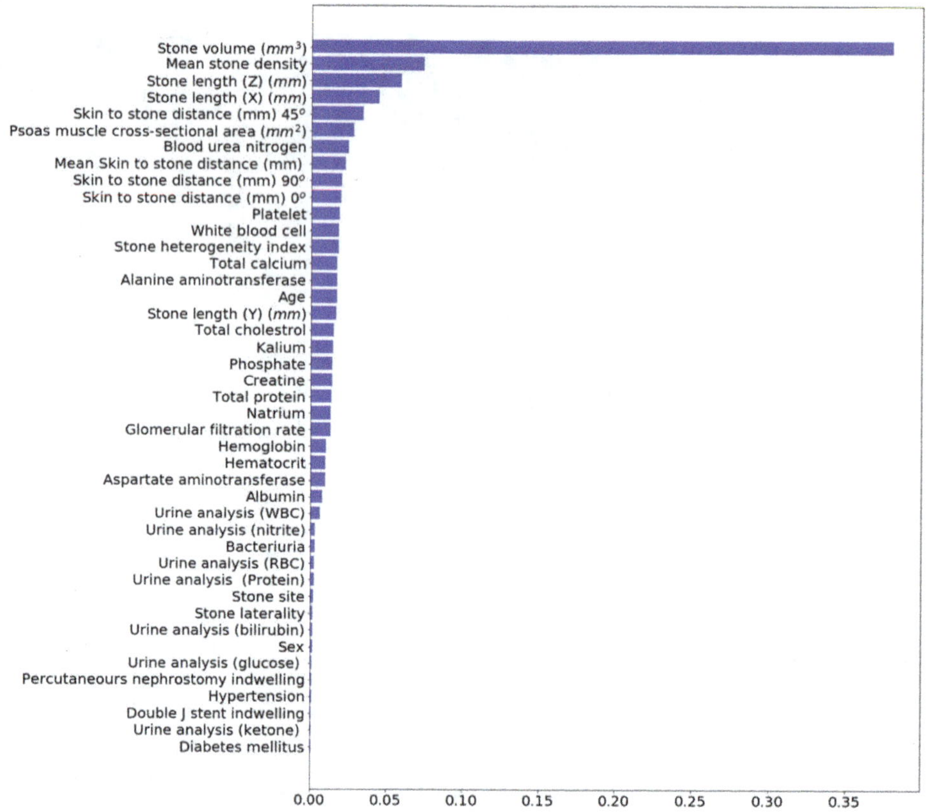

Fig. 2 Feature importance of Random Forest for one-session success prediction. One-session success was affected with stone volume, mean stone density, stone length, skin to stone distance, and psoas muscle cross-sectional area

together, although the predictive level of SHI seems to be lower than MSD, SHI can play a supplementary role in the prediction of SWL treatment outcomes.

The question of whether body mass index (BMI) affects the success rate of SWL treatment has been a controversial issue. Most of the studies have shown that BMI was an independent predictor of stone-free status after SWL [23, 24]. However, several studies took a different view [25, 26], so we tried to think about muscle mass, which is a factor that can indicate the whole-body health condition. No previous study has considered the relationship between muscle mass and the success rate of SWL treatment. Sarcopenia brings about mobility limitation and an inability to perform simple activities of daily life [27]. The psoas muscle cross-sectional area has been used in many studies to provide estimates of overall muscle mass and has been shown to be a simple and easily performed measure of a reliable marker of sarcopenia [28–30]. In this study, we found that the psoas muscle cross-sectional area was ranked as an important feature in the prediction of one-session success rather than in those of stone-free. That is, the higher the muscle mass, the higher the activity in daily life. Muscle mass can be regarded as an important factor in determining the extent of stone removal for a short period.

The results of blood and urine tests showed a generally low feature ranking. Among them, hemoglobin, glomerular filtration rate, and platelet count were judged to give a little meaning.

In the current study, there were some limitations. Its retrospective design may have introduced sampling bias. To compensate for its retrospective sampling bias and small sample size, we applied three machine learning methods, which can reduce bias from commonly used general statistical accesses. However, further studies with prospective data are needed to prove our monitoring on the relationship of feature importance.

MSD was the most significant in feature importance, and stone volume, SSD and stone length were the next most closely associated with stone-free prediction of SWL treatment outcomes in patients with urinary stone. In addition, stone volume was the most significant in feature importance, and MSD, stone length, SSD and psoas muscle cross-sectional area were the next most closely associated with the one-session success prediction in this study. Thus, these would be clinically useful parameters in order.

Conclusions

We analyzed the effect of SWL treatment by using three machine learning methods and confirmed that prediction accuracy can rise up to as much as 87.9% by using various patients and stone characteristics. We propose that the new machine learning based artificial intelligence and medical encounter are important. When further large studies, validated in a prospective group of urinary stone patients, become available, our machine learning methods might be useful for guiding SWL treatment selection and prediction of patients with urinary stone.

Abbreviations

SWL: Shock wave lithotripsy; NCCT: Non-contrast computed tomography; HU: Hounsfield units; PACS: Picture archiving and communication system; DM: Diabetes mellitus; HTN: Hypertension; SSD: Skin to stone distance; MSD: Mean stone density; SHI: Stone heterogeneity index; PCN: Percutaneous nephrostomy; RF: Random forest; XGBoost: Extreme gradient boosting trees; LightGBM: Light gradient boosting method; AUC: Area under the roc curve; PPV: Positive predictive value; BMI: Body mass index

Acknowledgements

The authors acknowledges the members of the department of Urology, Chungnam National University and National Institute for Mathematical Sciences.

Authors' contributions

YSW, HYK and SKH were involved in protocol, project development, data collection and management, data analysis, and manuscript writing and editing; NHS, JL, LJG, PJM, LJY, SJH, LJS, NYG and KJB was involved in data collection and analysis; JKW and HTY was performed statistical and machine learning analysis. All authors reviewed the results and approved the final version of the manuscript.

Author details

[1]Department of Urology, Chungnam National University College of Medicine, Chungnam National University Hospital, 282 Monwha-ro, Jung-gu, Daejeon, Republic of Korea 35015. [2]Division of Medical Mathematics, National Institute for Mathematical Sciences, 70 Yuseong-daero 1689beon-gil, Yuseong-gu, Daejeon, Republic of Korea 34047. [3]Department of Urology, Konyang University College of Medicine, Konyang University Hospital, 158 Gwanjeodong-ro, Seo-gu, Daejeon, Republic of Korea 35365.

References

1. Chaussy C, Brendel W, Schmiedt E. Extracorporeally induced destruction of kidney stones by shock waves. Lancet. 1980;2(8207):1265–8.
2. Ben Khalifa B, Naouar S, Gazzah W, Salem B, El Kamel R. Predictive factors of extracorporeal shock wave lithotripsy success for urinary stones. Tunis Med. 2016;94(5):397–400.
3. Bres-Niewada E, Dybowski B, Radziszewski P. Predicting stone composition before treatment - can it really drive clinical decisions? Cent European J Urol. 2014;67(4):392–6.
4. Zumstein V, Betschart P, Abt D, Schmid HP, Panje CM, Putora PM. Surgical management of urolithiasis - a systematic analysis of available guidelines. BMC Urol. 2018;18(1):25.
5. Cone EB, Eisner BH, Ursiny M, Pareek G. Cost-effectiveness comparison of renal calculi treated with ureteroscopic laser lithotripsy versus shockwave lithotripsy. J Endourol. 2014;28(6):639–43.
6. Pareek G, Armenakas NA, Fracchia JA. Hounsfield units on computerized tomography predict stone-free rates after extracorporeal shock wave lithotripsy. J Urol. 2003;169(5):1679–81.
7. Patel T, Kozakowski K, Hruby G, Gupta M. Skin to stone distance is an independent predictor of stone-free status following shockwave lithotripsy. J Endourol. 2009;23(9):1383–5.
8. Gupta NP, Ansari MS, Kesarvani P, Kapoor A, Mukhopadhyay S. Role of computed tomography with no contrast medium enhancement in predicting the outcome of extracorporeal shock wave lithotripsy for urinary calculi. BJU Int. 2005;95(9):1285–8.
9. Obermeyer Z, Emanuel EJ. Predicting the future - big data, machine learning, and clinical medicine. N Engl J Med. 2016;375(13):1216–9.
10. De Silva D, Ranasinghe W, Bandaragoda T, Adikari A, Mills N, Iddamalgoda L, et al. Machine learning to support social media empowered patients in cancer care and cancer treatment decisions. PLoS One. 2018;13(10): e0205855.
11. Kam HT, editor. Random decision forest. Proc of the 3rd Int'l Conf on Document Analysis and Recognition, Montreal, Canada, August; 1995.
12. Chen T, Guestrin C, editors. Xgboost: A scalable tree boosting system. Proceedings of the 22nd acm sigkdd international conference on knowledge discovery and data mining; 2016: ACM.
13. Ke G, Wang T, Chen W, Ma W, Ye Q, Liu TY, et al. LightGBM: A highly efficient gradient boosting decision tree. Adv neural inf proces syst Advances in Neural Information Processing Systems. 2017;2017-December: 3147–55.
14. Kevin PM. Machine learning: a probabilistic perspective. MIT Press, Cambridge, UK; 2012.
15. Hastie T, Tibshirani R, Friedman JH. The elements of statistical learning : data mining, inference, and prediction2017.
16. Wiesenthal JD, Ghiculete D, DAH RJ, Pace KT. Evaluating the importance of mean stone density and skin-to-stone distance in predicting successful shock wave lithotripsy of renal and ureteric calculi. Urol Res. 2010;38(4):307–13.
17. Cho KS, Jung HD, Ham WS, Chung DY, Kang YJ, Jang WS, et al. Optimal skin-to-stone distance is a positive predictor for successful outcomes in upper ureter calculi following extracorporeal shock wave lithotripsy: a Bayesian model averaging approach. PLoS One. 2015;10(12):e0144912.
18. El-Nahas AR, El-Assmy AM, Mansour O, Sheir KZ. A prospective multivariate analysis of factors predicting stone disintegration by extracorporeal shock wave lithotripsy: the value of high-resolution noncontrast computed tomography. Eur Urol 2007;51(6):1688–1693; discussion 93-4.
19. Weld KJ, Montiglio C, Morris MS, Bush AC, Cespedes RD. Shock wave lithotripsy success for renal stones based on patient and stone computed tomography characteristics. Urology. 2007;70(6):1043–1046; discussion 6-7.
20. Kacker R, Zhao L, Macejko A, Thaxton CS, Stern J, Liu JJ, et al. Radiographic parameters on noncontrast computerized tomography predictive of shock wave lithotripsy success. J Urol. 2008;179(5):1866–71.
21. Eisner BH, Kambadakone A, Monga M, Anderson JK, Thoreson AA, Lee H, et al. Computerized tomography magnified bone windows are superior to standard soft tissue windows for accurate measurement of stone size: an in vitro and clinical study. J Urol. 2009;181(4):1710–5.
22. Lee JY, Kim JH, Kang DH, Chung DY, Lee DH, Do Jung H, et al. Stone heterogeneity index as the standard deviation of Hounsfield units: a novel predictor for shock-wave lithotripsy outcomes in ureter calculi. Sci Rep. 2016;6:23988.
23. Ahmed MH, Ahmed HT, Khalil AA. Renal stone disease and obesity: what is important for urologists and nephrologists? Ren Fail. 2012;34(10):1348–54.
24. Hwang I, Jung SI, Kim KH, Hwang EC, Yu HS, Kim SO, et al. Factors influencing the failure of extracorporeal shock wave lithotripsy with Piezolith 3000 in the management of solitary ureteral stone. Urolithiasis. 2014;42(3):263–7.
25. Choi JW, Song PH, Kim HT. Predictive factors of the outcome of extracorporeal shockwave lithotripsy for ureteral stones. Korean J Urol. 2012; 53(6):424–30.
26. Hatiboglu G, Popeneciu V, Kurosch M, Huber J, Pahernik S, Pfitzenmaier J, et al. Prognostic variables for shockwave lithotripsy (SWL) treatment success: no impact of body mass index (BMI) using a third generation lithotripter. BJU Int. 2011;108(7):1192–7.
27. Janssen I, Heymsfield SB, Ross R. Low relative skeletal muscle mass (sarcopenia) in older persons is associated with functional impairment and physical disability. J Am Geriatr Soc. 2002;50(5):889–96.
28. Shen W, Punyanitya M, Wang Z, Gallagher D, St-Onge MP, Albu J, et al. Total body skeletal muscle and adipose tissue volumes: estimation from a single abdominal cross-sectional image. J Appl Physiol (1985). 2004;97(6):2333–8.
29. Cruz-Jentoft AJ, Baeyens JP, Bauer JM, Boirie Y, Cederholm T, Landi F, et al.

Sarcopenia: European consensus on definition and diagnosis: report of the European working group on sarcopenia in older people. Age Ageing. 2010; 39(4):412–23.

30. Jones KI, Doleman B, Scott S, Lund JN, Williams JP. Simple psoas cross-sectional area measurement is a quick and easy method to assess sarcopenia and predicts major surgical complications. Color Dis. 2015;17(1): O20–6.

30

Diabetic ketoacidosis complicated by emphysematous pyelonephritis

Yuanhao Song and Xingping Shen*

Abstract

Background: The management of emphysematous pyelonephritis (EPN) includes conservative medical treatment, percutaneous drainage, and surgical resection of the involved kidney. EPN with diabetic ketoacidosis(DKA) is very rare, in which the clinical management of refusing surgical drainage is inexperienced.

Case presentation: A 34-year-old woman presented with abdominal pain, chills, fever, nausea, vomiting, chest tightness, and shortness of breath. Blood test results were consistent with diabetic ketoacidosis. Urinary computed tomography scan showed multiple stones in the right kidney and lower ureter, with right hydronephrosis. Blood culture demonstrated *Escherichia coli* bacteremia, and EPN was diagnosed. Considering the need for a second percutaneous nephrolithotomy, the patient refused percutaneous drainage. After continuous intravenous infusion of small doses of insulin and antibiotic treatment, the ketoacidosis resolved. The patient's temperature returned to normal and abdominal pain was alleviated, and liver and kidney functions were also back to normal. After hospital discharge, the patient underwent two percutaneous nephrolithotomy in the department of urology.

Conclusions: EPN with diabetic ketoacidosis should be diagnosed as soon as possible. For patients with Class 1 and Class 2 EPN with diabetic ketoacidosis and urinary tract obstruction, if surgical drainage is refused, it is particularly important to rapidly correct diabetic ketoacidosis and intravenous use of sensitive antibiotics, so as to create conditions for follow-up percutaneous nephrolithotomy.

Keywords: Emphysematous pyelonephritis, Diabetes, Diabetic ketoacidosis, Kidney stones, Antibiotics

Background

Emphysematous pyelonephritis (EPN) is an acute, severe necrotizing infection affecting renal parenchyma, collecting system as well as surrounding tissue with hallmark of presence of gas within these structures [1]. Several large-scale retrospective studies have shown that affected patients commonly presented with fever, abdominal pain, nausea, and vomiting [1, 2]; although, occasionally, patients have experienced no obvious symptoms [3]. There has been no general consensus with respect to the diagnosis and treatment of EPN. A computed tomography (CT) scan is currently the gold-standard diagnostic test [4]. Treatment includes conservative medical therapy, with or without surgical drainage or nephrectomy [5].

At present, EPN with diabetic ketoacidosis is rare, only a few cases have been reported [6–10]. And diabetic ketoacidosis is an important predictor of death in patients with EPN [11]. Effective surgical drainage is a key measure for the management of EPN with diabetic ketoacidosis and urinary tract obstruction. In this case, the clinical management of patients refusing surgical drainage is inexperienced.

Case presentation

A 34-year-old woman was admitted to the hospital due to abdominal pain, chills, fever, chest tightness, and shortness of breath after eating contaminated food 2 days earlier. After admission, she became nauseated and vomited; but without dysuria, urinary frequency, or urgency. She had a medical history of type I diabetes for 19 months, with poor control of blood glucose due to non-compliance with the insulin treatments. One month

* Correspondence: sxpsxzlg@qq.com
Department of Endocrinology, Zhongshan Hospital Xiamen University, Xiamen 361004, Fujian, China

prior, she was found to have kidney stones. Physical examination revealed a temperature of 36.0 °C, pulse rate of 87 beats/minute, respiratory rate of 35 breaths/min, and a blood pressure of 105/66 mm of Hg. She had shortness of breath, dry skin, and dry mucous membranes and tongue; although her lungs sounded clear. There was an abdominal wall muscle strain in the epigastric area and right upper quadrant, with obvious tenderness. The right costovertebral angle also had tenderness.

Laboratory tests and imaging studies were as follows. Blood tests after admission showed a white blood cell count of 21.08×10^9/L, neutrophil count of 18.53×10^9/L, neutrophil percentage of 87.9%, platelet count of 107×10^9/L; and concentrations for albumin of 37.42 g/L, glucose of 35.95 mmol/L, urea of 10.54 mmol/L, creatinine of 145.1 μmol/L, bicarbonate of 2.2 mmol/L, potassium of 6.60 mmol/L, sodium of 122.10 mmol/L, β-hydroxybutyric acid of 10.08 mmol/L, lactic acid of 2.43 mmol/L, C-reactive protein of 448.39 mg/L, and procalcitonin > 100.000 ng/mL. Blood gas analysis showed a pH of 6.984, carbon dioxide partial pressure of 10.9 mm of Hg, oxygen partial pressure of 138.2 mm of Hg, measured bicarbonate of 2.5 mmol/L, calculated bicarbonate of 6.4 mmol/L, anion gap of 32.2 mmol/L, base excess of – 27.2 mmol/L, and carbon dioxide of 2.9 mmol/L. Urinalysis measurements were glucose, 4+; ketone body, 4+; leukocyte esterase, weakly positive; and white blood cell number, 41/μL; with negative results for urine culture. Blood culture identified *Escherichia coli.* Urinary CT scan revealed multiple stones in the right kidney and lower ureter, with right hydronephrosis; we therefore diagnosed EPN (Figs. 1, 2, and 3 reflect the CT scans during hospital admission).

After being admitted to the hospital for definite diagnosis, our endocrinology department cooperated with urology, nephrology, infection department and imaging department to formulate a treatment plan, which suggested that the patients should undergo percutaneous drainage but the patient refused. Hospital management and outcomes after admission included intravenous infusion of small doses of insulin to correct ketoacidosis. Liver and renal functions returned to normal after albumin infusion and hydration. Based upon blood culture results, Cefoperazone sulbactam was upgraded to meropenem. Inflammatory indicators and body temperature gradually returned to normal, and abdominal pain was relieved. Repeated blood cultures were negative, and urine culture remained negative. Repeated urinary CT

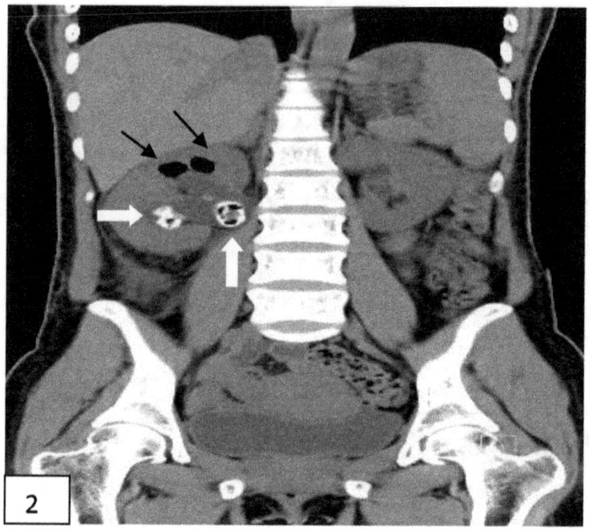

Fig. 2 Show the non-contrast urinary CT scans during hospital admission

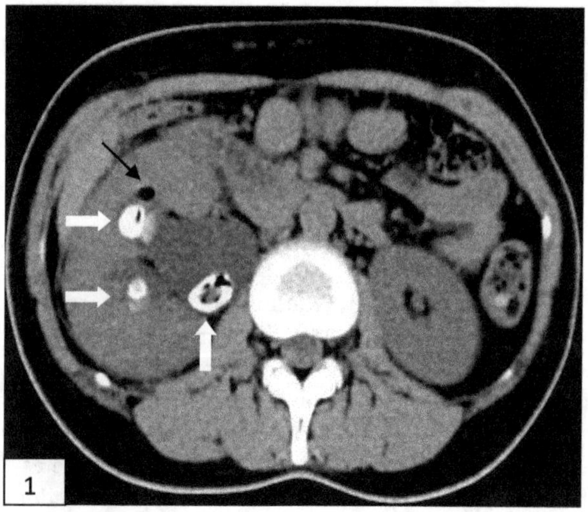

Fig. 1 Show the non-contrast urinary CT scans during hospital admission

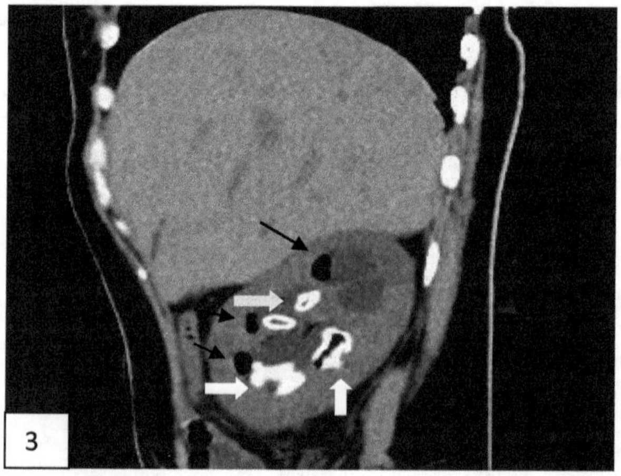

Fig. 3 Show the non-contrast urinary CT scans during hospital admission

scans revealed multiple stones in the right kidney with worsening right hydronephrosis and pyelonephritis, but with reduced gas accumulation (Fig. 4).

One month after discharge, the patient underwent percutaneous nephrolithotomy in the department of urology, and the urinary CT was reexamined after operation (Fig. 5).Two months after discharge, the patient underwent the second percutaneous nephrolithotomy in the department of urology, and the urinary CT was reexamined after operation (Fig. 6). Currently, three months after discharge, clinical follow-up checks detect normal renal function and stable blood glucose control.

Discussion and conclusions

In 1898, Kelly and MacCullum reported the first case of kidney infection with gas accumulation [12]. In 1962, Schultz and Klorfein described this disorder as emphysematous pyelonephritis [13]. Since then, there have been reports of various types of kidney infection with gas accumulation.

The pathogenesis of emphysematous pyelonephritis (EPN) is still unclear. It is believed that multiple factors, including diabetes, elevated glucose levels in kidney tissue, urinary tract obstruction, impaired renal circulation, decreased host immune function, and the presence of gas-producing microbial infections could cause EPN [1, 14]. EPN most commonly affects diabetic patients [2, 15–17]; and it is currently believed that the increased susceptibility to developing EPN in diabetic patients is due to impaired renal tissue perfusion [18]. Additionally, high blood glucose concentrations can also promote anaerobic growth and gas-producing metabolism [18].

CT scan is now considered to be the best method to diagnose EPN, and the most commonly accepted CT classification system for EPN was proposed by Huang and associates in 2000 [19]. These authors suggested 4 classes of EPN: Class 1, where gas is confined only to the collection; Class 2, where gas is located within the renal parenchyma and does not spread to the extrarenal space; Class 3A, where gas or an abscess spreads to the perinephric space; Class 3B, where gas or the abscess spreads to the pararenal space; and Class 4, depicting a bilateral or solitary kidney with EPN [19].. However, in one recent study, investigators attempted to re-correlate CT classification with clinical treatment options, analyzing 34 cases from 2009 to 2018. Their results showed that most Class 1 and Class 2 patients achieved satisfactory outcomes purely by conservative treatment. Only a small number of patients with urinary tract obstruction required combined percutaneous drainage, 2 of the 6 Class 3A patients required nephrectomy, and 2 Class 3B patients also required nephrectomy [16].

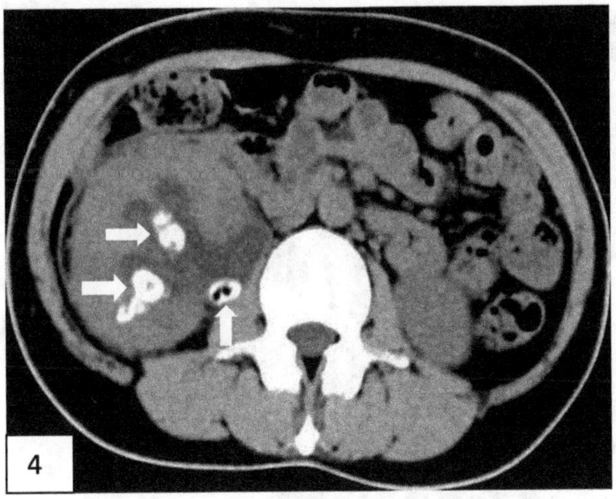

Fig. 4 Shows the repeat non-contrast CT scan before hospital discharge

Lu et al. retrospectively analyzed 51 patients with EPN and demonstrated that the most common bacteria were *Escherichia coli*, followed by *Streptococcus pneumoniae*, *Enterococcus*, and *Pseudomonas aeruginosa*; with a small number of patients showing mixed bacterial infections. The antibiotic-resistance rate was greater than 15% for fluoroquinolone, ampicillin, 1st- and 2nd-generation cephalosporins, and gentamicin; whereas the resistance rates for the 3rd- and 4th-generation cephalosporins were only 10.9 and 6.5%, respectively. These authors concluded that the 3rd-generation cephalosporins could be used routinely for most affected patients. However, carbapenem antibiotics such as meropenem should be selected if a patient carries high risk factors, including recent hospitalization, antibiotic use, or DIC [20]. At the present time, most studies depict *Escherichia coli* as the most common pathogenic bacterium [1, 17]; although there have been recent reports of EPN caused by *Candida albicans* [21]. Therefore, selection of antibiotics should be based upon the local epidemiology and antibiotic- resistance patterns. In addition, multiple blood and urine cultures should be performed. It is extremely important to then revise the antibiotics according to the disease severity and the antibiotic-susceptibility test results.

There is recent evidence that patients who received conservative management achieved satisfactory results [15]. However, a study of 17 patients with EPN also showed that patients who received conservative treatment tend to experience acute increases in the Sequential Organ Failure Assessment (SOFA) score after the beginning of treatment, even if transient, which presents a great risk of septic mortality [15]. Adequate surgical drainage combined with intravenous antibiotics have resulted in satisfactory results in patients with EPN and multiple organ failure who were not appropriate candidates for nephrectomy [17, 22, 23]. In another study researchers tried to evaluate the clinical prognosis and

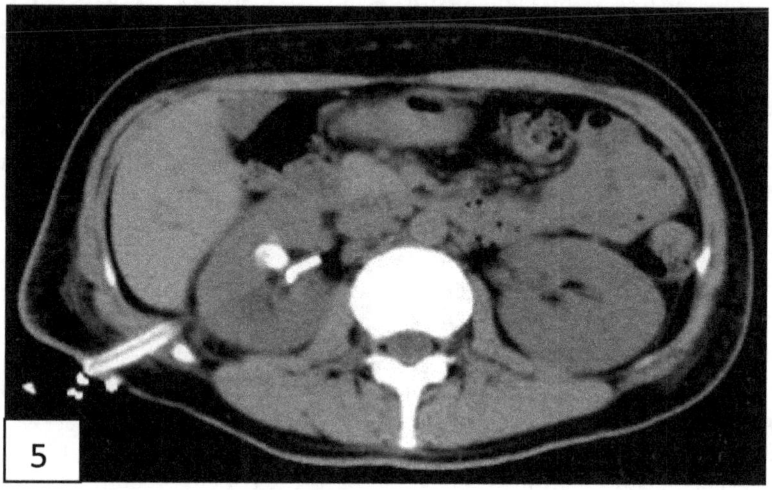

Fig. 5 Shows the repeat non-contrast CT scan after the first percutaneous nephroscopy

outcomes of this disorder by analyzing 74 patients with EPN [1]. Their results showed that 1. fever was the most common clinical presentation, which was followed by lower back pain; 2. most patients had diabetes, which was followed by urolithiasis; 3. *Escherichia coli* was still the most common pathogen; 4. older age, high body-mass index, impaired renal function, thrombocytopenia, sensory changes, and shock were associated with a poor prognosis; and 5. treatment mainly consisted of rapid hydration, maintenance of electrolyte balance, use of systemic antibiotics, strict control of blood glucose, effective urine drainage, and nephrectomy if necessary [1]. Sanford et al. have shown that mild EPN was treatable by conservative management that included infectious agent-susceptible antibiotics [24]. However, patients with severe infections required percutaneous renal puncture drainage and/or double-J stenting [24].

Nanki et al. successfully treated a 58-year-old woman with EPN caused by *Escherichia coli* complicated with diabetic ketoacidosis through nephrectomy, antibiotics and recombinant human granulocyte colony-stimulating factor(rhG-CSF) [8]. Harrabi et al. reported a 64-year-old woman with EPN complicated with diabetic ketoacidosis who died of septic shock without surgical drainage [6]. However, another patient with EPN with diabetic ketoacidosis who underwent percutaneous renal drainage combined with antibiotics died 7 days after admission [9]; Unlike our patient, according to CT, this patient belongs to class 3A EPN. Recently, it has been reported that EPN with diabetic ketoacidosis in the patient with allogeneic renal transplantation improved after conservative treatment with intravenous antibiotics without percutaneous drainage or nephrectomy [10]; But our patient is different from this successful case in that there are urinary tract

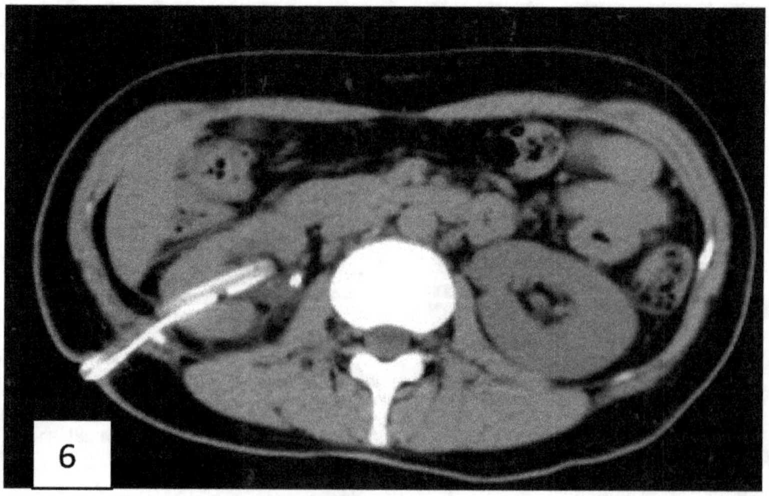

Fig. 6 Shows the repeat non-contrast CT scan after the second percutaneous nephroscopy

obstruction factors such as right kidney stone and right ureteral stone, and percutaneous drainage is more important in the treatment.

Our successful management of this patient lies in the following points: 1. We confirmed the diagnosis of EPN by urinary CT examination as soon as the patient was admitted to hospital; 2. Rapid correction of ketoacidosis by continuous intravenous infusion of low-dose insulin and fluid resuscitation; 3. We performed blood culture before using antibiotics and upgraded cefoperazone sulbactam to meropenem according to the results of blood culture and the antibiotic-susceptibility test results; 4. Our endocrinology department collaborated with urology, nephrology, infection and imaging departments to develop a treatment plan; 5. What is particularly important is that although the patient has sepsis, it belongs to Class 2 EPN. However, our treatment is also inadequate: the patient did not receive percutaneous drainage. Although the accumulation of gas in the kidney was less than before, the right hydronephrosis increased. In the end, the patient still underwent two percutaneous nephrolithotomy. Failed to achieve the goal that the patient wanted to have only one operation.

Our case report makes up for the gap in the clinical management of patients with EPN with diabetic ketoacidosis with urinary tract obstruction who refuse surgical drainage, but it is unclear whether our management experience can be extended to similar patients of EPN Class 3A,Class 3B and Class 4.

In conclusion, EPN with diabetic ketoacidosis should be diagnosed as soon as possible. For patients with Class 1 and Class 2 EPN with diabetic ketoacidosis and urinary tract obstruction, if surgical drainage is refused, it is particularly important to rapidly correct diabetic ketoacidosis and intravenous use of sensitive antibiotics, so as to create conditions for follow-up percutaneous nephrolithotomy.

Abbreviations

CT: Computed tomography; DKA: Diabetic ketoacidosis; EPN: emphysematous pyelonephritis; RHG-CSF: Recombinant human granulocyte colony-stimulating factor; SOFA: Sequential Organ Failure Assessment

Acknowledgements

Not applicable.

Authors' contributions

YHS made contributions to data collection, literature search. XPS was responsible for the patient's diagnosis and treatment. YHS drafted original manuscript and XPS reviewed and edited the manuscript. All authors read and approved the final manuscript.

References

1. Sokhal AK, Kumar M, Purkait B, Jhanwar A, Singh K, Bansal A, et al. Emphysematous pyelonephritis: changing trend of clinical spectrum, pathogenesis, management and outcome. Turk J Urol. 2017;43(2):202–9.
2. Karthikeyan VS, Manohar CMS, Mallya A, Keshavamurthy R, Kamath AJ. Clinical profile and successful outcomes of conservative and minimally invasive treatment of emphysematous pyelonephritis. Cent European J Urol. 2018;71(2):228–33.
3. Yeung A, Cheng CH, Chu P, Man CW, Chau H. A rare case of asymptomatic emphysematous pyelonephritis. Urol Case Rep. 2019;26:100962.
4. Mahesh HR, Padala KP, Swamy K, Pailoor a. A rare case of Pneumoureter: emphysematous Pyelitis versus emphysematous pyelonephritis. J Clin Diagn Res. 2015;9(11):TD03–5.
5. Boakes E, Batura D. Deriving a management algorithm for emphysematous pyelonephritis: can we rely on minimally invasive strategies or should we be opting for earlier nephrectomy? Int Urol Nephrol. 2017;49(12):2127–36.
6. Harrabi H, Marrakchi C, Daoud E, Elleuch E, Hammami B, Maaloul I, et al. Bilateral emphysematous pyelonephritis caused by Candida glabrata: an exceptional entity. Nephrol Ther. 2010;6(6):541–3.
7. Kirpekar M, Cooke KS, Abiri MM, Lipset RE. US case of the day. Emphysematous pyelonephritis. Radiographics. 1997;17(6):1601–3.
8. Nanki T, Ageishi Y, Iwama T, Murase H, Uchikawa T. Emphysematous pyelonephritis successfully treated with nephrectomy and granulocyte colony-stimulating factor. Intern Med. 1994;33(4):234–6.
9. Ghosh GC, Sharma B, Kamble U, Lamba BM. Vanishing kidney disease. BMJ Case Rep. 2013. https://doi.org/10.1136/bcr-2013-009117.
10. Crouter AJ, Abraham MK, Wilkerson RG. Emphysematous pyelonephritis in a renal allograft. Am J Emerg Med. 2017;35(3):520 e1- e2.
11. Wang JM, Lim HK, Pang KK. Emphysematous pyelonephritis. Scand J Urol Nephrol. 2007;41(3):223–9.
12. Kelly HA, WG MC. Pneumaturia. JAMA. 1898;31:375–81.
13. Schultz EH Jr, Klorfein EH. Emphysematous pyelonephritis. J Urol. 1962;87:762–6.
14. Arsene C, Saste A, Arul S, Mestrovich J, Kammo R, Elbashir M, et al. A case series of emphysematous pyelonephritis. Case Rep Med. 2014;2014:587926.
15. Ozawa M, Ichiyanagi O, Fujita S, Naito S, Fukuhara H, Suenaga S, et al. Risk of SOFA deterioration in conservative treatment for emphysematous pyelonephritis: pitfalls of current trends in therapeutics from multicenter clinical experience. Curr Urol. 2019;12(3):134–41.
16. Elawdy MM, Osman Y, Abouelkheir RT, El-Halwagy S, Awad B, El-Mekresh M. Emphysematous pyelonephritis treatment strategies in correlation to the CT classification: have the current experience and prognosis changed? Int Urol Nephrol. 2019:1709–13.
17. Kangjam SM, Irom KS, Khumallambam IS, Sinam RS. Role of conservative Management in Emphysematous Pyelonephritis - a retrospective study. J Clin Diagn Res. 2015;9(11):PC09–11.
18. Eswarappa M, Suryadevara S, John MM, Kumar M, Reddy SB, Suhail M. Emphysematous pyelonephritis case series from South India. Kidney Int Rep. 2018;3(4):950–5.
19. Huang JJ, Tseng CC. Emphysematous pyelonephritis: clinicoradiological classification, management, prognosis, and pathogenesis. Arch Intern Med. 2000;160(6):797–805.
20. Lu YC, Hong JH, Chiang BJ, Pong YH, Hsueh PR, Huang CY, et al. Recommended initial antimicrobial therapy for emphysematous pyelonephritis: 51 cases and 14-year-experience of a tertiary referral center. Medicine. 2016;95(21):e3573.
21. Ideguchi S, Yamamoto K, Ikeda A, Hashimoto K, Takazono T, Saijo T, et al. A case of bilateral emphysematous pyelonephritis caused by Candida albicans. J Infect Chemother. 2019;25(4):302–6.
22. Deoraj S, Zakharious F, Nasim A, Missouris C. Emphysematous pyelonephritis: outcomes of conservative management and literature review. BMJ Case Rep. 2018:bcr-2018-225931.
23. Tilden W, Valliani S, Chana HS. Severe emphysematous pyelonephritis: conservative management plus image-guided percutaneous drainage prior to successful elective nephrectomy. A case report and review of the literature. BJR Case Rep. 2015;1(1):20140004.
24. Sanford TH, Myers F, Chi T, Bagga HS, Taylor AG, Stoller ML. Emphysematous pyelonephritis: the impact of urolithiasis on disease severity. Transl Androl Urol. 2016;5(5):774–9.

Presepsin and procalcitonin as predictors of sepsis based on the new Sepsis-3 definitions in obstructive acute pyelonephritis

Mitsuhiro Tambo*, Satoru Taguchi, Yu Nakamura, Takatsugu Okegawa and Hiroshi Fukuhara

Abstract

Background: Acute pyelonephritis (APN) with obstructive uropathy often causes sepsis. Recently, sepsis was redefined using the sequential organ failure assessment (SOFA) score, based on the new Sepsis-3 criteria. We investigated predictors for sepsis using this new definition in patients with obstructive APN associated with upper urinary tract calculi.

Methods: We retrospectively evaluated patients who were admitted to our hospital for treatment of obstructive APN associated with upper urinary tract calculi. Blood and urine samples were collected before treatment of obstructive APN. Treatment included adequate antimicrobial therapy and emergency drainage to decompress the renal collecting system. We diagnosed sepsis using the new Sepsis-3 definition. We assessed predictors for sepsis by multivariate logistic regression analysis.

Results: Sixty-one patients were included in this study. Overall, all patients underwent emergency drainage, and 11 (18.0%) patients showed sepsis. There were no significant differences in performance status or comorbidities between sepsis and non-sepsis groups. Platelet count and serum albumin level were significantly lower in the sepsis group than in the non-sepsis group ($p = 0.001$ and $p = 0.016$, respectively). Procalcitonin (PCT) and presepsin (PSEP) levels were significantly higher in the sepsis group than in the non-sepsis group ($p < 0.001$ and $p < 0.001$, respectively). Multivariate analysis showed that PCT elevation (OR = 13.12, $p = 0.024$) and PSEP elevation (OR = 13.13, $p = 0.044$) were independent predictors for sepsis.

Conclusions: Elevation of PCT and PSEP levels before treatment might predict the development of sepsis in patients with obstructive APN.

Keywords: Acute pyelonephritis, Upper urinary tract calculi, Sepsis, Procalcitonin, Presepsin

Background

Sepsis is a major cause of morbidity and mortality among hospitalized patients, and its reported incidence is increasing [1]. Until recently, sepsis was defined as the presence of two or more positive systemic inflammatory response syndrome (SIRS) criteria and confirmed infection [2]. However, SIRS criteria are limited in that they exhibit inadequate specificity and sensitivity for dysregulated, life-threatening responses [3]. In 2015, sepsis was redefined (Sepsis-3 criteria) to emphasize the role of organ dysfunction, using the sequential organ failure assessment (SOFA) [4].

* Correspondence: tanbodes@ks.kyorin-u.ac.jp
Department of Urology, Kyorin University School of Medicine, Shikawa 6-20-2, Mitaka, Tokyo 181-8611, Japan

Urosepsis is commonly caused by obstructive disease of the urinary tract, such as urinary stones, stenosis, and tumor, and affects 20–30% of all septic patients [5]. A Japanese multicenter survey revealed that the rate of urosepsis based on SIRS criteria was 35.4% in patients with obstructive acute pyelonephritis (APN) secondary to urolithiasis [6]. A recent retrospective study showed that SOFA was more useful than SIRS for prediction of mortality in patients with APN associated with upper urinary tract calculi [7]. Most previous studies of sepsis have discussed biomarkers for sepsis and septic shock [8]; to the best of our knowledge, there have been no reports regarding markers for sepsis, based on the new definitions, in patients with obstructive APN. Thus, we investigated the predictors for sepsis based on the new definitions in patients with obstructive APN associated with upper urinary tract calculi.

Methods

This retrospective study was based on a medical chart review of patients who were admitted to our institution for the treatment of obstructive APN with upper urinary tract calculi between September 2015 and February 2018. The definition of APN and the regimen of antimicrobial treatment that we used were described in our previous report [8]. Patients who developed APN associated with surgical intervention were excluded from the final cohort to eliminate a potential bias. Prior to the initiation of treatment, blood samples were collected for biochemical and biomarker measurements, including procalcitonin (PCT) and presepsin (PSEP). Patients who had severe chronic kidney disease (estimated glomerular filtration rate [eGFR] < 30 mL/min/1.73 m^2) at baseline were also excluded from the final cohort to minimize the impact of kidney function on PCT and/or PSEP values. The severity of acute kidney injury (AKI) was graded according to the AKI network (AKIN) criteria [9]. Midstream urine and blood culture analyses with antimicrobial susceptibility tests were carried out for all patients. When a responsible bacterium showed resistance to the initial empirical treatment, the antibacterial agent was changed into another one to which the bacterium was susceptible. For the purpose of initial emergency drainage of the renal collecting system, retrograde ureteral stenting was generally carried out for most cases, whereas percutaneous nephrostomy was carried out for those who failed initial treatment or supposedly unfit cases for ureteral stenting (e.g. those who had histories of urinary tract abnormalities or severe hydronephrosis). Detailed procedures for retrograde ureteral stenting and percutaneous nephrostomy were described in our previous report [8].

Sepsis was defined based on the Sepsis-3 criteria. Briefly, patients with suspected infection were evaluated using the quick SOFA (qSOFA) (two or more of the following: respiratory rate ≥ 22/min, altered mental state, and systolic blood pressure ≤ 100 mmHg). Patients with positive for qSOFA and ≥ 2 SOFA score points were diagnosed with sepsis [4]. Performance status was classified in accordance with the Eastern Cooprative Oncology Group performance status classification. Cardiovascular or neurologic diseases and immunocompromised status were described in our previous report [8]. Risk stratification of comorbidity was classified using the Charlson Comorbidity Index [10]. The severity of hydronephrosis was categorized as low-grade and high-grade, as reported previously [8]. This study was approved by the Faculty of Medicine Research Ethics Committee, Kyorin University (approval No. H30–196). The review board waived the requirement for consent due to the retrospective nature of the study.

Statistical analysis

The variables were compared among groups using the Mann–Whitney U-test and Kruskal-Wallis test. The independence of categorical data was estimated by the chi-squared test or Fisher's exact test. Continuous variables (age, serum creatinine level, leukocyte counts, C-reactive protein (CRP) level, platelet count, serum albumin level, PCT level, and PSEP level) were used to divide the patients into two groups by receiver operating characteristic curve analysis. Independent predictors of sepsis were determined using logistic regression analysis. Differences with $p < 0.05$ were considered to be statistically significant. Statistical analyses were conducted using SPSS software (version 18.0, IBM Corp., Armonk, NY, USA).

Results

This study included 61 patients. Median patient age was 64 years, 24 patients were male and 37 patients were female. In total, five patients (8.2%) exhibited poor performance status (2–4). Of the 61 patients, there were 16, eight, six, three, and two with diabetes mellitus, cardiovascular diseases, neurologic diseases, immunocompromised status, and urinary tract abnormalities, respectively. Median serum creatinine was 1.22 mg/dL. Overall, 41 patients (67.2%) showed a large shift in leukocyte count (< 4000 or $> 12{,}000$/μL). Twenty and 19 patients exhibited reduced platelet count ($< 150{,}000$/μL) and reduced serum albumin level (< 3.1 g/dL), respectively. Median PCT and PSEP levels were 1.49 ng/mL and 445 pg/mL, respectively. PCT and PSEP levels increased significantly with the severity of AKI (Table 1). In total, 54 (88.5%) and 22 patients (36.1%) showed bacterial growth in midstream urine culture and blood culture, respectively.

Most stones were located in the ureter (90.2%). The median longest and shortest diameters of stones were 8.0 mm and 5.0 mm, respectively. Overall, 22 patients (36.1%) had high-grade hydronephrosis. Fifty-six (91.8%)

Table 1 PCT and PSEP stratified by AKI grade according to the AKIN criteria

Variables	AKI grade				*P*-value
	Grade 0 (*n* = 20)	Grade 1 (*n* = 34)	Grade 2 (*n* = 3)	Grade 3 (*n* = 4)	
PCT, median (ng/mL)	0.40	1.89	84.45	113.46	0.015
PSEP, median (pg/mL)	335	528	835	740	0.001

PCT Procalcitonin, *PSEP* Presepsin, *AKI* Acute kidney injury, *AKIN* Acute kidney injury network

and five patients (8.2%) underwent indwelling ureteral stenting and nephrostomy, respectively, to achieve decompression of the collecting system. The median duration from initial treatment to decompression of the collecting system was 1.0 days.

In total, 11 patients (18.0%) were positive for sepsis, using the Sepsis-3 criteria (Fig. 1). One patient (1.6%) died of the infection. Age did not significantly differ between sepsis and non-sepsis groups ($p = 0.209$). Performance status and underlying diseases did not significantly differ between sepsis and non-sepsis groups. With respect to laboratory data before treatment, platelet count and serum albumin level were significantly lower in the sepsis group than in the non-sepsis group ($p = 0.001$ and $p = 0.016$, respectively). However, inflammatory markers (leukocyte count and CRP level) and serum creatinine did not significantly differ between sepsis and non-sepsis groups ($p = 0.073$, $p = 0.586$, and $p = 0.058$, respectively). PCT and PSEP levels were significantly higher in the sepsis group than in the non-sepsis group ($p < 0.001$ and $p < 0.001$, respectively). There were no significant differences in stone characteristics between the sepsis and non-sepsis groups (Table 2).

Multivariate logistic regression analysis showed that elevated PCT and PSEP levels were predictors for sepsis in patients who had obstructive APN associated with upper urinary tract calculi (Table 3).

Discussion

The present study showed that elevated PCT and PSEP levels before treatment might be independent predictors for sepsis, based on the Sepsis-3 criteria, in patients with obstructive APN. Obstructive APN can be lethal, and a

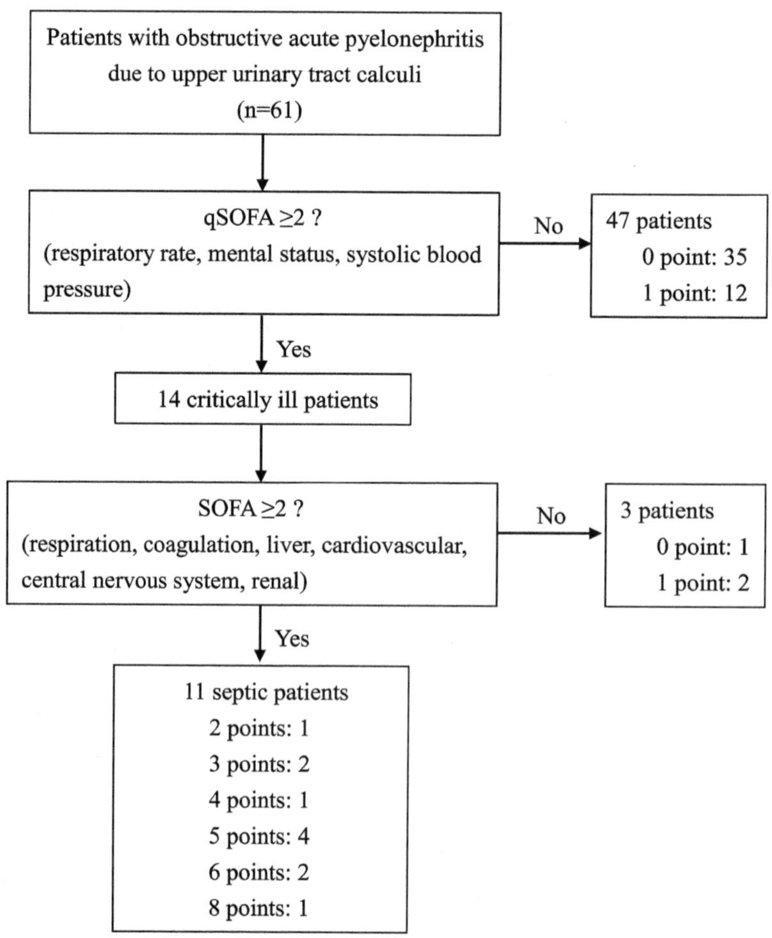

Fig. 1 Flow chart representing the diagnostic process of sepsis according to the Sepsis-3 criteria

Table 2 Characteristics of patients with and without sepsis

Variables			Sepsis group		Non-sepsis group		*P*-value
			n	%	n	%	
Patients			11		50		
Age (yr)		Median [IQR]	73 [55–77]		61 [52–76]		0.209
Gender		Male	3	27.3	21	42.0	
		Female	8	72.7	29	58.0	0.365
Performance status		0, 1	9	81.8	47	94.0	
		2, 3	2	18.2	3	6.0	0.182
Diabetes mellitus		Negative	8	72.7	37	74.0	
		Positive	3	27.3	13	26.0	0.931
Cardiovascular or neurologic disease		Negative	7	63.6	42	84.0	
		Positive	4	36.4	8	16.0	0.124
Immunocompromised status		Negative	10	90.9	48	96.0	
		Positive	1	9.1	2	4.0	0.480
CCI scores		0–2	8	72.7	47	94.0	
		≥3	3	27.3	3	6.0	0.066
Serum creatinine (mg/dL)		Median [IQR]	1.50 [1.22–2.14]		1.17 [0.78–1.70]		0.058
Leukocyte counts ($\times 10^3/\mu L$)		Median [IQR]	18.3 [10.0–22.3]		12.8 [10.1–15.5]		0.073
C-reactive protein (mg/dL)		Median [IQR]	14.17 [4.84–24.51]		10.72 [6.66–16.34]		0.586
Platelet counts ($\times 10^4/\mu L$)		Median [IQR]	10.1 [6.1–14.8]		19.2 [15.5–26.9]		0.001
Serum albumin (g/dL)		Median [IQR]	3.0 [2.6–3.5]		3.6 [3.2–4.0]		0.016
PCT (ng/mL)		Median [IQR]	31.57 [1.83–134.40]		0.54 [0.14–4.86]		< 0.001
PSEP (pg/mL)		Median [IQR]	1080 [696–1550]		387 [313–558]		< 0.001
Midstream urine culture		Negative	0	0.0	7	14.0	
		Positive	11	100.0	43	86.0	0.187
Blood culture		Negative	1	9.1	38	76.0	
		Positive	10	90.9	12	24.0	< 0.001
Hydronephrosis		Low-grade	7	63.6	32	64.0	
		High-grade	4	36.4	18	36.0	0.982
Laterality of stone		Right	5	45.5	25	50.0	
		Left	6	54.5	25	50.0	0.785
Position of stone		Renal pelvis or PUJ	2	18.2	4	8.0	
		Upper ureter	6	54.5	29	58.0	
		Mid ureter	1	9.1	8	16.0	
		Lower ureter	2	18.2	9	18.0	0.738
Size of stone (mm)	Longest diameter	Median [IQR]	7.0 [5.0–12.0]		8.0 [6.0–10.0]		0.806
	Shortest diameter	Median [IQR]	4.0 [3.0–8.0]		5.0 [4.0–7.0]		0.842
Drainage		Ureteral stent	10	90.9	46	92.0	
		Nephrostomy	1	9.1	4	8.0	0.905

CCI Charlson Comorbidity Index, *PCT* Procalcitonin, *PSEP* Presepsin, *PUJ* Pelvic ureteral junction

recent survey revealed a mortality rate of 2.3% [6]. Based on the new definition, a diagnosis of sepsis is associated [11]. Thus, patients who have obstructive APN and who have elevated PCT and PSEP levels before treatment might exhibit a risk of mortality. However, in adult patients with uncomplicated APN, Cleassens et al. reported that the performance of PSEP level for prediction of positive blood culture (area under the receiver operating characteristic curve [AUC] = 0.63) was similar to that of CRP level (AUC = 0.64) and less accurate than that of PCT level (AUC = 0.78, $p < 0.001$) [12]. The limitations of the study by Cleassens et al. included a low rate of bacterial

Table 3 Odds ratio for sepsis in relation to various factors by logistic regression analysis

Variables		Univariate			Multivariate		
		OR	95% CI	*p*-value	OR	95% CI	*p*-value
Age (yr)	64≥	Ref					
	64<	3.13	(0.74–13.20)	0.120			
Gender	Male	Ref					
	Female	1.93	(0.46–8.16)	0.370			
Performance status	0, 1	Ref					
	2, 3	3.48	(0.51–23.89)	0.204			
Diabetes mellitus	Negative	Ref					
	Positive	1.07	(0.25–4.64)	0.930			
Cardiovascular or neurologic disease	Negative	Ref					
	Positive	3.00	(0.71–12.69)	0.136			
Immunocompromised status	Negative	Ref					
	Positive	2.40	(0.20–29.10)	0.492			
History of urinary tract abnormalities	Negative	Ref					
	Positive	1.21	(0.15–9.82)	0.860			
CCI scores	0–2	Ref					
	≥3	5.87	(1.00–34.39)	0.050			
Serum creatinine (mg/dL)	1.26≥	Ref					
	1.26<	3.39	(0.80–14.32)	0.096			
Leukocyte counts (×10^3/μL)	13.1≥	Ref					
	13.1<	3.13	(0.74–13.20)	0.120			
C-reactive protein (mg/dL)	10.83≥	Ref					
	10.83<	1.20	(0.32–4.45)	0.785			
Platelet counts (×10^4/μL)	15.0≤	Ref			Ref		
	15.0>	15.95	(3.00–84.92)	0.001	3.23	(0.39–26.64)	0.276
Serum albumin (g/dL)	3.1≤	Ref			Ref		
	3.1>	5.54	(1.38–22.24)	0.016	1.21	(0.15–9.82)	0.860
PCT (ng/mL)	23.55≥	Ref			Ref		
	23.55<	30.67	(5.75–163.67)	< 0.001	13.12	(1.41–122.03)	0.024
PSEP (pg/mL)	515≥	Ref			Ref		
	515<	23.33	(2.73–198.87)	0.004	13.13	(1.07–161.45)	0.044

CCI Charlson Comorbidity Index, *PCT* Procalcitonin, *PSEP* Presepsin, *OR* Odds ratio, *CI* Confidence interval

detection in blood culture of sepsis patients, and low rate of sepsis in patients with uncomplicated APN.

A recent meta-analysis showed that PCT and PSEP levels had moderate diagnostic value for sepsis [13]. However, most previous studies reported that patients had SIRS and/or severe sepsis/septic shock. In addition, in a clinical study of sepsis based on the new definitions, multivariate analysis showed that patients who were admitted to the intensive care unit with high PSEP and PCT levels had significantly higher risk of sepsis, compared with that of patients with low PSEP and PCT levels [14]. The limitations of that study included the use of SIRS criteria for initial screening.

PCT is a prohormone of calcitonin; under normal conditions, it is only produced in C-cells of the thyroid gland. During infection, PCT can be produced by several cell types and many organs in response to pro-inflammatory cytokines (e.g., tumor necrosis factor-α and interleukin-6). Because it shows an early increase during infection, PCT is a useful biomarker for infection [15]. PSEP is the soluble form of CD14, a membrane-based receptor that is expressed by macrophages and monocytes. PSEP is a complex product of CD14 cleavage that is released into the general circulation by proteolysis and exocytosis, which occur following bacterial antigen binding. PSEP levels are presumed to increase during early stages of bacterial infections, and may depend on the intensity of innate immune induction [16]. In an animal model of sepsis, PSEP in the blood was detected within 2 h and peaked after 3 h, while PCT was elevated within 3–6 h and peaked at 6–8 h [17]. In contrast, elevated CRP levels have been found within 6–8 h of infection and peak after 36–50 h [18].

There were several limitations in this study. First, patients with severe chronic kidney disease (GFR < 30 mL/min/1.73 m^2) were excluded from analysis. PSEP levels inversely correlate with GFR, and PSEP levels in patients with GFR < 30 mL/min/1.73 m^2 were reportedly significantly higher than those in patients with GFR ≥ 30 mL/min/1.73 m^2 [19]. The evaluation of PSEP levels in patients with chronic kidney disease thus requires special considerations, such that the present results may not be generalizable to those patients. In the present study, three patients with GFR < 30 mL/min/1.73 m^2 demonstrated PSEP levels of 1150 pg/mL, 889 pg/mL, and 3620 pg/mL, respectively; all were negative for sepsis. Second, levels of PCT and PSEP could be influenced by acute kidney injury (AKI). Recently, a retrospective study in patients with AKI showed that different thresholds of PSEP and PCT levels might be useful markers of bacterial infections [20]. Another study demonstrated that the accuracy of sepsis diagnosis based on PCT level was significantly higher than that based on PSEP level in patients with severe AKI [21]. However, the values for cutoff levels, depending on renal function, remain controversial. Finally, our results were limited to a small number of enrolled patients and were retrospectively collected. Further studies should include larger prospective cohorts.

Conclusions

Elevated PCT and PSEP levels before treatment might predict the development of sepsis in patients with obstructive APN.

Abbreviations

AKI: Acute kidney injury; AKIN: Acute kidney injury network; APN: Acute pyelonephritis; CRP: C-reactive protein; PCT: Procalcitonin; PSEP: Presepsin; qSOFA: quick SOFA; SIRS: Systemic inflammatory response syndrome; SOFA: Sequential organ failure assessment

Acknowledgments

The authors thank Ryan Chastain-Gross, Ph.D., from Edanz Group (www.edanzediting.com/ac) for editing a draft of this manuscript.

Authors' contributions

MT performed project development, data collection, data analysis, and manuscript writing. ST contributed to data collection, data analysis, and manuscript editing. YN contributed to data collection and data analysis. TO and HF performed project development and manuscript editing. All authors read and approved the final manuscript.

References

1. Gaieski DF, Edwards JM, Kallan MJ, Carr BG. Benchmarking the incidence and mortality of severe sepsis in the unites states. Crit Care Med. 2013;41:1167–74.
2. Levy MM, Fink MP, Marshall JC, Abraham E, Angus D, Cook D, et al. 2001 SCCM/ESICM/ACCP/ATS/SIS international sepsis definitions conference. Intensive Care Med. 2003;29:530–8.
3. Churpek MM, Zadravecz FJ, Winslow C, Howell MD, Edelson DP. Incidence and prognostic value of the systemic inflammatory response syndrome and organ dysfunctions in ward patients. Am J Respir Crit Care Med. 2015;192:958–64.
4. Singer M, Deutschman CS, Seymour CW, Shankar-Hari M, Annane D, Bauer M, et al. The third international consensus definitions for sepsis and septic shock (Sepsis-3). JAMA. 2016;315:801–10.
5. Brun-Buisson C. The epidemiology of the systemic inflammatory response. Intensive Care Med. 2000;26(Suppl 1):64–74.
6. Hamasuna R, Takahashi S, Nagae H, Kubo T, Yamamoto S, Arakawa S, et al. Obstructive pyelonephritis as a result of urolithiasis in Japan: diagnosis, treatment and prognosis. Int J Urol. 2015;22:294–300.
7. Fukushima H, Kobayashi M, Kawano K, Morimoto S. Performance of quick sequential (sepsis related) and sequential (sepsis related) organ failure assessment to predict mortality in patients with acute pyelonephritis associated with upper urinary tract calculi. J Urol. 2018;199:1526–33.
8. Tambo M, Okegawa T, Shishido T, Higashihara E, Nutahara K. Predictors of septic shock in obstructive acute pyelonephritis. World J Urol. 2014;32:803–11.
9. Mehta RL, Kellum JA, Shah SV, Molitoris BA, Ronco C, Warnock DG, et al. Acute kidney injury network: report of an initiative to improve outcomes in acute kidney injury. Crit Care. 2007;11:R31.
10. Frenkel WJ, Jongerius EJ, Mandjes-van Uitert MJ, van Munster BC, de Rooij SE. Validation of the Charlson comorbidity index in acutely hospitalized elderly adults: a prospective cohort study. J Am Geriatr Soc. 2014;62:342–6.
11. Seymour CW, Liu VX, Iwashyna TJ, Brunkhorst FM, Rea TD, Scherag A, et al. Assessment of clinical criteria for sepsis: for the third international consensus definitions for sepsis and septic shock (Sepsis-3). JAMA. 2016;315:762–74.
12. Claessens YE, Trabattoni E, Grabar S, Quinquis L, Der Sahakian G, Anselmo M, et al. Plasmatic presepsin (sCD14-ST) concentrations in acute pyelonephritis in adult patients. Clin Chim Acta. 2017;464:182–8.
13. Wu CC, Lan HM, Han ST, Chaou CH, Yeh CF, Liu SH, et al. Comparison of diagnostic accuracy in sepsis between presepsin, procalcitonin, and C-reactive protein: a systematic review and meta-analysis. Ann Intensive Care. 2017;7:91.
14. Yamamoto T, Nishimura T, Kaga S, Uchida K, Tachibana Y, Esaki M, et al. Diagnostic accuracy of presepsin for sepsis by the new Sepsis-3 definitions. Am J Emerg Med. 2019;37(10):1936. https://doi.org/10.1016/j.ajem.2019.01.025.
15. Wacker C, Prkno A, Brunkhorst FM, Schlattmann P. Procalcitonin as a diagnostic marker for sepsis: a systematic review and meta-analysis. Lancet Infect Dis. 2013;13:426–35.
16. Chenevier-Gobeaux C, Borderie D, Weiss N, Mallet-Coste T, Claessens YE. Presepsin (sCD14-ST), an innate immune response marker in sepsis. Clin Chim Acta. 2015;450:97–103.
17. Maruna P, Nedelnikova K, Gürlich R. Physiology and genetics of procalcitonin. Physiol Res. 2000;49(Suppl.1):57–61.
18. Lelubre C, Anselin S, Zouaoui Boudjeltia K, Biston P, Piagnerelli M. Interpretation of C-reactive protein concentrations in critically ill patients. Biomed Res Int. 2013. https://doi.org/10.1155/2013/124021.
19. Nagata T, Yasuda Y, Ando M, Abe T, Katsuno T, Kato S, et al. Clinical impact of kidney function on presepsin levels. PLoS One. 2015;10:e0129159.
20. Takahashi G, Shibata S, Fukui Y, Okamura Y, Inoue Y. Diagnostic accuracy of procalcitonin and presepsin for infectious disease in patients with acute kidney injury. Diagn Microbiol Infect Dis. 2016;86:205–10.
21. Nakamura Y, Hoshino K, Kiyomi F, Kawano Y, Mizunuma M, Tanaka J, et al. Comparison of accuracy of presepsin and procalcitonin concentrations in diagnosing sepsis in patients with and without acute kidney injury. Clin Chim Acta. 2019;490:200–6.

Permissions

All chapters in this book were first published by BioMed Central; hereby published with permission under the Creative Commons Attribution License or equivalent. Every chapter published in this book has been scrutinized by our experts. Their significance has been extensively debated. The topics covered herein carry significant findings which will fuel the growth of the discipline. They may even be implemented as practical applications or may be referred to as a beginning point for another development.

The contributors of this book come from diverse backgrounds, making this book a truly international effort. This book will bring forth new frontiers with its revolutionizing research information and detailed analysis of the nascent developments around the world.

We would like to thank all the contributing authors for lending their expertise to make the book truly unique. They have played a crucial role in the development of this book. Without their invaluable contributions this book wouldn't have been possible. They have made vital efforts to compile up to date information on the varied aspects of this subject to make this book a valuable addition to the collection of many professionals and students.

This book was conceptualized with the vision of imparting up-to-date information and advanced data in this field. To ensure the same, a matchless editorial board was set up. Every individual on the board went through rigorous rounds of assessment to prove their worth. After which they invested a large part of their time researching and compiling the most relevant data for our readers.

The editorial board has been involved in producing this book since its inception. They have spent rigorous hours researching and exploring the diverse topics which have resulted in the successful publishing of this book. They have passed on their knowledge of decades through this book. To expedite this challenging task, the publisher supported the team at every step. A small team of assistant editors was also appointed to further simplify the editing procedure and attain best results for the readers.

Apart from the editorial board, the designing team has also invested a significant amount of their time in understanding the subject and creating the most relevant covers. They scrutinized every image to scout for the most suitable representation of the subject and create an appropriate cover for the book.

The publishing team has been an ardent support to the editorial, designing and production team. Their endless efforts to recruit the best for this project, has resulted in the accomplishment of this book. They are a veteran in the field of academics and their pool of knowledge is as vast as their experience in printing. Their expertise and guidance has proved useful at every step. Their uncompromising quality standards have made this book an exceptional effort. Their encouragement from time to time has been an inspiration for everyone.

The publisher and the editorial board hope that this book will prove to be a valuable piece of knowledge for researchers, students, practitioners and scholars across the globe.

List of Contributors

Yang Pan, Gang Chen, Han Chen, Yunxiao Zhu and Hualin Chen
Department of Urology, The First Affiliated Hospital of Chongqing Medical University, No. 1 Road Youyi, Yuzhong District, Chongqing, China

I. B. Osipov, D. A. Lebedev and M. V. Lifanova
Urology Department, State Pediatric Medical University, 2 Litovskaya Street, build.2, St. Petersburg, Russian Federation

Jindong Zhang, Liang Gao, Changlong Li, Xiaokang Yang, Yusheng Lei and Chuan Liu
Department of Urology, the Second Affiliated Hospital of Chongqing Medical University, Chongqing 400000, China

Stephen Fôn Hughes and Peter Ella-tongwiis
North Wales & North West Urological Research Centre, Betsi Cadwaladr University Health Board (BCUHB) Wrexham Maelor Hospital, Wrexham, Wales, UK
North Wales Clinical Research Centre, Betsi Cadwaladr University Health Board (BCUHB) Wrexham Maelor Hospital, Wrexham, Wales, UK

Alyson Jayne Moyes
North Wales & North West Urological Research Centre, Betsi Cadwaladr University Health Board (BCUHB) Wrexham Maelor Hospital, Wrexham, Wales, UK
School of Medical Sciences, Bangor University, Bangor, Wales, UK
Department of Biological Sciences, University of Chester, Chester, UK

Rebecca May Lamb
North Wales & North West Urological Research Centre, Betsi Cadwaladr University Health Board (BCUHB) Wrexham Maelor Hospital, Wrexham, Wales, UK
Department of Biological Sciences, University of Chester, Chester, UK

Christopher Bell and Ahmed Moussa
North Wales Clinical Research Centre, Betsi Cadwaladr University Health Board (BCUHB) Wrexham Maelor Hospital, Wrexham, Wales, UK
The Alan de Bolla Department of Urology, BCUHB Wrexham Maelor Hospital, Wrexham, Wales, UK

Iqbal Shergill
North Wales & North West Urological Research Centre, Betsi Cadwaladr University Health Board (BCUHB) Wrexham Maelor Hospital, Wrexham, Wales, UK
North Wales Clinical Research Centre, Betsi Cadwaladr University Health Board (BCUHB) Wrexham Maelor Hospital, Wrexham, Wales, UK
The Alan de Bolla Department of Urology, BCUHB Wrexham Maelor Hospital, Wrexham, Wales, UK

Katherine J. Cockerill, Amanda E. Kahn and David D. Thiel
Department of Urology, Mayo Clinic, 4500 San Pablo Road, Jacksonville, FL 32224, USA

Stacy M. Young
Department of Health Sciences Research, Mayo Clinic, Jacksonville, FL, USA

Colleen T. Ball
Division of Biomedical Statistics and Informatics, Mayo Clinic, Jacksonville, FL, USA

Martin L. Mai, C. Burcin Taner and Dana K. Perry
Department of Transplantation, Mayo Clinic, Jacksonville, FL, USA

Xiang Le, Hao Zhao, Ren-Fu Chen and Peng Ge
Department of Urology, the Affiliated Hospital of Xuzhou Medical University, Xuzhou, Jiangsu, China

Xiang-Bo Wang
Department of Pathology, the Affiliated Hospital of Xuzhou Medical University, Xuzhou, Jiangsu, China

Jonas Busch and Monika Jung
Department of Urology, Charité - Universitätsmedizin Berlin, corporate member of Freie Universität Berlin, Humboldt-Universität zu Berlin and Berlin Institute of Health, Berlin, Germany

Klaus Jung and Anja Rabien
Department of Urology, Charité - Universitätsmedizin Berlin, corporate member of Freie Universität Berlin, Humboldt-Universität zu Berlin and Berlin Institute of Health, Berlin, Germany
Berlin Institute for Urologic Research, Berlin, Germany

Sinisa Simonovic
Department of Urology, Charité - Universitätsmedizin Berlin, corporate member of Freie Universität Berlin, Humboldt-Universität zu Berlin and Berlin Institute of Health, Berlin, Germany
Berlin Institute for Urologic Research, Berlin, Germany
Max-Delbrück-Center for Molecular Medicine (MDC), Berlin, Germany

Christian Hinze
Max-Delbrück-Center for Molecular Medicine (MDC), Berlin, Germany

Kai M. Schmidt-Ott
Max-Delbrück-Center for Molecular Medicine (MDC), Berlin, Germany
Department of Nephrology and Medical Intensive Care, Charité - Universitätsmedizin Berlin, Berlin, Germany

Bin Yang, Haizhui Xia, Chuxiao Xu, Shudong Zhang, Guoliang Wang and Lulin Ma
Department of Urology, Peking University Third Hospital, 49 North Garden Road, Haidian District, Beijing 100191, People's Republic of China

Min Lu
Department of Pathology, Peking University Health Science Center, Beijing, China

Hongzeng Wu, Yi Zhao and Helin Feng
Department of Orthopedics, The Fourth Hospital of Hebei Medical University, 12 Health Road, Shijiazhuang, Hebei 050011, People's Republic of China

Ruoqi Han
Department of Breast Surgery, The Fourth Hospital of Hebei Medical University, 12 Health Road, Shijiazhuang, Hebei 050011, People's Republic of China

Qianqian Zhang
Department of Gynecology, Hebei Medical University Second Affiliated Hospital, 215 Heping Road, Shijiazhuang, Hebei 050011, People's Republic of China

Félix Couture and Patrick O. Richard
Division of Urology, Department of Surgery, Centre Hospitalier Universitaire de Sherbrooke, 3001, 12e avenue N, Sherbrooke, Quebec J1H 5N4, Canada

Antonio Finelli
Division of Urology, Department of Surgery, Princess Margaret Cancer Centre, University Health Network and the University of Toronto, Toronto, Canada

Amélie Tétu
Unité de recherche clinique et épidémiologique, Centre de Recherche, Centre Hospitalier Universitaire de Sherbrooke, Sherbrooke, Canada

Bimal Bhindi
Division of Urology, Department of Surgery, Southern Alberta Institute of Urology, Calgary, Canada

Rodney H. Breau and Luke Lavallée
Division of Urology, Department of Surgery, Ottawa Hospital, Ottawa Hospital Research Institute and University of Ottawa, Ottawa, Canada

Anil Kapoor
Division of Urology, Department of Surgery, Juravinski Hospital, St. Joseph Healthcare, McMaster University, Hamilton, Canada

Wassim Kassouf and Simon Tanguay
Division of Urology, Department of Surgery, McGill University Health Centre, McGill University, Montreal, Canada

Philippe D. Violette
Division of Urology, Department of Surgery, Woodstock Hospital, Woodstock, Canada

X. A. Sabaté Arroyo, J. L. Bauzà Quetglas, J. Guimerà Garcia and E. Pieras Ayala
Hospital Universitari Son Espases, Ctra. Valldemossa, 79, Palma de Mallorca, Spain

F. Grases Freixedas
Universitat de les Illes Balears. IUNICS, Ctra. de Valldemossa, Km. 7.5, Palma de Mallorca, Spain

G. Tsironis, M. Liontos, A. Kyriazoglou, K. Koutsoukos, A. Tsiara, M. Kaparelou, R. Zakopoulou, A. Cohen, E. Skafida, F. Zagouri, A. Bamias and M. A. Dimopoulos
Oncology Unit, Department of Clinical Therapeutics, Alexandra Hospital, Athens, Greece

S. Fontara
1st Department of Radiology, Aretaieio University hospital, Athens, Greece

Maximilian Pallauf, Christopher Steiner, Martin Drerup, Michael Mitterberger, Daniela Colleselli, Lukas Lusuardi and Thomas Kunit
Landeskrankenhaus Salzburg - Universitätsklinikum der Paracelsus Medizinischen Privatuniversität, Universitätsklinik für Urologie und Andrologie, Müllner Hauptstraße 48, 5020 Salzburg, Austria

Sabina Sevcenco
Abteilung für Urologie und Andrologie, Sozialmedizinisches Zentrum Ost – Donauspital, Langobardenstraße 122, 1220 Wien, Austria

Xiaobo Ding
Department of Radiology, First Hospital of Jilin University, Changchun, Jilin 130021, P.R. China

Gang Wang
Second Operating Room, First Hospital of Jilin University, Changchun, Jilin 130021, P.R. China

Tiejun Wang
Department of Orthopedic Traumatology, First Hospital of Jilin University, Changchun, Jilin 130021, P.R. China

Xiaobo Ma
Department of Pathology, First Hospital of Jilin University, Changchun, Jilin 130021, P.R. China

Yanbo Wang
Department of Urology, First Hospital of Jilin University, Changchun, Jilin 130021, P.R. China

Spencer Larkin and Jeremy Johnson
Department of Urology, University of Kentucky, Lexington, KY, USA

Trisha Venkatesh
Washington University in St. Louis, St. Louis, MO, USA

Joel Vetter and Ramakrishna Venkatesh
Division of Urology Surgery, Washington University School of Medicine, 4960, Children's place, Campus St. Louis, MO 63110, USA

Thiago Camelo Mourão and Walter H. da Costa
A.C. Camargo Cancer Center, Rua Antônio Prudente 211, Liberdade, São Paulo 01509-010, Brazil

Diego Abreu and Ricardo Decia
Pasteur Hospital, Montevideo, Uruguay

Gustavo F. Carvalhal
São Lucas Hospital - PUCRS, Porto Alegre, Brazil

Guillermo Gueglio
Italian Hospital, Buenos Aires, Argentina

Vinicius Fernando Calsavara
Epidemiology and Statistics Department, International Research Center, A.C.Camargo Cancer Center, São Paulo, Brazil

Luis Meza-Montoya
Instituto Nacional de Enfermedades Neoplásicas, Lima, Peru

Rubén G. Bengió
Urological Center Profesor Bengió, Cordoba, Argentina

Carlos Scorticati
Clinics Hospital José de San Martín, Buenos Aires, Argentina

Ricardo Castillejos-Molina and Francisco Rodríguez-Covarrubias
Instituto Nacional de Ciencias Médicas y Nutrición Salvador Zubirán (INCNSZ), Mexico City, Mexico

Ana María Autran-Gómez
Jiménez Díaz Foundation, Madrid, Spain

José Gadu Campos-Salcedo
Military Hospital, Mexico City, Mexico

Alejandro Nolazco
British Hospital, Buenos Aires, Argentina

Carlos Ameri
German Hospital, Buenos Aires, Argentina

Hamilton Zampolli
Instituto Arnaldo Vieira de Carvalho, São Paulo, Brazil

Raúl Langenhin and Diego Muguruza
Corporación Médica de Paysandú (COMEPA), Paysandu, Uruguay

Marcos Tobias Machado
Instituto Arnaldo Vieira de Carvalho, São Paulo, Brazil
16ABC Medical School, São Paulo, Brazil

Pablo Mingote
Policlinico Neuquén, Neuquen, Argentina

Jorge Clavijo
Clinics Hospital, Montevideo, Uruguay

Lucas Nogueira
Federal University of Minas Gerais, Belo Horizonte, Brazil

Omar Clark
Military Hospital, Montevideo, Uruguay

Agustín R. Rovegno
Centro de Educación Médica e Investigaciones Clínicas (CEMIC), Buenos Aires, Argentina

Fernando P. Secin
San Lázaro Foundation and FUNDES, Buenos Aires, Argentina

Gustavo C. Guimarães
Surgical Oncology Coordinator at Beneficencia Portuguesa Hospital, São Paulo, Brazil

Sidney Glina
ABC Medical School, São Paulo, Brazil
Ipiranga Hospital, São Paulo, Brazil

Oscar Rodríguez-Faba and Joan Palou
Puigvert Foundation, Barcelona, Spain

Stenio C. Zequi
A.C. Camargo Cancer Center, Rua Antônio Prudente 211, Liberdade, São Paulo 01509-010, Brazil
National Institute for Science and Technology in Oncogenomics and Therapeutic Innovation, AC Camargo Cancer Center, São Paulo, Brazil

Bashar Darayseh and Najla Aldaoud
Department of Pathology and Microbiology, Jordan University of Science and Technology, Irbid 22110, Jordan

Amer Hallak
Faculty of Medicine, Jordan University of Science and Technology, Irbid, Jordan

Liqa A. Rousan
Department of Diagnostic and Interventional Radiology and Nuclear Medicine, Jordan
University of Science and Technology, Irbid, Jordan

Omar Halalsheh
Department of Surgery and Urology, Jordan University of Science and Technology, Irbid, Jordan

Mousa A. Al-Abbadi
Department of Pathology, Microbiology and Forensic Medicine, School of Medicine, University of Jordan, Amman, Jordan

Wei Jia, Zikuan Zhang, Qian Chen and Yuan Shao
Shanxi Medical University, Taiyuan 030001, Shanxi, People's Republic of China

Bo Wu
Department of Urology, First Hospital of Shanxi Medical University, Taiyuan 030001, Shanxi, People's Republic of China

Dongwen Wang
Shanxi Medical University, Taiyuan 030001, Shanxi, People's Republic of China
National Cancer Center/National Clinical Research Center for Cancer/Cancer Hospital & Shenzhen Hospital, Chinese Academy of Medical Sciences and Peking Union Medical College, Shenzhen 518116, People's Republic of China

Mancheng Xia, Haosen Yang, Keqiang Yin and Yusheng Wang
First Clinical Medical College, Shanxi Medical University, No. 85, JieFang South Road, Yingze District, Taiyuan 030001, Shanxi, China

Chun Liu and Weibing Shuang
Department of Urology, The First Hospital of Shanxi Medical University, No. 85, JieFang South Road, Yingze District, Taiyuan 030001, Shanxi, China

Xunan Tong
Kidney Transplantation Centre, Shanxi Second People's Hospital, Taiyuan, Shanxi, China

Siyu Zhang
Department of Pathology, Shanxi People's Hospital, Taiyuan, Shanxi, China

Yuanfeng Zhang, Chengguo Ge, Junyong Zhang and Peihe Liang
Department of Urology, The Second Affiliated Hospital of Chongqing Medical University, Yuzhong, Chongqing 400010, China

Xirong Zhang
Department of Urology, The Second Affiliated Hospital of Chongqing Medical University, Yuzhong, Chongqing 400010, China
Department of Urology, Jiangmen Central Hospital, Jiangmen 529030, Guangdong, China

Naotaka Nishiyama, Takuya Kikushima and Hiroshi Kitamura
Department of Urology, Faculty of Medicine, University of Toyama, 2630 Sugitani, Toyama 930-0194, Japan

Megumi hirobe, Masahiro Matsuki and Naoya Masumori
Department of Urology, Sapporo Medical University School of Medicine, Sapporo, Japan

Atsushi Takahashi
Department of Urology, Hakodate Goryoukaku Hospital, Hakodate, Japan

Masahiro Yanase
Department of Urology, Sunagawa City Medical Center, Sunagawa, Japan

Keisuke Ichimatsu and Masayuki Egawa
Department of Urology, Tonami general hospital, Tonami, Japan

Norihiro Hayashi
Department of Urology, Takaoka city hospital, Takaoka, Japan

Takahito Negishi
Department of Urology, National Hospital Organization Kyushu Cancer Center, Fukuoka, Hakata, Japan

Jungyo Suh
Department of Urology, Seoul National University College of Medicine, Seoul, South Korea
Hospital Medicine Center, Seoul National University Hospital, Seoul, South Korea

Chang Wook Jeong, Ja Hyeon Ku, Hyeon Hoe Kim and Cheol Kwak
Department of Urology, Seoul National University College of Medicine, Seoul, South Korea

Seongmin Choi
Department of Medicine, Seoul National University College of Medicine, Seoul, South Korea

Kwangsoo Kim
Transdisciplinary Department of Medicine & Advanced Technology, Seoul National University Hospital, Seoul, South Korea

Wan-Zhang Liu, Ting Huang, Li Fang and Yue Cheng
Department of Urology, NingBo First Hospital, NingBo Hospital of ZheJiang University, #59 Liuting Street, NingBo City 315000, Zhejiang Province, China

Bruno Minotti
Emergency Department, Cantonal Hospital of St. Gallen, Rorschacher Strasse 95, CH-9007 St. Gallen, Switzerland

Giorgio Treglia
Heath Technology Assessment Unit, Ente Ospedaliero Cantonale, Bellinzona, Switzerland

Mariarosa Pascale
Clinical Trial Unit, Ente Ospedaliero Cantonale, Bellinzona, Switzerland

Samuele Ceruti
Department of Intensive Care Medicine, Clinica Luganese, Lugano, Switzerland

Laura Cantini, Luciano Anselmi and Andrea Saporito
Department of Anesthesia, Ospedale San Giovanni, Bellinzona, Switzerland

Wenyuan Zhuang, Ning Liu, Hongqian Guo and Weidong Gan
Department of Urology, Nanjing Drum Tower Hospital, Medical School of Nanjing University, Institute of Urology, Nanjing University, 321 Zhongshan Road, Nanjing 210008, China

Chunni Zhang
Department of Clinical Laboratory, Jinling Hospital, State Key Laboratory of Analytical Chemistry for Life Science, Jiangsu Engineering Research Center for MicroRNA Biology and Biotechnology, Nanjing University School of Medicine, Nanjing University, Nanjing, China

Zhu Wang, Ying Zhang, Qiong Deng, Rui Sun, Qi-yi Hu, Sheng-ping Zhang, Jian-wen Zhang and Hui Liang
Department of Urology, People's Hospital of Longhua, Southern Medical University, Shenzhen 518109, Guangdong, China

Ming-xing Li
Laboratory of Molecular Pharmacology, Department of Pharmacology, School of Pharmacy, Southwest Medical University, Luzhou 646000, Sichuan, China

Chang-zhi Xu
Department of Laboratory Medicine, Third Affiliated Hospital of Sun Yat-sen University, Guangzhou, Guangdong 510630, People's Republic of China

Nusret Can Cilesiz, Arif Ozkan, Arif Kalkanli and Burak Arslan
Department of Urology, GOP Taksim Education Training and Research Hospital, Karayolları Str. No:621 Gaziosmanpasa, İstanbul, Turkey

Ali Eroglu
Department of Urology, Yeniyüzyıl University Medicine Faculty, Gaziosmanpaşa Hospital, İstanbul, Turkey

Cem Tuğrul Gezmis
Bitlis State Hospital, Bitlis, Turkey 4 10 Sancaktepe State Hospital, İstanbul, Turkey

Berkan Simsek
Department of Urology, Sancaktepe State Hospital, İstanbul, Turkey

Giorgio Bozzini, Umberto Besana, Alberto Calori, Berti Lorenzo and Carlo Buizza
Department of Urology, ASST Valle Olona Busto Arsizio, Varese, Italy

Tahsin Batuhan Aydogan, Maria Chiara Sighinolfi and Bernardo Rocco
Department of Urology, University of Modena and Reggio Emilia, Modena, Italy

Alexander Müller
Department of Urology, Spital Limmattal, Schlieren, Switzerland

Alexander Govorov and Dmitry Y. Pushkar
Department of Urology, A.I. Evdokimov Moscow State University of Medicine and Dentistry, Moscow, Russia

Giovannalberto Pini
Department of Urology, San Raffaele Turro Hospital, Milan, Italy

Antonio Luigi Pastore
Department of Urology, ICOT Latina, Latina, Italy

Javier Romero-Otero
Department of Urology, Hospital Universitario 12 de Octobre, Madrid, Spain

Seung Woo Yang, Hyun Seok Na, Long Jin, Jae Geun Lee, Jong Mok Park, Ji Yong Lee, Ju Hyun Shin, Jae Sung Lim, Yong Gil Na and Ki Hak Song
Department of Urology, Chungnam National University College of Medicine, Chungnam National University Hospital, 282 Monwha-ro, Jung-gu, Daejeon, Republic of Korea

Yun Kyong Hyon, Kiwan Jeon and Taeyoung Ha
Division of Medical Mathematics, National Institute for Mathematical Sciences, 70 Yuseong-daero 1689beon-gil, Yuseong-gu, Daejeon, Republic of Korea

Jinbum Kim
Department of Urology, Konyang University College of Medicine, Konyang University Hospital, 158 Gwanjeodong-ro, Seo-gu, Daejeon, Republic of Korea

Yuanhao Song and Xingping Shen
Department of Endocrinology, Zhongshan Hospital Xiamen University, Xiamen 361004, Fujian, China

Mitsuhiro Tambo, Satoru Taguchi, Yu Nakamura, Takatsugu Okegawa and Hiroshi Fukuhara
Department of Urology, Kyorin University School of Medicine, Shikawa 6-20-2, Mitaka, Tokyo 181-8611, Japan

Index

www.ingramcontent.com/pod-product-compliance
Lightning Source LLC
LaVergne TN
LVHW081032210926
848485LV00004B/1004